# COGNITIVE THERAPY OF
# ANXIETY DISORDERS

# COGNITIVE THERAPY OF ANXIETY DISORDERS

## A Practice Manual and Conceptual Guide

Adrian Wells
*University of Manchester*

JOHN WILEY & SONS

Chichester · New York · Weinheim · Brisbane · Singapore · Toronto

*Other Wiley Editorial Offices*

John Wiley & Sons, Inc., 605 Third Avenue,
New York, NY 10158-0012, USA

WILEY-VCH Verlag GmbH, Pappelallee 3,
D-69469 Weinheim, Germany

Jacaranda Wiley Ltd, 33 Park Road, Milton,
Queensland 4064, Australia

John Wiley & Sons (Asia) Pte Ltd, 2 Clementi Loop #02-01,
Jin Xing Distripark, Singapore 129809

John Wiley & Sons (Canada) Ltd, 22 Worcester Road,
Rexdale, Ontario M9W 1L1, Canada

*Library of Congress Cataloging-in-Publication Data*

Wells, Adrian.
    Cognitive therapy of anxiety disorders : a practice manual and
conceptual guide / Adrian Wells.
        p.     cm.
    Includes bibliographical references and index.
    ISBN 0-471-96474-3 (cased). — ISBN 0-471-96476-X (paper)
    1. Anxiety.   2. Cognitive therapy.   I. Title.
RC531.W43   1997
616.85'2230651—dc21                                    96–46488
                                                          CIP

*British Library Cataloguing in Publication Data*

A catalogue record for this book is available from the British Library

ISBN 0-471-96474-3 (cased)
ISBN 0-471-96476-X (paper)

Typeset in 10/12pt Palatino from the authors disks by Dorwyn Ltd, Rowlands Castle, Hants
Printed and bound by CPI Antony Rowe, Eastbourne
This book is printed on acid-free paper responsibly manufactured from sustainable
forestation, for which at least two trees are planted for each one used for paper production.

# CONTENTS

# ABOUT THE AUTHOR

Adrian Wells is currently appointed as Senior Lecturer in Clinical Psychology and Consultant in the Department of Clinical Psychology at the University of Manchester. He is a leading cognitive therapist with an international reputation in the field. After receiving his PhD in 1987 he subsequently trained in clinical psychology. He was a post-doctoral fellow at the Center for Cognitive Therapy Philadelphia for the year 1989–1990 where he received his diploma in cognitive therapy from Aaron T. Beck. For the next five years he worked as Senior Research Clinical Psychologist at the University of Oxford Department of Psychiatry. There he collaborated with the Oxford Cognitive Therapy group in the development and evaluation of cognitive therapy of anxiety. He has been extensively involved in the training and supervision of cognitive therapists both nationally and internationally, and is the author of numerous published works on cognitive theory and treatment.

# PREFACE

There were two broad aims in writing this book. The first was to produce a comprehensive practical text of cognitive therapy of anxiety disorders. In order for a treatment guide to be of most value it should offer a detailed description of not only *what to do* in treatment but also an account of *how to do it*. This book does both. Through detailed analysis it has been possible to develop for the first time specific protocols of how to implement a range of basic and advanced cognitive modification procedures. The book is illustrated throughout with case examples and examples of therapeutic dialogues. All of the material used is based on actual cases.

Cognitive therapy represents many things to many clinicians. Often what clinicians do in treatment is determined by what their experience tells them should be effective. However, the principle on which this book is based is that if cognitive therapy is to advance and become increasingly effective in the hands of a range of therapists we need to develop a cognitive therapy of greater theoretical integrity. More specifically, the techniques used in treatment should be derived from a specific *cognitive* conceptualisation of a problem.

The second aim of this work, therefore, was to present a pure approach to cognitive therapy that makes a significant contribution to advancing theory and practice. The link between theory and practice and the influence of new ideas in 'cognitive therapy' is a recurrent theme. The practice of 'cognitive therapy' ranges from the more eclectic applications to more purist approaches in health settings; this book argues for a purer form of cognitive therapy.

## Structure of the book

The first chapters (1–4) of the book present a background to cognitive theory of anxiety disorders and an overview of assessment. The nature of cognitive therapy, and basic techniques are presented in Chapters 3 and 4. The first four chapters are indispensable reading and even experienced cognitive therapists should find new information here. The individual disorder chapters present detailed descriptions of the use of specific conceptualisations and strategies in treatment.

The book is written in a particular sequence so that fundamental skills are presented first and more advanced and complex concepts and strategies evolve as the work progresses. It is also written to reduce redundancy in the presentation of strategies across chapters. Each disorder chapter focuses on the application of some of the most useful techniques for the specific disorder under consideration. Nevertheless, many of the techniques reviewed in earlier chapters should be considered. In this way the book presents a comprehensive coverage of a wide range of cognitive therapy case conceptualisations and techniques.

The panic disorder chapter follows the influential cognitive theory and treatment developed by David M. Clark, and colleagues. The hypochondriasis chapter follows the theory and treatment developed by Paul Salkovskis, David Clark, Hilary Warwick and colleagues. These chapters contain some new material devised by the author. The rest of the book is based on the author's theoretical, research and practical experience.

## Training and supervision in cognitive therapy

While this book offers a comprehensive guide to cognitive therapy of anxiety, appropriate training and continued supervision by appropriately trained therapists are essential for the development of effective cognitive therapy skills. It is recommended that therapists should attend recognised workshops and pursue cognitive therapy training at centres that offer suitable courses.

Adrian Wells

Chapter 1

# COGNITIVE THEORY AND MODELS OF ANXIETY: AN INTRODUCTION

There is no single cognitive theory or model of anxiety disorder. This book focuses primarily on the approach of Beck and allied approaches, which are among the most influential and are supported by data from rigorous experiment and self-report studies. Since the concept of cognition is central in this volume it is necessary to define what is meant by this term in the present context. In its broadest sense cognition refers to the full range of processes and mechanisms that support thinking, and also the content or products of these processes, namely thoughts themselves. The basic premise of cognitive theories of emotional disorder is that dysfunction arises from an individual's interpretation of events. Moreover, behavioural responses emerging from particular interpretations are also important factors involved in the maintenance of emotional problems.

Ellis's (1962) cognitive approach is based on the principle that 'irrational beliefs' are the source of disturbed emotional and behavioural consequences. These beliefs predominantly consist of unconditional *shoulds*, *musts*, *commands* and *demands* which lead to illogical cognitions and emotional disturbances. Ellis (1962) initially documented 11 beliefs which he considered predisposed to negative emotional reactions. For example: 'A person must be perfectly competent, adequate and achieving to be considered worth while; it is essential that a person be loved or approved of by virtually everyone in the community'. Because these belief systems are reinforced by society, by self-indoctrination, and may even have an inherited basis, they should be disputed vigorously in therapy.

Beck's cognitive theory of emotional disorders (Beck, 1967; 1976) asserts that emotional disorders are maintained by a 'thinking disorder' in which anxiety and depression are accompanied by distortions in thinking. Dysfunctional processing of this kind is manifest at a surface level as a stream of negative automatic thoughts in the patient's consciousness. Distortions in processing and negative automatic thoughts reflect the operation of underlying beliefs and assumptions stored in memory. Beliefs and assumptions are relatively stable representations of knowledge stored in memory structures that cognitive psychologists have termed schemas (Bartlett, 1932). Once activated schemas influence information processing, shape the interpretation of experience, and affect behaviour. While the behaviour or thinking of an anxious individual may superficially seem 'irrational' it is derived logically from the beliefs and assumptions held. Dysfunction in information processing in emotional disorder is evident in the patient's beliefs, cognitive distortions, and negative automatic thoughts.

## COGNITIVE THEORY OF ANXIETY DISORDERS

In anxiety disorder the disturbance in information processing which underlies anxiety vulnerability and anxiety maintenance can be viewed as a preoccupation with or 'fixation' on the concept of danger, and an associated underestimation of personal ability to cope (Beck, Emery & Greenberg, 1985). The theme of danger in anxiety is evident in the content of anxious schemas (i.e. assumptions and beliefs) and the content of negative automatic thoughts. The predominance of danger-related thoughts in the stream of consciousness of anxiety patients (e.g. Beck, Laude & Bohnert, 1974a; Hibbert, 1984; Rachman, Lopatka & Levitt, 1988), contrasts with the themes of loss and self-devaluation in depressive negative automatic thoughts (e.g. Beck, Rush, Shaw & Emery, 1979; Beck, 1987), and is the basis of the content-specificity hypothesis in which anxiety and depression are distinguishable in terms of thought content.

The overestimation of danger and underestimation of ability to cope with situations in anxiety disorder reflects the activation of underlying danger schemas: 'The locus of the disorder in the anxiety states is not in the affective system but in the hypervalent cognitive schemas relevant to danger that are continually presenting a view of reality as dangerous and the self as vulnerable' (Beck, 1985, p. 192). Once danger appraisals are activated a number of vicious circles maintain anxiety. Particular anxiety symptoms may themselves pose a threat. For example, they may impair performance or be interpreted as a sign of serious physical or mental disorder. These effects increase the subjective sense of vulnerability, and as appraisals of danger increase so do primal anxiety responses which in turn contribute to un-favourable responses and appraisals, and so on.

## Dysfunctional schemas

The term schema refers to a cognitive structure. However, in the schema theory of emotional disorder it is the content of these structures which is given most consideration. Two types of informational content or knowledge at the schema level are considered in Beck's theory: *beliefs* and *assumptions*. Beliefs are 'core' constructs that are unconditional in nature (e.g. 'I'm a failure; I'm worthless; I'm vulnerable; I'm inferior'), and are taken as truths about the self and the world. Assumptions are conditional and may be thought of as instrumental, insomuch as they represent contingencies be-tween events and self-appraisals (e.g. 'if I show signs of anxiety then people will think I'm inferior; having bad thoughts means I am a bad person; unexplained physical symptoms are usually a sign of serious illness; if I can't control anxiety I am a complete failure'). Beliefs are typically expressed as unconditional self-relevant statements (e.g. 'I am a failure'), whereas assumptions are expressed as 'if–then' propositions (e.g. *if* I show signs of anxiety *then* everyone will reject me').

The maladaptive schemas that characterise emotional disorder are hypoth-esised as more rigid, inflexible and concrete than schemas of normal individ-uals (Beck, 1967). The content of a schema is purported to be specific to a disorder. Therefore, anxiety schemas contain assumptions and beliefs about danger to one's personal domain (Beck et al., 1985) and of one's reduced ability to cope. Specific models of disorders such as panic (Clark, 1986), Social phobia (Clark & Wells, 1995), and Generalised Anxiety Disorder (Wells, 1995), identify more specific themes in appraisal and schemas associ-ated with problem maintenance. In generalised anxiety, for example, a disorder characterised by chronic worry, beliefs about general inability to cope, and positive and negative beliefs about worrying itself, have been implicated (Wells, 1995). In panic disorder, in which patients show a tend-ency to misinterpret bodily sensations in a catastrophic way, appraisals and assumptions concerning the dangerous nature of anxiety symptoms and other bodily events predominate (Clark, 1986). In the specific phobias indi-viduals associate a situation or object with danger and hold assumptions concerning the negative events that could occur when exposed to the phobic stimulus (Beck et al., 1985).

Although dysfunctional assumptions and beliefs may form as a result of early experience this is not always the case. In panic disorder, for example, dysfunctional assumptions may not pre-date the first panic attack, but may develop as a consequence of how the attack was dealt with (Clark, personal communication). If, for example, the individual is led to believe that panic attacks can lead to negative events such as fainting, or the person is presented with ambiguous information concerning his or her state of health, dysfunctional assumptions are likely to be established. In generalised anxiety, patients seem to hold positive and negative beliefs about worrying (Wells, 1995). Positive beliefs in some cases are derived from early experience, and negative beliefs about worrying only develop after an extended time period, perhaps when attempts to control worry seem impaired. In social phobia, some patients may function well most of their lives but develop specific negative assumptions about the social self only after they fail to meet up to personal rules for social self-regulation (Clark & Wells, 1995; Wells & Clark, 1997). In other cases negative beliefs about the social self may be longstanding and are associated with shyness and timidity since childhood.

Assumptions or 'rules' in anxiety influence the conclusions individuals draw from situations and also the manner in which they behave. For example, a socially anxious patient with the *assumption* 'Showing anxiety will lead people not to take me seriously' may reach the *conclusion* 'I had better say as little as possible in order to conceal my anxiety'; this may lead to the *self-instruction* 'Don't say a lot; try and look relaxed'. In this scenario the linkages between assumptions, situational appraisals and behavioural imperatives are observable. As discussed later in this chapter, behavioural responses emerging from dysfunctional appraisals and assumptions are often involved in the maintenance of belief in danger appraisals, assumptions, and beliefs (Salkovskis, 1991; Wells et al., 1995b).

## Negative automatic thoughts, worries and obsessions

The content of cognition in emotional disorders has been given various labels, such as automatic thoughts (Beck, 1967), self-statements (Meichenbaum, 1977), and worry (Borkovec, Robinson, Pruzinsky & De Pree, 1983a). In Beck's schema theory of anxiety, negative automatic thoughts represent the surface cognitive features of schema activation. Negative automatic thoughts (NATs) are appraisals or interpretations of events, and can be tied to particular behavioural and affective responses. A strong cognitive position would argue that negative automatic thoughts cause anxiety, however, in schema theory they are considered to reflect cognitive mechanisms that modulate and maintain anxiety.

The description of negative automatic thoughts provided by Beck and colleagues (e.g. Beck et al., 1985) suggests that they are rapid negative thoughts that can occur outside of the focus of immediate awareness although they are amenable to consciousness. They occur in verbal or imaginal form, and are believable at the time of occurrence. Distinctions can be made between different types of thought in anxiety disorders. More specifically, negative automatic thoughts can be distinguished from worry, and obsessions. Wells (1994a) suggests that it may be useful to distinguish between all these varieties of thought. For example, negative automatic thoughts can be distinguished from worry, and both worry and negative automatic thoughts can be distinguished from obsessions (Wells, 1994a; Wells & Morrison, 1994). Worry is described by Borkovec and colleagues (Borkovec et al., 1983) as a chain of negatively affect laden thoughts aimed at problem solving. Borkovec et al. (1983a) contend that worry is predominantly a verbally based thought process; however, negative automatic thoughts can occur in a verbal and an imaginal form. Obsessions tend to be of shorter duration than worries, but most relevant of all they are ego-dystonic whereas worries and NATs are not—that is, they are experienced as senseless and alien to the self-concept. For example, a mother may have thoughts of harming her newborn baby although she has no desire to do so. In general, NATs and worries represent appraisals of events in cognitive models of anxiety, while obsessions are intrusive mental experiences that are the focus of appraisals. Obsessions occur as urges or impulses as well as thoughts (e.g. Parkinson & Rachman, 1981). Worries are normal phenomena (Wells & Morrison, 1994), as are obsessions (Rachman & de Silva, 1978; Salkovskis & Harrison, 1984), and automatic thoughts are also likely to be a normally occurring type of cognition. Wells and Morrison (1994) compared the attributes of normally occurring worries and obsessions over a two-week period in non-patient subjects. Their data showed significant self-rated differences between these two types of thought. Worries were rated as significantly more verbal and obsessions as more imaginal; worries were also of longer duration (overall mean = 9 minutes for worries and 2 minutes for obsessions), worries were less involuntary, and more realistic than obsessions. These data suggest that distinctions between different types of thought are possible. In Chapters 8 and 10 the theoretical and practical relevance of potential distinctions is considered in detail.

## The role of behaviour

When a danger appraisal is made the cognitive system facilitates caution by eliciting a series of self-doubts, negative evaluations, and negative predictions. The somatic manifestation of this consists of a range of feelings such as unsteadiness, faintness, and weakness. Beck et al. (1985) assume that this is part of a primal survival mechanism that exists to terminate risk-taking behaviour and orient behaviour towards self-protection. In some circumstances such as social performance situations these responses can increase the danger they are designed to avert (i.e. they interfere with social performance).

Apart from automatic and reflexive anxiety responses highlighted in the schema model, behavioural reactions that are more volitional in nature are an important influence in the maintenance of dysfunction. Wells and Matthews (1994) suggest that many of the cognitive and behavioural responses to threat reflect strategies or plans of action that are actively (at least initially) executed and modified by the individual to protect against danger. Unfortunately some of these responses are counterproductive because they maintain preoccupation with threat and prevent unambiguous disconfirmation of dysfunctional thoughts and assumptions (Salkovskis, 1991; Wells et al., 1995b). For example, a social phobic fearful of babbling and talking incoherently in a social situation may focus more attention on the self and monitor his/her spoken words closely. In addition to this cognitive self-monitoring strategy there may be attempts to pronounce words in a clear and controlled way, and rehearse mentally the material to be spoken before speaking in order to check that it sounds acceptable. These subtle and covert responses constitute 'safety behaviours' (Salkovskis, 1991) that are intended to avert feared events. Safety behaviours play a significant role in the maintenance of anxiety. For example, a person having a panic attack who believes that a catastrophe such as fainting is imminent is likely to engage in behaviour designed to prevent the catastrophe, such as sitting down or trying to relax. Whilst the behaviour may relieve anxiety it unintentionally preserves the belief in the catastrophe. Under these conditions each panic becomes an example of a 'near-miss' rather than a disconfirmation of belief, and danger may seem subsequently more evident. In some instances safety behaviours not only prevent exposure to disconfirmatory experiences, but exacerbate symptoms in a way that enhances belief in danger appraisals. In social phobia, attempts to monitor one's own speech and mentally censor sentences before saying them interferes with processing important aspects of the situation and interferes with subjective verbal fluency, thereby contributing to appraisals of poor performance (e.g. Wells et al., 1995b). Similarly, attempts to suppress certain types of thought, have been shown to increase the frequency of the unintended thought (Wegner, Schneider, Carter & White, 1987). This effect has implications for disorders characterised by unwanted intrusive thoughts, in particular obsessional problems and generalised anxiety disorder. In these cases individual attempts to control or suppress obsessions or worries may exacerbate these thoughts. In summary, it is likely that safety behaviours maintain anxiety via a number of pathways:

1. Safety behaviours exacerbate bodily symptoms — an effect that may be interpreted as evidence for feared catastrophes. For example, controlling one's breathing may lead to hyperventilation and the symptoms associated with respiratory alkalosis. Controlling certain thoughts may contribute to paradoxical effects of increased preoccupation with thoughts and concomitant diminished appraisals of control.
2. The non-occurrence of feared outcomes can be attributed to the use of the safety behaviour rather than correctly attributed to the fact that catastrophe will not occur.
3. Particular safety behaviours, such as increased vigilance for threat, reassurance seeking, etc., enhance exposure to danger-related information that strengthens negative beliefs. For example, the health-anxious patient may seek reassurance from numerous medical consultations, increasing the likelihood of exposure to contradictory and ambiguous information. This information may then be interpreted as evidence that 'doctors tend to miss serious illness' which strengthens danger appraisals and disease conviction.
4. Safety behaviours may contaminate social situations and affect interactions in a manner consistent with negative appraisals. The social phobic who elects to say little about the self and avoid eye contact in order to reduce a risk of appearing 'foolish' is difficult to make conversation with. This may lead people to interact less with the social phobic and exclude them from conversation. This effect could then be interpreted by the social phobic as evidence that people really think he or she is foolish. Wells et al. (1995b) document a range of safety behaviours tied to specific fears of social phobics (see Chapter 7 and the rating scales in the Appendix for examples).

## Cognitive biases

Once activated, danger schemata introduce biases in the processing of information. These biases are often distortions that affect interpretations of events in a way that is consistent with the content of dysfunctional schemas. As a result, negative beliefs and appraisals are maintained. Biases in processing include attentional phenomena such as selective attention for threat-related material, and biases in the interpretation of events.

Beck and associates, and Burns (1989) have labelled a range of interpretive biases as 'thinking errors' or 'cognitive distortions' (Beck et al., 1979, 1985; Beck, 1967; Burns, 1989). Common errors or distortions include the following:

- *Arbitrary inference:* Drawing a conclusion in the absence of sufficient evidence.

- *Selective abstraction:* Focusing on one aspect of a situation while ignoring more important (and more relevant) features.
- *Overgeneralisation:* Applying a conclusion to a wide range of events or situations when it is based on isolated incidents.
- *Magnification/minimisation:* Enlarging or reducing the importance of events. Minimisation is similar to *discounting* the positives—insisting that positive experiences don't count.
- *Personalising:* Relating external events to the self when there is no obvious basis to do so.
- *Catastrophising:* Dwelling on the worst possible outcome of a situation and overestimating the probability that it will occur.
- *Mind reading:* Assuming people are reacting negatively to you when there is no definite evidence for this.

To illustrate how cognitive biases can maintain belief in negative interpretations, consider the example of a socially phobic person involved in a conversation with a work colleague. The colleague suddenly cuts short the conversation and leaves the situation. The social phobic may interpret this as: 'I must be so boring' or 'he thinks I'm an idiot, he doesn't like me'. These appraisals are examples of *'arbitrary inference'* and *'mind reading'*. In the next encounter with the colleague the social phobic is pre-occupied with negative thoughts about 'appearing boring and idiotic', he/she selectively attends to his/her own anxious performance, and fails to notice positive signals from the work colleague, or discounts these as evidence that he is 'just trying to be nice'. In this example biases of attention and inference serve to maintain belief in negative appraisals, as negative information is abstracted, and positive information is not processed, or is discounted.

## SUMMARY OF THE GENERAL SCHEMA THEORY

The central principles of schema theory of anxiety were outlined in the previous sections. In summary, anxiety is associated with appraisals of danger. Some individuals are more susceptible to appraising situations as dangerous because they possess schemas containing information about the dangerous meaning of situations and about their diminished ability to deal effectively with threat. Once 'danger schemas' are activated, appraisals are characterised by negative automatic thoughts about danger. These thoughts reflect themes of physical, social or psychological catastrophes directly or indirectly involving the self. Biases in processing associated with schema activation maintain belief in negative automatic thoughts, assumptions and beliefs by distorting interpretations in a manner that is consistent with dysfunctional beliefs and appraisals. Individuals typically try to reduce danger

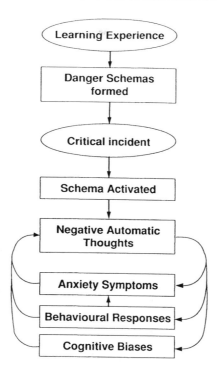

**Figure 1.0**   Generic cognitive theory of anxiety disorder

through their behavioural responses of avoidance or safety-behaviours. These behaviours cause their own problems in anxiety disorders by intensifying anxiety symptoms, and preventing disconfirmation of belief in danger cognitions. The basic features of this generic cognitive theory are depicted diagrammatically in Figure 1.0.

## EVIDENCE FOR THE SCHEMA THEORY OF ANXIETY

Predictions based on schema theory have been tested with a range of paradigms: interviews, questionnaires, and information-processing tasks. Early work on the nature of automatic thoughts in anxiety focused on the content of appraisals in patients with anxiety neurosis—a disorder category now outmoded but one that consisted of both panic and generalised anxiety disorder. Beck et al. (1974) conducted open-ended interviews with patients with anxiety and showed that all patients reported the experience of thoughts and/or visual fantasies concerned with themes of death, disease, and social humiliation occurring just prior to or during anxiety attacks. Hibbert (1984) replicated this finding with generalised anxiety or panic patients, and concluded that thoughts in panic could be understood as a reaction to somatic symptoms. Patients reported that their thoughts were more credible, more intrusive, and harder to dismiss when anxiety was most severe. Ottaviani and Beck (1987) showed that patients with panic disorder had thoughts about physical catastrophes such as dying, having a heart attack, suffocating and having a seizure. However, patients also feared psychological catastrophes such as losing control or going crazy. Almost half of the patients also feared social humiliation as a result of appraised physical or mental catastrophes. Rachman et al. (1988) exposed panic patients to their feared situation and obtained similar thoughts concerning personal catastrophe. These data combined with results from similar studies (see Wells, 1992, for review) provide evidence consistent with a central prediction of schema theory that anxiety disorders are associated with negative thoughts about danger. Moreover, depression can be differentiated from anxiety by the predominance of particular types of cognition. In depression negative thoughts are predominantly concerned with themes of loss and self-devaluation while in anxiety themes of danger predominate (Beck, Brown, Steer, Eidelson & Riskind, 1987). There are, of course, limitations with self-report data of this kind; it may be contaminated by subjects ability to report covert events, by the accuracy of memory processes or by demand characteristics. However, a source of evidence for schema theory comes from the use of more objective measures of cognitive processes, that are not subject to the problems of self-report. A number of information-processing paradigms have been adopted in this context.

## Information-processing tasks

The schema theory of emotional disorders asserts that anxiety and depression result from the activation of specific dysfunctional schemas, and once activated they direct attention towards schema congruent information (e.g. Beck, 1987). Attentional bias has been investigated with a variety of experimental tasks that may be loosely divided into three groups: *encoding, filtering* and *Stroop task* paradigms. Wells and Matthews (1994) have critically reviewed in detail results of anxiety and depression studies using these paradigms, and a summary of the main findings are presented here for brevity.

Encoding tasks require subjects to recognise or make a decision about a single stimulus; there are no other stimuli competing for attention. For example, threat-related or neutral words may be briefly presented on a tachistoscope and subjects are required to recognise them accurately as positive or negative. Another task, the lexical decision task, depends on recognising a string of letters as a valid word. Anxiety effects on these types of task appear limited (e.g. Mathews, 1988; Watson & Clark, 1984). However, one task that has been successful in demonstrating bias is homophone spelling. Homophones are words that sound the same but can be spelled in two different ways. The spelling determines the meaning, as for example with the words *dye* and *die*. The prediction is that subjects will attend to one or other meaning of the word. Thus in anxiety disorders, if danger and threat schemas are active, there should be an increased tendency to write threatening versions of the word rather than non-threatening versions. In a study using this paradigm Mathews, Richards and Eysenck (1989) demonstrated that anxious patients produced more threat homophones than did controls.

Filtering tasks typically consist of the presentation of two or more stimuli or channels of information that are discriminated by a simple physical cue. The task requires subjects to attend to only one channel while ignoring the other. Usually emotional information is presented on the unattended channel and the extent to which this 'captures' attention is inferred from disruptions in performance on the focal task. In the dichotic listening task, for example, subjects repeat aloud or 'shadow' a message presented to the attended channel of a stereo headset while ignoring material presented on the other channel. The extent to which the unattended material (often threat and neutral words) attracts attention is determined from the number of errors in shadowing. Mathews and MacLeod (1986) used a dichotic listening task in conjunction with a reaction time task in which subjects responded by pressing a key in response to a visual 'press' command during shadowing. Both threat and non-threat words were presented on the unattended channel and their relative impact on reaction time was assessed. Anxious subjects were slower than non-anxious subjects at performing the reaction time task when the unattended words were threatening rather than neutral. Tests of recognition memory showed that neither anxious nor non-anxious groups could recognise words presented on the unattended channel. However, when a higher control for momentary awareness of the unattended channel was used by Trandell and McNally (1987) to investigate attentional bias in Post-Traumatic Stress Disorder, no significant bias was obtained.

An innovative task used frequently in anxiety research is the 'dot-probe detection task' devised by MacLeod, Mathews and Tata (1986). This task requires that subjects attend to one spatial location on a VDU while ignoring another location. An emotion-related stimulus may be present in either of the two locations, and a probe stimulus in the form of a dot then appears in place of one of the original stimuli. Response time for detection of the dot-probe is measured to determine if attention remained fixed on the initial location or shifted to the other location. In one study MacLeod et al. (1986)

paired social and physical threat words with neutral words, and these word pairs were presented simultaneously at upper and lower positions on a computer screen. Subjects were required to name the upper word, and attentional bias was assessed using a key-press response on detection of a dot which appeared in the location of one of the words immediately after a brief display of the words was terminated. By examining the effect of word type on reaction time it was possible to determine if subjects' attention had shifted away from a particular word or had been maintained on the word. They compared the responses of individuals with generalised anxiety disorder with non-anxious controls. Results showed that anxious subjects consistently shifted attention towards threat words while control subjects tended to shift attention away from threat words. Mogg, Mathews and Eysenck (1992) report a replication of this effect. This paradigm has been employed to examine state and trait influences on attentional bias. Since schemas are relatively stable structures, attention biasing effects associated with dysfunctional schemas should be a relatively stable phenomenon rather than a transitory effect of anxiety state. Consistent with this prediction, several studies show that trait anxiety is a stronger predictor of bias than state-anxiety (MacLeod & Mathews, 1988; Broadbent & Broadbent, 1988). However, Mogg, Mathews, Bird and MacGregor-Morris (1990, study 2) report a failure to replicate this effect.

The third type of task used in attention research is the Stroop test. In its original form (Stroop, 1935) the test consists of rows of X's printed in coloured inks which serve as control stimuli, with the names of colours printed in different coloured inks which serve as experimental stimuli (e.g. the word BLUE printed in red ink). The task requires subjects to name as quickly as possible the ink colour that the control and experimental stimuli are printed in. Subjects are consistently slower at naming the ink colour of colour words than of X's, an effect that has been interpreted as evidence of the automatic and involuntary processing of word meaning which interferes with colour naming. The Stroop test has been modified to test for involuntary processing of danger-related information in anxious individuals. Mathews and MacLeod (1985) asked subjects who had been referred by their physician for anxiety-management training to name the colours of physical threat (e.g. disease, coffin), social threat (e.g. failure, lonely), and neutral words. Anxious subjects were slower than non-anxious subjects with all words but they were particularly slow in colour-naming threat words. Mogg, Mathews and Weinman (1989) provided further support for threat words interfering with performance in generalised anxiety but not in non-anxious controls. In an interesting study of Stroop interference in spider phobics, Watts, McKenna, Sharrock and Trezise (1986) found that interference for spider-related words was eliminated after systematic desensitisation treatment.

In summary, research on attentional bias in anxiety demonstrates a reliable bias effect across a range of paradigms and a range of anxiety disorders. These attention data are consistent with predictions based on Beck's general theory of anxiety disorder. Individuals with anxiety show attentional bias for schema congruent danger information. Nevertheless, the underlying mechanisms for bias effects requires systematic evaluation.

## Judgement, evaluation, and memory tasks

Biased processing has been assessed in a range of other tasks that involve complex judgements and evaluations, and in tasks involving memory. Butler and Mathews (1983, 1987) showed that anxious patients and individuals high in trait-anxiety just before an exam reported elevated likelihood estimates for hypothetical negative events. MacLeod, Williams and Bekerian (1991) gave chronic worriers a range of future negative outcomes (e.g. 'your health will deteriorate') and asked them to rate how likely it was that each outcome would happen to them. Chronic worriers produced higher subjective probability estimates than control subjects. These results imply biased reasoning in anxiety and worry-prone subjects. Biased reasoning is also a feature of other forms of anxiety. For example, patients with panic disorder or agoraphobia are prone to endorse negative interpretations of bodily events (Clark, 1988).

Although the results of biased attention studies and studies of interpretations and judgement are consistent with the predictions of schema theory of anxiety, the results of studies of biased memory seem less consistent with initial predictions based on the theory. If individuals selectively process schema-congruent information it would be reasonable to predict that they should show a memory bias in favour of schema-congruent information. While memory bias has been found in depression it is less reliable across anxiety studies, and this has led some theorists to predict that anxiety is associated with attentional biasing while depression is associated more with memory biases. However, as discussed by Wells and Matthews (1994), support for this distinction is inconclusive.

## A QUESTION OF CAUSALITY

Tests of predictions from schema theory have provided support for biases of information processing in attentional tasks, and tasks involving interpretations and judgement, and for a preponderance of danger-related appraisals in anxiety. However, questions of causality in the relationship between cognition and anxiety remain unresolved. Studies of state and trait effects on anxiety, longitudinal studies and studies of recovered patients shed some light on this question. Wells and Matthews (1994) review these data and conclude that the cognition–emotion relationship is bi-directional. That is, cognitive factors appear to predispose to emotional disorder, and emotional disorder effects cognition in a way that is likely to maintain dysfunction.

## FROM SCHEMA THEORY TO DISORDER SPECIFIC MODELS

Schema theory presents a general theoretical framework for exploring and conceptualising cognitive-behavioural factors in the maintenance of anxiety. However, for cognitive therapy to evolve and for treatment effectiveness to increase, specific models of cognitive-behavioural factors associated with vulnerability and problem maintenance are required. Specific models based on generic schema theory principles have been advanced for panic disorder (Clark, 1986), social phobia (Clark & Wells, 1995), health anxiety (Warwick & Salkovskis, 1990), generalised anxiety disorder (Wells, 1995), and obsessional problems (Salkovskis, 1985; Wells & Matthews, 1994). These approaches have attempted to integrate schema theory with other psychological concepts considered to be important in specific disorders. The aim in all of these cases is the construction of a model that can be used for individual case conceptualisation for guiding the focus of interventions, and for generating testable model-based hypotheses. Even when specific models are lacking, case conceptualisation and treatment may be based on operationalising basic constructs of the general theory on a case by case basis. Armed with basic principles such as the use of positive feedback cycles, negative automatic thoughts, and an understanding of the role of behaviours, and beliefs in maintaining anxiety, effective cognitive therapy is possible.

Specific cognitive models are presented in detail in the relevant chapters. However, as an orientation the general principles of these models and related concepts in the literature are briefly reviewed in the rest of this chapter.

### Panic disorder and health anxiety

There are a number of cognitive approaches to panic disorder and agoraphobia. These models tend to be variants of the 'fear of fear' concept in which panic patients fear the experience of bodily symptoms, predominantly those symptoms associated with anxiety itself. In an early cognitive model Goldstein and Chambless (1978) elaborate on the interoceptive conditioning (Razran, 1961) concept, in which bodily sensations become the conditioned stimuli for the conditioned response of panic. They assert that once an individual experiences one or more panic attacks, a hyperalertness for sensations develops and sensations are interpreted as a sign of oncoming panic. As the feared sensations are integral to the individual they occur in a wide range of situations, and fear generalises widely so that external situations become anxiety provoking. The approaches of Clark (1986) and Beck et al. (1985) also emphasise that panic patients fear the experience of certain bodily sensations.

Clark's (1986) model of panic is one of the most influential and comprehensive approaches, and is supported by data from self-report studies and rigorous experiment (Clark et al., 1988; Clark & Ehlers, 1993; Clark, 1993). His model asserts that panic attacks result from the catastrophic misinterpretation of bodily sensations and, once established, misinterpretations are maintained by selective attention to bodily events, avoidance and safety behaviours. Normal bodily sensations and anxiety symptoms are typical targets for misinterpretations. There are a number of differences in predictions derived from the cognitive model and the interoceptive conditioning model. First the cognitive model predicts that anxiety only leads to panic when symptoms are misinterpreted, while the interoceptive conditioning model assumes that anxiety sensations always automatically lead to a conditioned response of panic. Second, the interoceptive model assumes that anxiety sensations are conditioned stimuli for panics, however panic attacks occur that do not result from the perception of anxiety related sensations. The cognitive model predicts that any sensations, whether or not they are anxiety responses, can lead to panic if they are misinterpreted as a sign of an immediate physical, mental, or social catastrophe.

The central cognitive theme in health anxiety or hypochondriasis is the misinterpretation of bodily symptoms as signs of illness. Warwick and Salkovskis (1990) offer a cognitive model in which the misinterpretations differ from those in panic in two ways. First, hypochondriacal patients are likely to misinterpret signs and symptoms such as skin blemishes and lumps in addition to the sensations misinterpreted by panickers. Second, the time course of the appraised catastrophe in hypochondriasis is more protracted than the time course of appraised catastrophe in panic. However, panic attacks and hypochondriasis do co-occur suggesting that in these cases both types of appraisal operate. Important variables thought to maintain misinterpretation include bodily checking, avoidance, and reassurance seeking. Bodily checking is problematic because it maintains preoccupation with symptoms and signs, and self-examination can traumatise delicate body tissues. Avoidance reduces exposure to experiences that could disconfirm misinterpretations, and reassurance seeking leads to short-term anxiety reduction but longer term problems as the individual is exposed to conflicting explanations for symptoms. Recently, Wells and Hackmann (1993) have elaborated on the role of beliefs in health anxiety and propose that dysfunctional beliefs about death, illness, and the self combine and predispose to misinterpretation.

## Social phobia

Cognitive accounts of social phobia tend to emphasise two themes; the first is the role of *fear of performance failure* and *fear of negative evaluation*, and the second is the role of *self-focused attention* in exacerbating symptoms and interfering with performance (Hartman, 1983; Beck et al., 1985; Clark & Wells, 1995; Wells & Clark, 1997). There is a tradition in some psychological approaches of conceptualising the difficulties experienced by social phobics in terms of deficits in social skills. However, there is inadequate support for a skills deficit approach. Recent cognitive models, such as the model proposed by Clark and Wells (1995) emphasise the role of interference with social processing rather than deficit. Beck et al. (1985) propose that the social phobic is hypersensitive to signals from other people regarding personal acceptability, and autonomic arousal symptoms activate fears of failed performance. It is the fear of failed or diminished performance that maintains anxiety associated with exposure to the phobic situation. The fear is particularly problematic in social anxiety because it may actually contribute to problems in performance. Hartman (1983) also suggests that certain types of processing can interfere with satisfactory social functioning. In this case, the socially anxious individual is conceptualised as engaged in too much self-focused attention in social situations. This interacts with a negative self-view in producing anxiety. Hope, Gansler and Heimberg (1989) also assign an important role to self-focus in the maintenance of social anxiety. In addition to impairing performance, they draw on the evidence linking self-focus to a tendency to make internal attributions, and propose that even if no negative feedback is encountered in social situations the social phobic is likely to make internal attributions for neutral or ambiguous feedback, while discounting positive feedback to an external cause.

Clark and Wells (1995) have advanced a detailed cognitive model of social phobia that offers a unique and new synthesis of existing concepts and is based on a self-regulation framework of emotional vulnerability (Wells & Matthews, 1994). The central theme in this model is that social phobics are concerned about conveying a favourable impression to others but are insecure about their ability to do so. This insecurity is marked by negative self-appraisal of performance, avoidance and safety behaviours. Rather than focusing on the social situation, and on feedback from others, the social phobic focuses on the self in social situations and uses interoceptive information to construct an unrealistic impression of how they think they appear to others. Dysfunctional processing of the self as a social object is a central feature of the model, rather than the concept of processing of other peoples reaction to the self. Self-directed attention plus safety and avoidance behaviours prevent disconfirmation of negative self-appraisals, and contaminate the social situation in a way that leads others to view the social phobic in a negative way. Empirical support for the model comes from studies of social phobic imagery, manipulations of safety behaviours, and attentional bias tasks (Wells & Clark, 1997, for review).

## Generalised anxiety disorder

In comparison with disorders such as panic, health anxiety and social phobia the central cognitive theme in generalised anxiety disorder (GAD) is more diffuse and appears at the surface level not to be tied to a particular theme. Beck et al. (1985) assert that individuals with generalised anxiety have assumptions about a general inability to cope, and appraise a variety of situations in a threatening way. A key cognitive feature of generalised anxiety is recurrent and persistent worry that is experienced as excessive and uncontrollable (DSM-IV; APA, 1994). Borkovec and Inz (1990) suggest that individuals with generalised anxiety use verbal conceptual activity, namely worry, as a means of distraction from more upsetting thoughts that are likely to be more anxiogenic. One problem with the use of such a strategy is that it blocks emotional processing (e.g. Foa & Kozac, 1986) and thus intrusive thoughts become more likely as a symptom of failed emotional processing. Borkovec, Shadick and Hopkins (1991) suggest that the activity of worrying in generalised anxiety is negatively reinforced by its anxiety-reducing effects and thus control of the activity diminishes.

Wells (1994a, 1995) proposed a detailed and specific cognitive model of generalised anxiety in which a central theme is that worry is used as a coping strategy but it is also appraised negatively. Worrying becomes problematic when the individual develops negative beliefs about worrying, at which point worry about worry develops as worrying itself is appraised as dangerous and uncontrollable. In this model two types of worry are distinguished: Type 1 and Type 2. Type 1 worries are worries about external events and internal non-cognitive events. Type 2 worries are worries about cognition itself, in particular worries about the occurrence of worry. Negative beliefs and worry about worry are associated with monitoring for unwanted thoughts, thought control attempts, and avoidance of triggers for worry. These responses in turn exacerbate intrusions and prevent disconfirmation of dysfunctional beliefs. Preliminary empirical findings support predictions that worry incubates intrusions (Wells & Papageorgiou, 1995), negative and positive beliefs are associated with proneness to pathological worry (Cartwright-Hatton, 1996), and when the content and frequency of worries are statistically controlled, worrying about worry significantly predicts the extent to which worrying is a problem (Wells & Carter, submitted).

## Obsessive-compulsive disorder

Several cognitive models of obsessive compulsive disorder have been advanced. McFall and Wollersheim (1979) propose that obsessional patients make inflated risk appraisals and in particular hold dysfunctional beliefs about the unacceptability of certain types of thought. More specifically, these beliefs concern the possibility that having certain thoughts could lead to catastrophe, or consist of assumptions that disasters can be averted by the execution of magical rituals or by ruminating. Salkovskis (1985; Salkovskis, Richards & Forrester, 1995) extends the concept of appraisal of intrusive thoughts in a more coherent and detailed cognitive-behavioural model. Following from the observation that obsessions are normally occurring phenomena, he proposes that clinical obsessions are intrusive thoughts, the occurrence and content of which patients interpret as an indication that they might be responsible for harm to themselves or others unless they take action to prevent it (Salkovskis, 1989). Obsessional patients attempt to reduce their level of appraised responsibility through neutralising responses. Such responses along with strategies such as reassurance seeking, and thought suppression, reduce anxiety in the short term but prevent extinction of anxiety and maintain preoccupation with intrusive thoughts.

Wells and Matthews (1994) advance a prototypical model of obsessions based on a general self-regulation framework of emotional disorder. The model integrates features of Salkovskis's model with information-processing concepts. In particular, they emphasise the role of meta-cognitive beliefs (beliefs about the meaning of one's own thoughts) in the interpretation of intrusions. In the model responsibility appraisals are emergent properties of meta-cognitive beliefs, such as believing that particular thoughts can make bad events happen, or believing that certain negative thoughts signal the commission of uncontrollable negative actions. The role of meta-cognitive beliefs is also emphasised in the reformulation of obsessional problems presented by Clark and Purdon (1993). Wells and Matthews (1994) suggest that negative appraisals of obsessional thoughts in the form of perseverative worry (rumination) may be more relevant to problem maintenance than negative automatic thoughts about intrusions.

## OVERLAPPING AND DISTINCT CONSTRUCTS

Each of the models reviewed here have common features: (1) positive feedback cycles between cognition, symptoms, and behaviour; (2) dysfunctional appraisals; (3) cognitive biases; and (4) avoidance and safety behaviours. Differences between models occur at the level of the exact content of appraisals, and beliefs, and in terms of some specific effects of the disorder on feared stimuli/situations.

All cognitive models are based on the principle that appraisal processes intervene between stimuli and emotional responses. These appraisals occur as negative automatic thoughts, misinterpretations or worries, to name a few labels. Behaviour resulting from appraisals is often problematic because it leads to a failure to confront new information that could challenge belief in appraisals or assumptions. Some safety behaviours exacerbate arousal responses and bodily sensations, or exaggerate cognitive symptoms such as the frequency of intrusive thoughts. Safety behaviours also support an attributional bias in that the non-occurrence of negative events can be attributed to the use of avoidance or safety behaviours, rather than to the fact that catastrophes cannot happen or are very unlikely. Thinking errors such as: mental filtering, dichotomous thinking, catastrophising, and personalisation can be identified with most anxiety disorders. Equipped with the core set of constructs that permeate most disorder-specific models in cognitive therapy, it is possible to conceptualise in a preliminary way disorders for which specific models have not yet been developed, such as stress syndromes that do not resemble specific diagnoses, or disorders in which theoretical perspectives are still underdeveloped such as Post Traumatic Stress Disorder.

As discussed in Chapter 10, it may be possible to identify a core dysfunction of cognition that exists in all anxiety disorders and that can be targeted for treatment before constructing disorder-specific profiles. While this idea is still in its infancy, it is nevertheless an exciting possibility for the future.

## CONCLUSION

The basic principle of cognitive approaches to anxiety is that anxiety reactions are maintained by appraisals of danger. Beck's general theory offers an overarching framework for conceptualising specific anxiety disorders and for generating idiosyncratic case conceptualisations. An overall general model presenting a synthesis of key concepts from this approach was presented. Subsequent developments have focused on modelling the specific cognitive and behavioural characteristics of individual anxiety disorders. Specific models illustrate unique variations in concepts and their interactions involved in the maintenance of problems. For example: in generalised anxiety disorder general worry is distinguished from worry about worry; in panic disorder negative appraisals are viewed predominantly as catastrophic misinterpretations of bodily sensations; and in social phobia appraisals centre on a negative impression of the publicly observable self. In all models positive feedback cycles of varying complexity and quantity serve to link appraisals with anxiety responses and behaviour in a reciprocal fashion.

In this book each chapter on individual disorders presents in detail a leading cognitive model and shows how the model is used to generate idiosyncratic case conceptualisations. In the final chapter (Chapter 10), new developments in theory and research are discussed in connection with attempts to build more comprehensive and parsimonious general models of information processing and vulnerability to emotional disorder.

Chapter 2

# ASSESSMENT: AN OVERVIEW

Different methods of assessment include: interviews, questionnaire measurements, observational techniques, and self-monitoring. The interview is
the most frequently used assessment method. Two types of interview can
be generally distinguished: the *standardised diagnostic* interview, and the
*clinical assessment* interview. A standardised diagnostic interview is a
structured rule-based interview schedule based on a symptom classifica-
tion system. An example is the Structured Clinical Interview for DSM-IV
(SCID IV; APA, 1994). The aim is to determine a specific diagnosis for a
problem or combination of problems. In contrast, the clinical assessment
interview is a more general semi-structured interview that does not aim to
generate a specific diagnostic label for a presenting complaint. The content
of this interview is more flexible and is informed by a particular theoretical
framework from which it is derived, such as learning theory or cognitive
therapy.

This chapter focuses on the use of questionnaire measurements, the clinical
assessment interview, and exposure tests, which are among the most widely
used strategies in cognitive therapy assessment.

## AIMS OF ASSESSMENT

Several aims are served by assessment: identification of problems; elicitation of information for case conceptualisation; determination of past and
present level of patient functioning; monitoring treatment outcome. An
initial aim of assessment is the identification and *objectification* of

presenting problems. Presenting problems can be objectified by defining them in concrete measurable terms, such as ratings of symptoms and behaviours on standardised questionnaires, or through self-monitoring of problem behaviour or symptom frequency using diary measures. Assessment also aims to determine specific *goals* for treatment, and such goals should present tangible targets for therapeutic change. Two categories of treatment goal are relevant: general outcome goals that are collaboratively generated between patient and therapist (e.g. eliminating panic attacks, being able to eat in public without intense fear) and process-linked goals derived from a conceptualisation of factors maintaining patient problems and which guide the content of treatment (e.g. goals to modify belief in negative automatic thoughts, reduce attentional bias, strengthen new beliefs). Measurement should be used to determine progress in meeting treatment goals, and should be used as a guide to modifying components of treatment in a way that maximises the probability of cognitive-behavioural change. For purposes of formulation and to aid the therapist in determining if treatment is affecting key theoretical variables as intended, several rating scales are presented in the Appendix. These scales reflect the types of process ratings typically constructed or used to assess progress in cognitive therapy. They are also useful as a means of reducing therapist drift in treatment when used as intended on a sessional basis. Measurement, a particular form of assessment, therefore aims to monitor treatment outcome as well as to determine if specific processes involved in the maintenance of disorder are successfully modified.

## Measurement

Two categories of measurement most frequently used are *standard* or global measures, and *specific target* measures. Standard measures are measures that are developed for particular populations and problems and have good psychometric properties (validity and reliability). Examples of standard measures often used in cognitive therapy are: Beck Anxiety Inventory; Beck Depression Inventory; Beck Hopelessness Scale; Agoraphobic Cognitions Questionnaire; Fear of Negative Evaluation Scale/Social Avoidance and Distress Scale; Maudsley Obsessional-Compulsive Inventory. In contrast, specific target measures are developed for use in individual cases and include measures of panic attack frequency; belief ratings; diary measures, duration of exposure; frequency of checking behaviour, etc.

The Beck scales (Anxiety and Depression Inventories) and specific target measures such as the rating scales presented in this book are typically administered on a sessional basis in cognitive therapy.

*Beck Depression Inventory (BDI)*

The BDI (Beck, Ward, Mendelson, Mock & Erbaugh, 1961), is a 21-item self-report scale measuring severity of depressive symptoms. Each item comprises four statements reflecting gradations in the intensity of depressive symptoms. Respondents are asked to choose the statement that best describes the way they have felt over the past week. Each statement corresponds with a score (0–3) and the overall score is derived from a summation of individual items. The score may be interpreted as follows: 0–9, normal range; 10–15, mild depression; 16–19, mild–moderate depression; 20–29, moderate–severe depression; 30–63, severe depression.

Items 2 and 9 on the BDI should be examined independently since they provide an indication of degree of hopelessness and suicidality (respectively). High scores on these items indicate the need for detailed assessment of suicidal risk, and indicate the need to challenge hopelessness, and reduce suicidal risk in treatment.

*Beck Anxiety Inventory (BAI)*

The BAI (Beck, Epstein, Brown & Steer, 1988) is a 21-item self-report instrument designed to measure the severity of physiological and cognitive anxiety symptoms (e.g. numbness or tingling; feeling hot; wobbliness in legs; fear of worst happening) over the preceding week including the day of administration. Subject responses to each item are required on a 4-point scale consisting of the points: 'not at all, mildly, moderately, severely', corresponding to individual scores of 0–3. Total score is achieved by summating the ratings of individual symptom items.

*Hopelessness Scale (HS)*

Hopelessness can interfere with engagement in treatment, and the Hopelessness Scale (Beck, Weissman, Lester & Trocler, 1974) is a predictor of suicide intent, and suicide in outpatients. Assessment and treatment of hopelessness when present is therefore crucial. The Hopelessness Scale measures negative appraisals about the future, and consists of 20 items requiring a True/False response. A score of 1 is allocated to each response indicating pessimism concerning the future, and a total score is obtained from a summation of such responses. Interpretation of the total score is as follows: 0–3, no/minimal hopelessness; 4–8, mild hopelessness; 9–14, moderate hopelessness; 15–20, severe hopelessness.

The Beck scales are published by the Psychological Corporation (contact: The Psychological Corporation, Foots Cray High Street, Sidcup, Kent DA14 4BR, UK).

*State–Trait Anxiety Inventory (STAI)*

The STAI (Spielberger, Gorsuch, Lushene, Vagg & Jacobs, 1983) measures two anxiety constructs each on a separate subscale: *state-anxiety* and *trait-anxiety*. State-anxiety is the intensity of an emotional state of anxiety at a given moment in time and is characterised by tension, apprehension, nervousness, worry and autonomic arousal. Trait-anxiety is a relatively stable individual difference in anxiety-proneness, and as such is conceptualised as a personality characteristic. Individuals high in trait-anxiety are more likely to experience high state-anxiety in threatening situations. Both the state- and trait-anxiety subscales consist of 20 items with a 4-point response scale. The state-anxiety response scale consists of the responses 'not at all; somewhat; moderately so; very much so', and asks for responses referring to feelings 'right now, at this moment' on items such as 'I feel calm; I am tense; I feel strained'. Some items are reverse scored.

The trait-anxiety subscale elicits responses on a 4-point scale with the options 'almost never; sometimes; often; almost always', and is presented with the instruction to 'indicate how you *generally* feel'. Examples of items are: 'I feel nervous and restless; I feel like a failure; I feel rested.'

The STAI has been used extensively in research; its psychometric properties are well established, and norms are available. (The STAI is published by Consulting Psychologists Press, and the distributor in UK and Ireland is: Oxford Psychologists Press, Lambourne House, 311–321 Banbury Road, Oxford, OX2 7JH, UK.)

## RECOMMENDED ADDITIONAL MEASURES FOR SPECIFIC DISORDERS

In this section measures that are useful in the assessment and treatment of particular anxiety disorders are considered.

### Panic disorder and agoraphobia

*Agoraphobic Cognitions Questionnaire (ACQ)*

The ACQ (Chambless, Caputo, Bright & Gallagher, 1984) is a measure of thoughts (catastrophic misinterpretations) about the negative consequences of anxiety. It consists of 14 items (thoughts) and asks respondents to rate 'how often each thought occurs when you are nervous'. Responses are required on a 5-point scale ranging from 1 (thought never occurs) to 5 (thought always occurs). Items of the ACQ are presented in Table 2.0.

**Table 2.0**   Items of the Agoraphobic Cognition Questionnaire*

I am going to throw up
I am going to pass out
I must have a brain tumour
I will have a heart attack
I will choke to death
I am going to act foolish
I am going blind
I will not be able to control myself
I will hurt someone
I am going to have a stroke
I am going to go crazy
I am going to scream
I am going to babble and talk funny
I will be paralysed with fear

* ACQ: Chambless, Caputo, Bright and Gallagher (1984)

A useful modification of the questionnaire incorporates belief rating for each item, i.e. 'How much do you believe each thought when you are anxious': (0–100 per cent). The modified version has been developed and used by the Oxford Group (Clark & Salkovskis). The ACQ is an indispensable tool in the assessment and cognitive treatment of panic. Some of the items are also useful in the assessment of other anxiety disorders (e.g. Chambless & Gracely, 1989).

### Fear Questionnaire

The Fear Questionnaire (Marks & Mathews, 1979) is a 15-item instrument with the items corresponding to the 15 commonest phobias. Three phobia subscores (agoraphobia; blood-injury phobia; social phobia) can be derived each from the sum of 5 items. Respondents are asked to rate on a 9-point scale ranging from 0 (would not avoid it) to 8 (always avoid it) a range of situations. The situations are listed in Table 2.1.

Marks and Mathews (1979) report test–retest reliabilities (n=20 phobic patients) over a one-week period for the subscales agoraphobia = 0.89, blood injury = 0.96, social = 0.82, with a total score of 0.82. The scale appears to be sensitive to treatment. In summary the Fear Questionnaire offers a valuable self-report assessment of types of phobic avoidance, and is useful in the assessment and treatment of most anxiety disorders. A copy of the full scale is reproduced in the Marks and Mathews (1979) paper.

### Diary measures

Diary records for monitoring the daily frequency and intensity of panic attacks, and for monitoring triggers for panic, provide valuable assessment

**Table 2.1**   Items of the Fear Questionnaire*

*Agoraphobia*
  4. Travelling alone by bus or coach
  5. Walking alone in busy streets
  7. Going into crowded shops
  11. Going alone far from home
  14. Large open spaces

*Blood injury phobia*
  1. Injection or minor surgery
  3. Hospital
  9. Sight of blood
  12. Thought of injury or illness
  15. Going to the dentist

*Social phobia*
  2. Eating or drinking with other people
  6. Being watched or stared at
  8. Talking to people in authority
  10. Being criticised
  13. Speaking or acting to an audience

\* Marks and Matthews (1979)
*Note:* Numbering represents ordering of items on the original questionnaire

information and data for gauging treatment effects. These diaries also include columns for noting misinterpretations and responses to misinterpretations for use later in the treatment (see Chapter 5).

## Health anxiety

There are few well-validated self-report instruments relevant to assessment of health anxiety. Existing published measures tend not to be targeted at assessing specific disease convictions or underlying beliefs. Some potentially useful measures are presented here.

### Symptom Interpretation Questionnaire (SIQ)

The SIQ (Robbins & Kirmayer, 1991) measures causal attributions for common physical symptoms. A total of 13 somatic symptoms are presented followed by three items addressing different possible causes (physical illness, emotional/stress, and an environmental/normalising cause). For example:

A. If I got dizzy all of a sudden, I would probably think it is because:
  1. There is something wrong with my heart or blood pressure.

2. I am not eating enough or I got up too quickly.
3. I must be under a lot of stress.

For each possible cause respondents are required to indicate its appraised likelihood on a 4-point scale; 'not at all; somewhat; quite a bit; or a great deal'. The questionnaire is scored by summating the scores on items belonging to each category of attribution. A copy of the questionnaire is produced in the Robbins and Kirmayer (1991) article.

*Private body consciousness*

Private body consciousness (Miller, Murphy & Buss, 1981) is a subcategory of body consciousness, the tendency to focus attention on one's body. The private body consciousness subscale consists of 5 items assessing awareness of internal bodily sensations in non-affective states. Items include: 'I can often feel my heart beating; I know immediately when my mouth or throat get dry.' Responses to these items are made on a 5-point scale ranging from 'extremely uncharacteristic' (0) to 'extremely characteristic' (4). Total score is derived from summating individual item scores. Miller et al. (1981) report test–retest reliabilities over a two month period for the subscale of 0.69.

*Illness Attitude Scale (IAS)*

The IAS (Kellner, 1986) is a 29-item self-report measure of: worry about health; death; bodily preoccupation; illness behaviour; concern about pain; and hypochondriacal beliefs. The scale can be useful for highlighting areas that need to be covered in treatment. The scale measures nine areas with three questions tapping each one:

1. *Worry about illness* (e.g. 'Do you worry about your health?')
2. *Concern about pain* (e.g. 'If you have a pain, do you worry that it may be caused by serious illness?')
3. *Health habits* (e.g. 'Do you avoid habits which may be harmful to you such as smoking?')
4. *Hypochondriacal beliefs* (e.g. 'Do you believe that you have a physical disease but the doctors have not diagnosed it correctly?')
5. *Thanatophobia* (e.g. 'Does the thought of death scare you?')
6. *Disease phobia* (e.g. 'Are you afraid that you may have cancer?')
7. *Bodily preoccupation* (e.g. 'When you notice a sensation in your body, do you find it difficult to think of something else?')
8. *Treatment experience* (e.g. 'How often do you see your doctor?')
9. *Effects of symptoms* (e.g. 'Do your bodily symptoms stop you from working?')

*The Health Anxiety Questionnaire (HAQ)*

The HAQ (Lucock & Morley, 1996) is a 21-item measure of symptoms of health anxiety based on items of the IAS (Kellner, 1986). Responses are made on a 4-point scale. Four clusters of items were obtained in the analysis reported by Lucock and Morley (1996): fear of illness and death; interference with life; reassurance-seeking behaviours; health worry and preoccupation. Factor analysis of items in which four factors were extracted with eigenvalues greater than 1 revealed that health worry and preoccupation, and interference with life loaded on the same factor, the fourth factor appeared to be largely redundant. Test–retest correlations over a 4–7-week period for the total scale score was 0.53 for medical outpatients ($n=46$) and 0.95 for clinical psychology outpatients ($n=17$) presenting with anxiety problems. The scale distinguishes patients with a diagnosis of hypochondriasis ($n=23$) from a group ($n=26$) of other anxiety disorders (GAD, panic, social phobia). Correlation between HAQ and the BDI for 41 clinical psychology patients (with diagnoses of panic, social phobia, GAD, hypochondriasis, or mixed diagnoses) is reported at 0.42. Further evaluations are required of the properties of the scale but it appears promising for delineating areas for treatment.

## Social phobia

*Fear of Negative Evaluation (FNE), and Social Avoidance and Distress (SAD) scales*

These two scales were developed to measure the cognitive (FNE), and affective/behavioural (SAD) components of social anxiety (Watson & Friend, 1969). The instruments have been widely used in social phobia treatment research, although limitations of the instruments exist. More specifically, some items are reversed which can cause confusion, and the response format is 'True/False' which diminishes the potential sensitivity of the scales. The FNE scale consists of 30 items, while the SAD scale consists of 28 items. Example items from the scales are:

FNE:  I worry that others will think I am not worthwhile.
I am afraid that people will find fault with me.

SAD:  I often find social occasions upsetting.
I tend to withdraw from people.

*Social Cognitions Questionnaire (SCQ)*

The SCQ (Wells, Stopa & Clark, unpublished) was developed to assess a wide range of negative self-appraisals, fear of negative evaluation by others, and negative beliefs in social phobia. Responses are required on a 0–100 scale of belief ranging from 0 (I do not believe this thought) to 100 (I am completely convinced this thought is true). Original items for the scale were derived from clinical interviews with social phobics. While the scale is used to derive an overall score clinically, factor analysis (with non-anxious subjects) suggest the scale may have three dimensions of: (1) negative self-beliefs; (2) fear of performance failure and showing anxiety; (3) fear of negative evaluation and attracting attention. However, some items overlap and subscale intercorrelations are high. Psychometric properties of the SCQ are presented in Table 2.2. Further research is needed to explore the psychometric properties of the questionnaire with patient groups. However, the scale provides a useful clinical tool for identifying and monitoring thoughts and beliefs. The scale appears to be sensitive to treatment effects.

**Table 2.2** Psychometric properties of the SCQ (non-anxious subjects)

| Subscale | Alpha | Test–retest (4–6 weeks $n$ = 38) | Subscale correlations ($n$ = 334) with | |
|---|---|---|---|---|
| | | | FNE | SAD |
| 1. Negative self-beliefs | 0.72 | 0.81* | 0.60* | 0.37* |
| 2. Fear performance failure/showing anxiety | 0.84 | 0.61* | 0.46* | 0.37* |
| 3. Fear negative evaluation/attracting attention | 0.81 | 0.71* | 0.56* | 0.36* |
| Total score | – | 0.79* | 0.59* | 0.36* |

*Source:* Stopa (1995)
FNE and SAD: Fear of Negative Evaluation and Social Avoidance and Distress Scales (Watson & Friend, 1989).
* $p < 0.001$

Items from the SCQ are reproduced in Table 2.3 for reference purposes.

*Social Interaction Anxiety Scale (SIAS) and Social Phobia Scale (SPS)*

These two scales (Mattick & Clark, 1989) assess social phobia with particular reference to two types of situation: situations involving social interactions, and situations in which the individual may be observed by others. The SIAS assesses social interaction anxiety, and the SPS observational anxiety. Each scale is composed of 20 items. Validation data for the scale are reported by Heimberg, Mueller, Holt, Hope and Liebowitz (1992).

**Table 2.3**   Items of the SCQ factors

*Negative self-beliefs*
  I am vulnerable
  I am foolish
  I am inferior
  I am inadequate
  People are not interested in me

*Fear of performance failure/showing anxiety*
  I am unlikeable
  I will babble or talk funny
  I will be unable to speak
  I will drop or spill things
  I am going to tremble or shake uncontrollably

*Fear of negative evaluation/attracting attention*
  I will be unable to concentrate
  People will stare at me
  People won't like me
  I am going to be sick
  I will be unable to write properly
  People will reject me

## Generalised anxiety disorder (chronic worry)

*Anxious Thoughts Inventory (AnTI)*

The AnTI (Wells, 1994b) is a 22-item questionnaire measure of three dimensions of worry. These dimensions and corresponding subscales are: social worry, health worry, and meta-worry. The three subscales are replicable and reflect measures of worry content and process. Social and health subscales assess purely content dimensions, while the meta-worry subscale assesses worry about worry (content) and process characteristics such as the involuntary and uncontrollable nature of worrying. Meta-worry is a central concept in the cognitive model of GAD (Wells, 1995) reviewed in Chapter 8. The scale and subscales have very good psychometric properties (Table 2.4). Single case treatment data shows that the AnTI is responsive to treatment effects. Wells (1994b) showed that the health-worry subscale differentiated between panic patients, and other groups of depressed, social-phobic, and non-clinical subjects. In unpublished work, health worry discriminated GAD patients from depressed patients and meta-worry discriminated GADs from mixed panic and social phobics, with GADs reporting the highest scores in these cases.

The AnTI is reproduced in the Appendix for practical purposes. In order to score the subscales, individual subscale items are summated. Summating the three subscales gives an overall worry score. The scoring key is as follows:

**Table 2.4**    Psychometric properties of the AnTI (non-anxious subjects)

| Subscale | Alpha | Test–retest (six weeks *n* = 64) | Subscale intercorrelations | | Correlations with | | |
|---|---|---|---|---|---|---|---|
| | | | Health | Meta | Trait Anxiety | EPI | PSWQ |
| | | | | | Neuroticism | | |
| | | | | | (*n* = 96) | (*n* = 96) | (*n* = 105) |
| 1. Social worry | 0.84 | 0.76† | 0.30* | 0.54* | 0.63† | 0.62† | 0.58† |
| 2. Health worry | 0.81 | 0.84† | | 0.39† | 0.36† | 0.52† | 0.39† |
| 3. Meta worry | 0.75 | 0.77† | – | – | 0.68† | 0.60† | 0.50† |
| Total score | – | 0.80† | – | – | 0.72† | 0.73† | 0.61† |

*Source:* Wells (1994)
EPI = Eysenck Personality Inventory (Eysenck & Eysenck, 1976).
PSWQ (unpublished data) = Penn State Worry Questionnaire (Meyer et al., 1990).
* $p < 0.001$, † $p < 0.0001$

| *Subscale* | *Item number* |
|---|---|
| Social worry | 1,2,8,9,12,14,17,18,20 |
| Health worry | 4,5,7,10,15,19 |
| Meta-worry | 3,6,11,13,16,21,22 |

*Meta-Cognitions Questionnaire (MCQ)*

The MCQ (Cartwright-Hatton & Wells, 1997) is a measure of beliefs about worrying thoughts, and attitudes and processes associated with cognition. Five replicable subscales have been derived through factor analysis:

1. Positive beliefs
2. Beliefs about uncontrollability and danger of thoughts
3. Cognitive confidence
4. Need for control, responsibility, and punishment
5. Cognitive self-consciousness

Psychometric properties of the MCQ and subscales are presented in Table 2.5.

The scoring key for the MCQ is as follows (* reverse scored items):

**Table 2.5**   Psychometric properties of the MCQ

| Subscale | Alpha | Test–retest (five weeks) ($n$ = 47) | Subscale intercorrelations ($n$ = 306) | | | | Correlations with ($n$ = 104) | |
|---|---|---|---|---|---|---|---|---|
| | | | 2 | 3 | 4 | 5 | Trait anxiety | AnTI Total |
| 1. Positive beliefs | 0.87 | 0.85‡ | 0.08 | 0.14* | 0.26* | −0.01 | 0.26† | 0.41† |
| 2. Uncontrollability | 0.89 | 0.89‡ | – | 0.40* | 0.43* | 0.27* | 0.73† | 0.66† |
| 3. Cognitive confidence | 0.84 | 0.84‡ | – | – | 0.29* | 0.10 | 0.50† | 0.54† |
| 4. Need for control | 0.74 | 0.76‡ | – | – | – | 0.30* | 0.47† | 0.49† |
| 5. Cognitive self-consciousness | 0.72 | 0.89‡ | – | – | – | – | 0.36† | 0.36† |
| Total score | – | 0.94‡ | – | – | – | – | 0.68† | 0.74† |

*Source:* Cartwright-Hatton and Wells (1997)
AnTI = Anxious Thoughts Inventory (Wells, 1994b)
* $p < 0.05$;   † $p < 0.01$;   ‡ $p < 0.001$

| Subscale | Item number |
|---|---|
| Positive beliefs | 1,9,12,22,26,27,30,32,35,38,44*,46,52,54, 56,60,62,63,65 |
| Control beliefs | 2,5,8,11,13,18,21,31,33,36,40,42,45,48, 53,64 |
| Cognitive confidence | 3,10,16,24,28,43,47,51,57,58 |
| Need for control, responsibility and punishment | 7,15,17,19,29,34,37,39,41*,49,50,55,59 |
| Cognitive self-consciousness | 4,6,14,20*,23,25,61 |

To obtain individual subscale scores summate subjects responses. A total score is obtained by summating subscale scores. A copy of the MCQ is included in the Appendix.

*Fear Questionnaire*

This instrument (Marks & Mathews, 1979) was outlined previously. It is useful in GAD since it offers a measure of avoidance, an often overlooked component of this disorder.

## Obsessive-compulsive disorder

A range of measures are available for assessing dimensions of obsessive-compulsive disorder (OCD). For more details the reader is referred to the reviews by Clark and Purdon (1993), Tallis (1995) and Steketee (1993).

### Maudsley Obsessive-Compulsive Inventory (MOCI)

The MOCI (Hodgson & Rachman, 1977) is a 30-item questionnaire consisting of a True/False response format. Respondents are asked to indicate their responses to a series of self-referent statements relating to symptoms. The MOCI provides a total obsessional score, or four subscale scores: checking, cleaning, slowness, and doubting. Coefficient alphas for the subscales are within the range 0.7–0.8, and test–retest reliability is good (0.8; Kendall's Tau).

### Padua Inventory (PI)

The (Sanavio, 1988) PI is a 60-item questionnaire utilising a 0–4 point rating scale for degree of disturbance. Factor analysis of the scale produced a four-factor structure consisting of: (1) impaired control over mental events; (2) contamination fears; (3) checking behaviours; and (4) urges and worries of losing control over motor behaviour. Correlations between the impaired control of mental events subscale and measures of worry such as the Penn State Worry Questionnaire (PSWQ: Meyer, Miller, Metzger & Borkovec, 1990) are high suggesting that the subscale is tapping dimensions of worry as well as obsessional thinking. Sanavio (1988) reports an alpha coefficient of 0.90 in male subjects and 0.94 in females for the overall scale. Test–retest correlations over 30 days were 0.78, and 0.83 for males and females respectively. The scale differentiates OCD patients from a mixed neurotic disorder group. In an American college sample alpha coefficients for the individuals subscales ranged from 0.77 to 0.89 (Sternberger & Burns, 1990). A copy of the PI is presented in the Sanavio (1988) article.

### Diary measures

Self-monitoring of compulsions and avoidance provides data on the extent of these symptom dimensions, and offers a means of establishing a baseline index of symptoms against which treatment effects can be evaluated. Self-monitoring often includes a measure of frequency, and duration of obsessions and compulsions. The degree of discomfort or anxiety associated with these symptoms is also rated on a scale from 0 (no discomfort/anxiety) to 100 (extreme discomfort/anxiety). An example of a self-monitoring diary is presented in Figure 2.0.

Date:

Please record the daily occurrence of rituals, make a note of the time when the ritual occurred, the situation in which it occurred, and describe the type of ritual (e.g. washing, checking oven). Rate your discomfort on a scale of 0 (no discomfort/anxiety) to 100 (extreme/discomfort anxiety - the worst I have had) and put the number in the discomfort column.Record the length of time taken in your ritual. Finally, at the end of each day record the total number of rituals.

| Time | Situation | Description of ritual | Discomfort (0-100) | Duration of ritual |
|------|-----------|-----------------------|--------------------|--------------------|
| A.M. | | | | |
| P.M. | | | | |

Total number of rituals today:

**Figure 2.0**   Diary of obsessive-compulsive rituals

While this monitoring sheet is configured for monitoring rituals it can be readily modified for recording obsessional thoughts, by substituting the term 'obsessional thought' for 'ritual' on the form.

## SPECIFIC RATING SCALES

Specific target measures offer a valuable source of information, particularly if the measures are aimed at assessing the cognitive and behavioural factors central to models of problem maintenance. In this case they provide information for conceptualisation, allow quantification of key maintenance processes that can be targeted for intervention, and the effectiveness of treatment on individual variables can be monitored. In view of this, and in view of the fact that specific measures can be used to guide the focus of treatment sessions, a number of specific anxiety disorder rating scales have been constructed for inclusion in this book, and should be used on a sessional basis. The rating scales measure dimensions that are central in the cognitive models of anxiety presented in the different chapters of this book. Included here are scales for panic, social phobia, health-anxiety and generalised anxiety. Refer to the Rating Scales section at the back of the book.

## COGNITIVE THERAPY ASSESSMENT INTERVIEW

The Cognitive Therapy Assessment Interview consists of three broad components: (1) detailed description of the presenting problem; (2) analysis of cross-sectional symptom, cognitive, and behavioural details; (3) details of aetiology (longitudinal assessment).

### Detailed description of the presenting problem

A detailed description of the presenting problem consists of a description of the main affective, physiological, behavioural and cognitive symptoms. Base-rates for target symptoms should be established following operationalisation and objectification. For example, an agoraphobic patient reported recurrent panic attacks and avoidance of 'going-out'. Initially, she was encouraged to describe the symptoms of recent panic attacks, and panics were clearly defined as sudden increases of anxiety in which at least four symptoms were experienced (in accordance with DSM-IV). Once panics were defined an initial impression of the frequency of such attacks in the preceding week, and preceding month was established. A similar analysis of the nature of her avoidance was undertaken. It transpired that she travelled alone away from home twice a week, but she would not venture beyond a 'safe' zone within striking distance of home or a relatives house. Treatment outcome measures of panic frequency, distress associated with panics, and distance travelled from home were established.

### Cross-sectional cognitive-behavioural analysis

A cross-sectional analysis is intended to extend the general description and quantification of symptoms by assessing cognitive-behavioural factors contributing to the maintenance of the problem, and exploring modulating influences. This analysis ranges from an interview intended to construct a simple A-B-C cross-sectional formulation to an interview in which the questions are driven by a disorder-specific model (e.g. the cognitive model of social phobia). An A-B-C analysis is the most basic form of cognitive analysis which should be superseded by a more specific model-driven analysis as assessment evolves. This facilitates the development of an idiosyncratic theory-based case conceptualisation. Techniques for accomplishing this are discussed in each of the disorders chapters.

The A-B-C analysis refers to antecedents (A), appraisals and beliefs (B), and emotional/behavioural consequences (C), and is broadly translated into three categories of question:

(A) What was the trigger for anxiety?
(B) What thoughts were activated when anxious?
(C) What were the emotional and behavioural responses in the situation?

*Antecedents* or triggers (A) for anxiety include: internal and external stimuli. Examples of internal stimuli are: bodily sensations, emotional responses or symptoms of intrusive thoughts/mental experiences. External triggers include the behaviour of others, environmental stressors, exposure to feared situations, etc. The *appraisal* (B) of such stimuli and the meaning attached to them influence emotional and behavioural responses (C). Appraisals are labelled negative automatic thought, or catastrophic misinterpretations in schema theory of anxiety, and Clark's (1986) cognitive model of panic. In eliciting appraisals it is crucial that their *idiosyncratic meaning* is clearly established. Particular care should be taken in assessing the full range of behavioural responses. While some forms of avoidance or escape behaviours are obvious, subtle forms of avoidance and in-situation safety behaviours may not be so apparent to the patient, and it is therefore necessary to undertake a detailed analysis of behaviour.

An illustrative A-B-C profile of a social phobic patient is presented in Figure 2.1.

In the example depicted in Figure 2.1 the person concerned feared signing his name in public (A). The negative automatic thought (B) was: 'What if I shake?', the idiosyncratic meaning (i.e. implication of shaking) was determined (e.g. everyone will look at me), and the emotional and typical behavioural responses (C) derived. Note for purposes of developing an integrative conceptualisation that some of the behavioural responses are likely to exacerbate anxiety symptoms, and all of them are capable of preventing disconfirmation of belief in negative thoughts, thus a number of vicious cycles are established that maintain the problem (see Chapters 1 and 7).

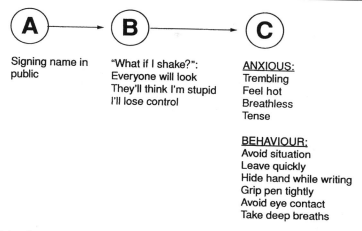

**Figure 2.1** A social phobic idiosyncratic A-B-C diagram

## Longitudinal analysis

The longitudinal analysis sets out to determine aetiological details, and information concerning the development of a problem over a longer time course. One of the central aims of longitudinal assessment is elicitation of historical details that may contribute to an understanding of the patient's vulnerabilities, and the present problem. This includes discussion of past stresses, nature of relationships, childhood factors, and how the individual has coped in the past.

## Underlying assumptions and beliefs

Apart from assessment of situational appraisals, a basic formulation of underlying assumptions and beliefs associated with presenting problems is necessary for a full conceptualisation. Techniques such as the vertical arrow, identifying themes in negative-automatic thoughts, and other strategies discussed in Chapter 3 should be used for this purpose. In anxiety disorders without concurrent personality problems, schemas underlying anxiety vulnerability may be readily elicited or inferred through questioning the meaning and significance of events. In cases of anxiety and concurrent personality disorder the content of personality disorder schemas may be obscured by situational negative thoughts associated more closely with the anxiety disorder. In this case the clinician may generate hypotheses concerning the possible content of patients personality schemas and the hypotheses may be tested following symptomatic improvement.

## Use of behaviour tests

Behaviour tests offer a strategy for eliciting information at assessment. Two types of information are generally obtained: (1) overt indices of problem status; (2) subjective data. Overt data are observable, such as the frequency of checking, duration of contact (exposure) to the phobic situation, distance from a phobic object, etc. Subjective information includes the content of thought/beliefs activated in the situation and belief ratings (0–100), rating of urges, discomfort/anxiety, and use of safety behaviours (some of which may be observable). Behaviour tests used at assessment and post-treatment provide a measure of treatment outcome. In cases where the acquisition of information from retrospective self-report is difficult, an exposure test can be used to activate and access relevant data for conceptualisation. For example, a social phobic patient with a long history of avoiding drinking and writing in public was unable to report discrete negative thoughts or safety behaviours. He was asked to drink out of a full cup and saucer during assessment. The task activated his anxiety and safety behaviours such that his anticipatory negative appraisals, in-situation negative appraisals, and safety behaviours became accessible.

## STRUCTURE OF THE ASSESSMENT INTERVIEW

An absence of a basic structure and outline for the assessment interview can lead to uneconomical usage of time and failure to elicit important information. The following structure is suggested:

1. *Review objective measures.* When the patient arrives at the assessment interview it is helpful to administer basic questionnaire measures. Suggested measures are the BAI and BDI, and a more specific measure selected on the basis of any pre-assessment information concerning the nature of the patient's problem (e.g. if panic or agoraphobia is indicated administer the Agoraphobic Cognitions Questionnaire and the panic rating scale). The first task during the interview proper is a brief review of objective measures. These data serve to direct the therapist's attention to potential problems of depression (suicidability/hopelessness: BDI items 2 and 9) and give an overall impression of problem severity and content.
2. *Explain the structure and goal of assessment.* In order to reduce drift in the assessment session, provide a brief outline of the purposes of assessment and its nature at the outset. An explanation like the following could be used:

'The aim of today's interview is to determine the nature of your problem. I'm going to ask you a range of questions about how you've been feeling recently over the past month or so. Then I'll ask you about background details to your problem. Try to be as clear and open as you can with your answers, some people feel embarrassed about disclosing their fears and anxieties, but anxiety is a common problem. This session will take 1 to 1½ hours. Hopefully, at the end of that time we will have a clear impression of the nature of your problem and be in a better position to determine what to do about it.'

3. *Ask patient to describe present problem.* The clinical interview should begin by asking the patient to describe the present problem as it has presented over a recent time period: the *past month*. This may be introduced as follows:

    'I'd like to begin by asking you to describe your problem. How has it been recently over the past month?'

4. *Determine cross-sectional details.* Follow-up questions should aim to establish the nature of main symptom clusters (affective, cognitive, physiological, behavioural) and determine base rates. The therapist should then proceed in directing questions aimed at building a cross-sectional model of the patient's problem (e.g. A-B-C analysis).

5. *Determine longitudinal details.* Use questions directed at elucidating the development of the problem to identify historical triggers (critical incidents), modulating variables, and factors that may contribute to vulnerability (e.g. childhood trauma). Elicit underlying assumptions and beliefs or, if inaccessible, form hypotheses about their content.

6. *Check for remaining issues and feedback.* Determine if there are areas that the patient thinks have been overlooked, and explore any areas. The interview is concluded by a therapist summary of patient problems and an accuracy check of the summary. The therapist should provide feedback concerning an initial conceptualisation of the problem and an impression of suitability for cognitive therapy is presented.

7. *Preparation for the first therapy session.* At the end of assessment a preparation for the first treatment session offers continuity of therapist–patient contact and increases the likelihood of continued patient attendance. Preparation should consist of:
   - describing the nature and methods of cognitive therapy;
   - discussing the role of the patient in the treatment process (e.g. homework, commitment, an active role);
   - introducing self-monitoring strategies (e.g. panic diary, thoughts record, symptom monitoring);
   - eliciting and challenging doubts about cognitive therapy (e.g. use engagement methods: present treatment as a no-lose experiment).

## MULTIPLE PRESENTING PROBLEMS

Patients frequently present with multiple problems. The aim of assessment is then to assess the full range of problems, determine any interrelationship between them, and prioritise problems for intervention. The prioritisation of problems for intervention is determined through a combination of *patient* and *therapist factors*. Initially the therapist should ask the patient what the main problem is, and determine if problems would remain if the main problem were effectively treated. If there are multiple problems that require treatment in their own right, these should appear as items on a *problem list*. The patient can then be asked to assign priorities to different problems.

Prioritisation of problems may be based on degree of impairment caused, such that problems causing most distress/impairment may be treated first. However, some problems have to be dealt with *immediately*. In particular, severe hopelessness, suicidality, and self-harm behaviours should be given priority. For example, a 43-year-old male panic-disorder patient presented with weekly panic attacks, health-anxiety, morbid jealousy and alcohol abuse. His main priority was elimination of panic; however, his alcohol use was potentially self-damaging and was conceptualised as a self-medication strategy that had counter-productive effects of contributing to panic triggers (bodily sensations) during the withdrawal phases of his drinking behaviour. This model was presented to the patient and a negotiated initial target for intervention was alcohol consumption. This was accomplished as a behavioural experiment to test out the effect of alcohol use on panic. After two weeks of decreased alcohol consumption, panic frequency also decreased.

Some difficulties appear to be secondary to other primary problems, although they may contribute to the maintenance of primary problems, as in the alcohol and panic problem just reviewed. In this case the limitation of alcohol use was an initial therapeutic aim. However, in other cases a secondary problem may not contribute to maintenance of a primary problem and may not be an initial therapeutic target. For example, an agoraphobic patient was also depressed. She conceded that her depression was a consequence of her panic and agoraphobia and the restricted lifestyle imposed by these problems. Since she was not suicidal or hopeless and her depression was not severe enough to require treatment itself (i.e. did not interfere with her ability to think or engage in treatment), panic and agoraphobia were primary treatment targets. It was hypothesised that as anxiety receded, and the patient became more active, depression should improve automatically, The therapist closely monitored depression (BDI score) during treatment to ensure that this prediction was upheld. (Note: When high hopelessness and suicidality are present, hopelessness and depression should be treated in their own right as an *immediate* priority.)

Prioritisation of problems relies on discriminating between different problems in co-morbid cases. Structured clinical interviews (e.g. Structured Clinical Interviews for DSM-IV: SCID-IV) offer standardised criteria for accomplishing this. Discrimination can be more difficult without a knowledge or use of structured interviews. It is recommended that therapists at least have a basic knowledge of diagnostic features of different anxiety disorders.

## CONCLUSION

This chapter presented an overview of key issues related to effective general assessment of presenting anxiety problems. The use of disorder-specific anxiety models in guiding a fine-grained assessment and conceptualisation of anxiety is reviewed in each disorder chapter.

In summary, assessment aims to define, objectify, and measure patient problems. Most of all, it is intended to derive information necessary for developing a rudimentary understanding of problem maintenance, and factors contributing to patient vulnerability. The therapist should utilise information from a range of sources in assessment. Key sources are: cognitive-behavioural interviews; structured diagnostic interviews; global and specific questionnaire measures, behaviour tests, and self-monitoring. The cognitive-behavioural interview is the most commonly used assessment device and is based on an initial cross-sectional A-B-C analysis of problems, and an exploration of underlying vulnerabilities. While the A-B-C analysis is the most basic unit of conceptualisation, it delivers information that can be built into a more comprehensive conceptualisation of disorder maintenance incorporating feedback cycles between components, such as the generic cognitive model of anxiety presented in Chapter 1, or preferably, more specific models where these exist (e.g. panic, GAD, social phobia).

Assessment should be a continuing process throughout treatment. The sessional use of questionnaire and self-report measurement provides a main source of treatment outcome data. These instruments facilitate the identification of factors that should be the target of treatment and they are helpful in providing a consistent focus for treatment. For example, the treatment of panic should focus on challenging belief in catastrophic misinterpretations of bodily sensations. This can be systematically achieved if the therapist monitors the extent to which the goals of treatment are being met (e.g. with the panic rating scale). Failure to meet goals may require a more detailed reassessment and reconceptualisation of patient problems.

Chapter 3

# COGNITIVE THERAPY: BASIC CHARACTERISTICS

Cognitive therapy of anxiety is a time-limited, problem-focused approach to treatment based on the cognitive model of anxiety disorders. Treatment relies on 'collaborative empiricism' in which patient and therapist work together with a scientific ethic aimed at treating concrete target problems. Continuous measurement and evaluation of patient problems is used to test hypotheses concerning problem maintenance and to assess treatment efficacy. Mini-experiments in the form of behavioural strategies are employed as a means of socialising patients in a cognitive conceptualisation, and as a means of challenging dysfunctional thoughts and beliefs. Homework is an essential part of treatment and patients are encouraged to undertake specific homework assignments between sessions. Cognitive therapy is a conceptually driven treatment that proceeds according to the therapist's case conceptualisation. A wide range of cognitive, interpersonal, and behavioural techniques are used in treatment. Many of the strategies used are familiar techniques of other orientations such as behaviour therapy. However, their use in cognitive therapy is not excluded if they can be justified within the cognitive formulation of a disorder. Nevertheless, these procedures are often presented with particular rationales and are modified in ways that maximise cognitive change at the level of beliefs or appraisals.

Cognitive therapy is educational, and new information may be presented didactically, although the preferred mode of delivery is through the socratic dialogue. The socratic method relies on a format of questioning to explore the patient's understanding and experience and to restructure interpretations and beliefs. Advantages of the socratic dialogue include the maintenance of a collaborative framework, and it offers a means to acquire a detailed understanding of the patient's 'internal reality'—an essential preliminary step in the effective modification of cognition. Of particular importance, the socratic method primes dysfunctional knowledge and allows the individual to be active in the modification of behaviour and cognition.

## COGNITIVE TECHNIQUES

Cognitive therapy is concerned with identifying negative automatic thoughts and dysfunctional appraisals, with the aid of recall, affect shifts, role plays, imagery induction, exposure tasks, diaries, and questionnaires. Guided discovery is used to determine the meaning and nature of automatic thoughts and interpretations, and to elicit and define underlying assumptions and beliefs. Belief in dysfunctional automatic thoughts, assumptions and beliefs are modified through collaborative empiricism which involves techniques such as questioning the evidence for thoughts, examining counter-evidence, reviewing alternative explanations, education, and strategies for combating cognitive biases.

## BEHAVIOURAL TECHNIQUES

Behavioural strategies are in some instances aimed at modifying symptoms directly (e.g. relaxation, distraction techniques), however, their key use is in the form of experiments to challenge belief at the automatic thought and schema levels. Some early cognitive-behavioural interventions tended to use behavioural techniques and cognitive techniques as components of eclectic treatment packages. A criticism of such approaches is that they lack theoretical integrity, and may be combining strategies in a suboptimal way. In this book a more conceptually coherent approach is advocated that uses behavioural strategies tailored specifically to modify cognition with the aim of challenging dysfunctional thoughts and beliefs. Use of a behavioural strategy, like any other strategy, should be defensible in terms of the therapeutic aims specified by an individual cognitive case conceptualisation. For example, the cognitive model of panic suggests that treatment should focus on modifying belief in symptom misinterpretations. Teaching panic patients relaxation and distraction techniques are unlikely to produce optimal changes in belief in misinterpretations since patients could attribute the non-occurrence of catastrophe to use of their relaxation strategy. Behavioural attempts to maintain anxious sensations and reduce self-control behaviours to discover that misinterpretations are false is likely to be a better strategy. Problems of selecting behavioural strategies are diminished if the strategies are primarily selected on the basis that they will modify cognition that is central in the anxiety model being implemented. Typical behavioural strategies include, exposure experiments, mini-surveys, activity monitoring and scheduling, manipulation of safety behaviours, attentional manipulations, and symptom inductions.

In the next chapter basic techniques such as use of socratic dialogue, guided discovery, verbal reattribution and behavioural experiments are presented. The remainder of this chapter is devoted to a detailed account of the characteristics of cognitive therapy, beginning with structure and then focusing on the therapy process.

## THE STRUCTURE OF THERAPY

A typical course of cognitive therapy of anxiety consists of between ten and fifteen sessions of treatment. Sessions are usually held weekly and the duration of a session is between 45 and 60 minutes. In certain cases of multiple presenting problems, such as major depression and anxiety disorders, or anxiety disorders with personality disorder, treatment may consist of a greater number of sessions. However, in some uncomplicated cases of panic disorder, social phobia, and generalised anxiety fewer than ten sessions may be required for effective treatment.

In a course of treatment, the initial sessions focus on assessment, conceptualisation, engagement, and socialisation. As treatment progresses more emphasis is placed on modifying behaviours and cognition involved in the maintenance of anxiety. Initially this is symptom-focused work, aimed at alleviating the symptoms of the presenting problem. When symptom relief is accomplished treatment focuses on underlying issues that are conceptualised as risk factors for subsequent anxiety problems or relapse. This focus is typically a component of the later stages of treatment, consisting of relapse prevention work. The termination of weekly therapy sessions is followed by scheduled 'booster sessions' of two or three therapy contacts within a four- to five-month period. Follow-up appointments at six and twelve months post-treatment are desirable in order to ensure that treatment gains have been maintained. A guiding structure for a twelve-week course of therapy is presented in Figure 3.0. Individual factors will of course modify timing.

### Case conceptualisation (Formulation)

Following a full assessment, the early treatment sessions are predominantly devoted to conceptualisation based on a cognitive model. Conceptualisation

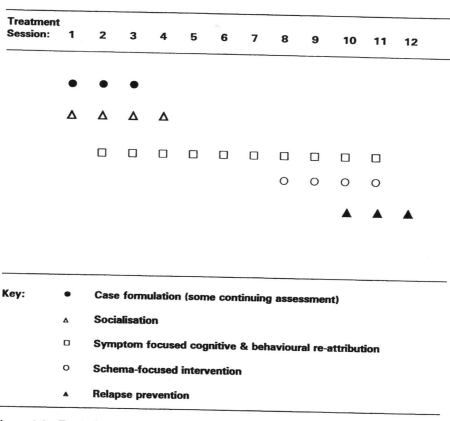

Figure 3.0    Typical structure of a course of treatment

and assessment are ongoing throughout treatment, however they occupy most of the session time during the first session of treatment. Goal setting is a component of the initial treatment session: armed with a conceptualisation and a clear set of therapeutic goals, treatment proceeds with socialisation and symptom-focused interventions. Strategies for building individual case conceptualisations are presented in each of the anxiety disorder chapters.

## Socialisation

Socialisation refers to 'selling' the cognitive model and providing a basic mental set for understanding the nature of treatment. Typically, this involves educating the patient about cognitive therapy, discussing the patient's own role in treatment, and presenting the case conceptualisation.

Reading material (bibliotherapy) is provided to assist socialisation, and demonstrations of the model are used, in particular demonstrations of the links between cognition, anxiety and behaviour. Aims of socialisation include laying the foundations for a psychological explanation of presenting problems, providing a general rationale for understanding the content of treatment, and providing accurate expectations concerning the type and level of patient involvement in the treatment process.

## Symptom and schema-focused intervention

The most part of cognitive therapy of anxiety disorders should consist of modifying the cognitive and behavioural variables involved in the maintenance of the presenting anxiety problem. In most cases schema-focused interventions should be introduced only after symptomatic relief is accomplished, or when there is reason to believe that underlying assumptions or beliefs are interfering with engagement in therapy or with progress.

Primary schemas in anxiety disorders are beliefs and assumptions that are hypothesised to contribute to anxiety vulnerability. These schemas tend to be modified in the latter part of treatment as a component of relapse prevention work. The same techniques that are used for modifying automatic thoughts are also used for modifying cognition at the schema level.

## Relapse prevention

Relapse prevention strategies other than schema modification are undertaken in the last few sessions of treatment. Relapse prevention typically consists of checking for residual beliefs in negative automatic thoughts and challenging them. The reversal of any remaining avoidance behaviours tied to target fears is also undertaken. Information acquired during therapy is summarised and consolidated by drawing up a detailed therapy 'blueprint' that covers details of the model, cognitive and behavioural strategies for overcoming the problem, summaries of alternative responses, etc. Booster sessions are scheduled for monitoring progress and dealing with any emerging difficulties.

## SESSION STRUCTURE

Each session of cognitive therapy has a core structure involving the following elements:

1. Review self-report data (BDI, BAI, Target measures). Check patient's reaction to last session.
2. Agenda setting.
3. Feedback from homework.
4. Implementation of specific strategies.
5. Provision of new homework.
6. Summary and patient feedback.

## Review of objective measures

Since cognitive therapy is a problem-focused and scientific approach to treatment, measurement is a crucial component of hypothesis testing and treatment outcome assessment. Mood, anxiety, the intensity and frequency of specific symptoms, base rates for behaviour, and so on, are typical measures in treatment. (Specific measures were reviewed in more detail in Chapter 2.) Self-report questionnaires are completed on a sessional basis and diaries are provided for monitoring of thoughts and symptoms on a daily basis between therapy sessions. The initial task of the patient is to complete relevant self-report instruments just before the therapy session or during the first few minutes of therapy. The measures are reviewed collaboratively and the therapist looks for changes in anxiety, symptoms, behaviours, etc. A decrease in target measures is used to encourage the patient and signals the exploration of factors that have contributed to improvement. The factors that have been useful may be isolated for continued development. An increase in symptoms or problem status or no change signals the need to explore exacerbatory and blocking processes in treatment. Measurement is essential because it provides information that is not readily available from the patient's general verbal account of his/her problem. Two to three minutes should be devoted to reviewing measures at the beginning of each session.

## Agenda setting

Cognitive therapy is guided by a session agenda. Following the review of objective scores the agenda is collaboratively established. Initially in the course of treatment this process may have to be less collaborative as the patient knows little of what to expect from therapy. Later on, most of the responsibility for agenda setting may rest with the patient. The agenda offers a means of reinforcing a collaborative working agreement between patient and therapist. It makes both therapist and patient responsible for deciding targets in treatment, and it allows flexibility to work on problems as they emerge. The agenda should be used to maintain a focus to therapy that is consistent with the case conceptualisation and with specific goals.

The content of the agenda is influenced by the stage of treatment. However, it typically incorporates the following:

1. Review of homework. Examples:
   - reaction to bibliotherapy
   - feedback from thought monitoring
   - results of mini-experiments
   - problems with homework
2. Identification of automatic thoughts/assumptions and implementation of cognitive and behavioural re-attribution. Examples:
   - recall of recent anxiety episodes
   - questioning the evidence for thoughts and generating counter-evidence
   - behavioural experiments
   - labelling thinking errors.
3. Discussion of the role of emerging thoughts and behaviours in the overall case conceptualisation. Examples:
   - effect of safety behaviours on symptoms
   - role of avoidance in preventing disconfirmation
   - influence of danger appraisals on behaviour
   - effects of negative thoughts on emotion.
4. Setting new homework. Examples:
   - give dysfunctional thoughts record
   - exposure plus dropping safety-behaviours
   - mini-surveys
   - worry-postponement strategies.

## Use of feedback

Two broad classes of feedback are distinguishable in cognitive therapy: feedback from homework and continuous in-session feedback. Feedback from homework assignments normally consists of a review of the nature and aims of the homework, and reviews and consolidates information learned through completion of assignments. In particular, the results of homework should be discussed within the context of disconfirming or confirming particular beliefs. Difficulties encountered with the execution of homework or emerging from the homework are normally discussed. Within-session feedback consists of inviting the patient to comment on therapy itself, and consists of comprehension checks during sessions. This type of feedback is helpful for keeping 'on-track', and allows the therapist to gauge the patient's level of understanding in treatment.

## Implementation of specific strategies

The majority of time in session is devoted to the use of cognitive, behavioural, or interpersonal techniques aimed at modifying affect, behaviour, and cognition. Cognitive techniques involve: identifying automatic thoughts, assumptions and beliefs; and the use of guided discovery to elicit meanings and facilitate the acquisition of new meanings. Collaborative empiricism is used to evaluate evidence for and against particular beliefs and automatic thoughts, and 'thinking errors' may be identified in challenging thoughts. The cognitive therapist normally uses a combination of different cognitive techniques. Specific techniques are considered in detail in the disorder chapters of this book. Behavioural techniques include mini-experiments, exposure-related exercises, survey techniques, and procedures such as relaxation practice to modify affective experience. Interpersonal techniques include role-plays, practise in appropriate expression of emotion, assertiveness techniques. Many of these strategies are constituents of behavioural experiments in therapy.

The choice of strategy is largely determined by the aims of the therapy session and the stage of treatment. However, issues such as degree of patient impairment, level of motivation, concurrent depression/hopelessness, and level of patient insight are considerations at different stages of strategy selection. Factors affecting strategy choice are considered in detail in the next chapter.

## Provision of new homework

The generation of homework should be collaborative where possible. Assignments should not be hurriedly selected at the end of a treatment session. The content of each session should be used to suggest homework assignments on an ongoing basis throughout the session. Ideally, assignments should be presented as no-lose experiments—that is, whatever the outcome, it may be used to guide therapeutic change. The rationale for homework should generally be made explicit since this increases patient motivation, enhances understanding of the cognitive model, and presents the patient with a cognitive set for interpreting and assimilating disconfirmatory experiences. In cognitive therapy of anxiety, homework assignments typically consist of self-monitoring, exposure to anxiety-provoking stimuli/situations plus abandonment of safety behaviours, mini-surveys, and paradoxical procedures.

## Ending a session

Closure of sessions is normally marked by asking the patient to summarise the main points that have been learned (e.g. 'We are drawing to the end of today's session. Can I ask you to summarise for me the main things that you have discovered today?'). The therapist should assist in this process by offering capsule summaries. Finally, the therapist should check that the patient has a clear note of the homework, and determine the patient's overall reaction to the session.

## THE FIRST TREATMENT SESSION

The first treatment session is most likely to deviate from the structure out-lined above. Unless homework in the form of self-monitoring (e.g. diary measures) have been implemented at the assessment session there will be no homework to review. The first session tends to differ from other sessions in another fundamental way in its focus on determining *GOALS* for therapy.

The general structure and content of a first treatment session should be as follows:

1. Review self-report data
2. Set agenda
3. Check problem list and begin goal setting
4. Begin building an idiosyncratic formulation based on a cognitive model(s)
5. Commence socialisation in the model
6. Check patient expectancies about therapy and educate about therapy
7. Set homework
8. Summarise and feedback.

## Problem list and goal setting: issues of problem primacy

If a problem list has been derived at assessment a task in the first treatment session is to review the problem list and use this to set specific goals for treatment. If a problem list has not been elicited, an initial task in the first session is to review the range of the patient's difficulties. The problem list is particularly useful when there is more than one presenting problem (e.g. a combination of panic attacks, depression and relationship difficulties). When multiple problems exist they should be *prioritised*. Prioritisation can be achieved in a variety of ways: based on patient accounts of the most distressing or disruptive problems which are given priority over less distressing problems; therapist priorities based on hypotheses concerning the interrelationship between problems. For example, depression may be a consequence of disability due to panic attacks and a restricted lifestyle. In this case panic attacks would be given first priority in treatment, unless depression or related problems were of sufficient severity to warrant treatment in its own right. For example, in cases of anxiety with concurrent depression in which the individual is suicidal, the primary interventions must focus on harm-limitation techniques such as elicitation and reinforcement of deterrents, reframing the problem in soluble terms, and behavioural strategies that counteract hopelessness and depressive inertia (see Beck, Rush, Shaw & Emery, 1979, pp. 209–24 for more details).

Once problems have been prioritised they should be *reframed* as goals. The problem list provides details of *'what is wrong'* and this should be changed into a goal or a statement of *'what the patient would like to happen'*. Goals should be *operationalised* in concrete terms. Vague patient goals such as 'I want to feel better; I want to be able to relate to people more easily' require operationalising. In operationalising goals it is helpful to question the patient's meaning: *'What does the patient mean by* (e.g. feeling better; relate to people)?' The next step is *concretisation* of the operationalised goal, meaning that the goal has to be tied to an observable or assessable outcome (e.g. What will you be able to do when you relate better that you cannot do now?). A central aim of treatment is progress towards meeting the concrete goal.

Goals often shift and require revision during the course of treatment as further information is gathered and as problems change. In addition to explicit goals, the therapist has implicit goals or aims that guide the content of treatment. These aims are derived from the conceptualisation of the patient's problem and are usually made explicit when they are activated in treatment.

## THE PROCESS OF THERAPY: ESSENTIAL BASICS

### Pacing and efficient time use

In order to use the 45–60 minute therapy time efficiently it is helpful for the therapist to generate a list of aims before meeting with the patient. These aims vary in their level of detail, and may be general such as: continue with socialisation; elicit key negative automatic thoughts and illustrate their linkages with emotion. In other circumstances they will be more specific. For example, in the treatment of health anxiety the aim of a mid-term session could be: check evidence for residual belief in heart disease; continue behavioural experiments involving exercise; begin to explore underlying assumptions about health.

Approaching each treatment session with aims in mind increases the ease with which the contents of the agenda are determined. However, it is necessary for the therapist to maintain flexibility, and be able to reformulate aims based on the patient's needs. A basic conception of aims in conjunction with a clear agenda helps to ensure a tight focus for treatment sessions and reduces the risk of *therapeutic drift*. Therapeutic drift is commonly the result of: (1) poorly defined goals or aims of treatment sessions; (2) conflict between therapist and patient expectancies or goals; (3) cognitive-emotional avoidance; (4) lack of a coherent and focused case conceptualisation. If there is a persistent failure to maintain focus on target issues in treatment, particular attention should be given to these four problem areas.

## The socratic dialogue

The socratic method depends on the use of questions and summary statements. The aim of using this technique is both to explore the content and meaning of the patient's experience and to modify behaviour and cognition. While use of the socratic dialogue is simple in principle it requires practise in order for the process to become automatic. A frequent question asked by trainee cognitive therapists is: 'What are the best questions to ask when a patient says . . . ?' There is no definitive answer to this question, and it is better not to be preoccupied with asking *the* 'best' question. Instead, attention should be devoted merely to keeping a socratic dialogue flowing and extracting *relevant information* from it. There are at least five basic requirements for extracting relevant information:

1. The therapist is able to ask questions that the patient is able to respond to.
2. The questions selected offer a means of approaching a particular implicit or explicit goal (examples of goals include: eliciting key negative thoughts; exploring meanings; reframing thoughts).
3. The questions used open up subject areas rather than close them down.
4. The patient should not feel interrogated by the therapist.
5. The therapist genuinely seeks to understand the patient's experience.

In order to maximise the likelihood of patient responses to questions, questions should be as direct and uncomplicated as possible. Normally *general questions* are combined with more specific *probe questions* in socratic sequences. Probe questions are directed at clarifying issues and gaining more detail. In practice, a socratic dialogue combines these two classes of questioning with therapist *reflections*. Reflections consist of repeating back aspects of a patient's answer to questions often in the form of another question. An illustration follows:

T:   What did you feel in the situation? (*General question*)
P:   I felt scared and couldn't stop shaking.
T:   When you felt *scared* and *shaky* (*reflection*) what thoughts went through your mind?
P:   I don't know. I just felt awful.
T:   Did you think anything bad could happen when you felt like that? (*probe*)
P:   Yes, I thought I looked stupid.
T:   What do you mean by stupid? (*probe*)
P:   I thought everyone would notice and think I was an alcoholic or something.

### General questions

General questions are initial questions intended to open up a particular area of exploration—useful general questions include:

1. When was the last time you felt anxious?
2. What was the first thing you noticed?
3. What did that feel like?
4. What symptoms did you notice?
5. What thoughts went through your mind?
6. What images did you have?
7. How did you cope with the situation?
8. What is the worst thing that could have happened?
9. What did you do?

### Probe questions

Probe questions are used to follow-up on answers of general questions with the aim of eliciting more detailed information and checking that the initial response is accurate. Probe questions often search for *worst scenarios* or the appraised *consequences* of not coping or not using safety behaviours. For example:

1. What is the worst that could have happened if you'd felt more anxious?
2. Could anything bad happen?

3. If you had not done (safety behaviour) what is the worst that could have happened?
4. What's so bad about that?
5. What would it mean to you if (catastrophe) happened?
7. If you couldn't leave the situation what's the worst that could happen?
8. What would it look like if (e.g. you lost control; looked nervous)?
9. How would people respond if that happened?
10. How much do you believe that (0–100 per cent)?

The following vignettes illustrate an interweaving of general questioning with probes and reflection to produce a continuous socratic dialogue aimed at elucidating the patient's feelings, thoughts and behaviours in a recent problematic situation. The first vignette is based on a dialogue with a patient suffering from social phobia, and the second dialogue is based on an obsessional case.

*Vignette 1*

T: Can you think of the most recent time that you were socially anxious?
P: Yes. It was yesterday when I had to go shopping for new shoes.
T: How did you feel?
P: I was up-tight about going on my own
T: Going on your own seems to have been an issue. What was bad about that?
P: It isn't right to go on your own.
T: What do you mean by that?
P: Most people you see in town are with someone
T: So what's the worst that can happen if you go on your own?
P: Everyone will notice and think there's something wrong with me.
T: If everyone did notice you what would that be like?
P: I'd feel embarrassed and self-conscious.
T: What would be bad about that?
P: I don't know what you mean. It feels bad.
T: What actually happened when you went out?
P: Well I didn't really do it in the end.
T: What do you mean?
P: I looked around the shops but I didn't try any shoes on.
T: What would have happened if you had tried some on?
P: Nothing really.
T: You don't sound too convinced about that. What's the worst that could have happened at the time?
P: I could have had a panic attack and made a fool of myself.

*Vignette 2*

T: What symptoms bother you most?

P: I don't want to have these thoughts anymore.

T: Which particular thoughts bother you most?

P: When I get a picture of men kissing.

T: You don't want to have the thoughts. But what if you continue to have them?

P: They will ruin my life. I can't cope with them like this.

T: It's not pleasant to be bothered by thoughts. Could anything bad happen if you continue to have them?

P: They could affect me in some way.

T: When you say they could affect you what do you mean by that?

P: I'm worried in case they make me gay.

T: So you think that having them could make you gay. How much do you believe that on a scale of 0 to 100 per cent?

P: About 50 per cent. But I know I'm not gay.

T: When you get the thoughts what do you do to cope with them?

P: There's nothing I can do. They just happen anyway.

T: Is there anything you do to try and stop them?

P: I tell myself that I'm not gay and I try to focus on something else.

T: Do you do anything to stop yourself becoming gay or to prove that you're not?

P: I cancel the thought out by replacing one of the men with a woman, and I look at pretty girls to see if I still find them attractive.

These two vignettes illustrate use of the socratic dialogue. It is clear from these illustrations that *open-ended* questions, that is, questions that cannot be answered with a simple 'yes' or 'no' response, constitute most of the questioning used. Occasionally the therapist used *closed-ended* questions. These questions are generally regarded as less effective since they can be answered with simple 'yes' or 'no' responses. It is better therefore to concentrate on asking open-ended rather than closed-ended questions. Open-ended questions are those that begin with: What, Where, When, and How?. Why? is also open ended but is often met with the response 'I don't know', since an answer relies on a level of insight that is normally unavailable to the patient early in treatment. In most cases a why question can be replaced with the question: 'For what reason?' (e.g. What was your reason for checking the light switch?), or can be reframed as a question concerning the implications of not engaging in a particular behaviour (e.g. 'What's the worst that could have happened if you hadn't checked the light switch?').

It is difficult to adequately convey in writing the subtle nature of socratic dialogues when they are used expertly. A fear expressed by cognitive therapists in training when they are introduced to the concept of the socratic method is that it will lead to the patient feeling interrogated. Typically this is not the case, since most patients are reassured by the therapist taking so much care over the details of their problem. However, caution should be exercised in eliciting certain types of material such as information relating to memories of trauma and abuse. This material can be particularly traumatic, and the therapist should respect the patients boundaries of disclosure at any one time. Moreover, exploration of such material is most often initially unwarranted within the context of a particular cognitive model of a presenting anxiety disorder. Generally, an air of interrogation is avoidable if questions are paced appropriately and the non-verbal demeanour of the therapist conveys genuine interest, warmth, and a desire to understand and help with the problem.

### Using the socratic method as guided discovery

Not all cognitive therapists are in agreement about what constitutes good socratic questioning. In some cases the therapist knows where s/he is guiding the patient and has a clear impression of the desired end point or reinterpretation. Padesky (1993) suggests that this strategy of 'changing patients beliefs' may not be the best strategy, and cognitive therapists can guide without knowing where the patient will end up. According to Padesky (1993), this latter style is closer to true collaborative empiricism in so much as it prompts the patients to examine and evaluate their own thoughts and behaviours. My own view on guided discovery and the socratic dialogue at the time of writing is that a combination of both knowing where to go, but allowing time to explore the patient's evidence for thoughts and for the patient to generate solutions is desirable. As we shall see in the next chapter, verbal reattribution is easier to accomplish if time is permitted to explore the patient's evidence and reasoning associated with negative automatic thoughts and beliefs. In these circumstances a range of entry points for re-attribution present themselves to the therapist. However, a danger of not guiding patients to a particular endpoint is that therapy time may be considerably extended.

## CONCLUSION

The basic characteristics of cognitive therapy were reviewed in this chapter. A structure to sessions was also outlined. Together these characteristics and the overall structure function to preserve a focus on developing a clear case conceptualisation of specific target problems, and offer a framework for active cognitive-behavioural change.

Chapter 4

# COGNITIVE THERAPY: BASIC TECHNIQUES

In this chapter a range of cognitive therapy techniques are presented and illustrated with examples. The material presented here is intended to serve as an introduction to cognitive and behavioural reattribution methods, and a source from which the therapist may build and strengthen a repertoire of techniques. The techniques presented are general strategies that can be used in treating anxiety. Collectively they are fundamental and indispensable components of treatment. The chapters of this book on specific disorders present additional and individually tailored examples of cognitive and behavioural strategies.

The chapter begins with a review of techniques for eliciting negative automatic thoughts (NATs), and for identifying thoughts that are most relevant to a problem. Verbal and behavioural reattribution techniques are then considered. Finally, methods for eliciting and modifying underlying beliefs and assumptions are discussed.

## ELICITING NEGATIVE AUTOMATIC THOUGHTS

Anxiety is accompanied by different types of thought, and it is necessary to distinguish between types of thought in correctly targeting NATs. For more information on this differentiation refer to Chapter 1. For present purposes, it is important to distinguish between *primary NATs* and *secondary thoughts* in anxiety. Secondary thoughts concern themes of escape, avoidance and neutralisation of danger, whereas primary NATs concern themes of danger. For example, when asked 'What thought did you have when you felt anxious?' a social phobic could answer 'I thought I'd better not say much'. Clearly this is not a danger-related cognition but represents a secondary response to some primary and implicit NAT. Other examples of secondary thoughts include: 'I just wanted to escape; I didn't want to be there; I had to get out; I must get a drink.' To elicit a primary NAT, questions should be directed at elucidating the consequences of not engaging in coping or avoidance responses. In the example of the NAT 'I thought I'd better not say much', follow-up probe questions like the following could be used: 'If you did say things, what's the worst that could happen?' or in cases where thoughts concern escape and avoidance the probe question 'What's the worst that could happen if you were unable to leave the situation?' could be used. Some thoughts articulated by patients are neither primary NATs or secondary thoughts, but are what we might call surface thoughts. An example of a surface thought in panic disorder is: 'I thought I was going to panic.' The thought is representative of a primary NAT but the precise nature of the danger is obscure. In order to determine the primary NAT the meaning of the thought should be determined (e.g. 'What's the worst that could happen if you panicked in the situation?' or 'What does having a panic attack mean to you?').

In summary, NATs can be distinguished from other forms of anxious thought such as obsessions and worries (see Chapter 1). In the conceptualisation of problems of intrusive thoughts (i.e. chronic worry and obsessions) it is the NAT or negative appraisal of the obsession or worry that is of central significance. In treating anxiety disorders it is necessary to ensure that the focus of conceptualisation and intervention is directed at *relevant* NATs. Primary NATs should be distinguished from secondary coping-related appraisals, or surface thoughts. Some NATs are implicit and occur as 'silent' thoughts, which are accessible by exploring the consequences of not coping, not escaping, and not avoiding situations, or by asking about the worst consequences in a situation. With this distinction in mind we now consider ten methods for accessing NATs.

## Ten ways of eliciting relevant NATs

*Worst consequences scenario*

One of the most effective questions for eliciting NATs in the therapeutic dialogue is '*What's the worst that could happen if . . .*'? This question stem can be completed with a number of different items depending on the context in which it is used. It is advisable that the therapist seeks the worst consequences scenario in response to more general negative appraisals. We saw earlier in this chapter how a combination of questions targeted at worst scenarios and questions focused on determining meanings can be used to elicit primary NATs. The technique is illustrated in the following example of social phobia:

P: I just felt very self-conscious in the group.
T: What thoughts did you have when you felt that way?
P: I wasn't aware of having any thoughts, it was just a feeling.
T: What were you most aware of when you were self-conscious? Was it a feeling?
P: My mind goes blank, I don't know what to say in the situation.
T: What's the worst that can happen if you have nothing to say and your mind is blank?
P: People will think there is something wrong with me.
T: What's the worst they could think?
P: They'll think I'm boring and stupid. (*primary NAT*)
T: When you were in the group were you aware of thinking that?
P: That's the usual worry I have.

In this example the patient was initially unaware of negative thoughts in recounting the situation. However, by questioning for *worst consequences*, a key negative automatic thought was elicited: 'They'll think I'm boring and stupid.' Notice that the therapist followed up elicitation of the thought with a question to check the validity of the NAT in the patient's case: 'When you were in the group were you aware of thinking that?'

*Re-counting specific episodes*

Recent occurrences of anxiety, such as panic attacks or worry episodes, can be discussed in detail to elicit negative automatic thoughts and appraisals. Typically, it is most efficient to select a concrete recent and specific episode rather than focusing the review on episodes in general. Initial aspects of the review focus on a description of the situation in which anxiety occurred or the events leading to anxiety or particular symptoms. The individual's appraisals of these events is elicited, and the emotional reaction accompanying such appraisals is sought. Emotional reactions are often determined first, and then NATs accompanying emotion are often more accessible. The following example demonstrates the use of this technique in a patient with agoraphobia.

T: When was the last time you felt anxious in public?
P: I had a bad day at the weekend.
T: Tell me about that. Where were you?
P: We were getting ready to go out on Sunday, and I began to feel nervous.
T: What did that feel like? (*elicitation of feelings*)

P: Horrible, my legs were weak and I was unsteady.

T: What thoughts went through your mind when you felt that?

P: I thought I didn't want to go out. (*secondary thoughts*)

T: Were you afraid something bad could happen if you went out feeling like that? (*probe for danger*)

P: I often feel like it, I don't want to feel like that any more.

T: It feels unpleasant. Did you go out after all? (*continues exploring the episode in search of a NAT*)

P: Yes, we drove to the garden centre and that's when it really hit me.

T: What really hit you?

P: I came over all weak and trembly, and my legs were shaking.

T: When you felt that way what thought went through your mind?

P: I just wanted to get back in the car and go home. (*secondary thought*)

T: When you noticed those symptoms did you think anything bad could happen? (*probe for danger*)

P: I thought my legs would give way, and I'd collapse. (*a primary NAT*)

T: How much did you believe that at the time?

In this example, the patient reports a period of anticipatory anxiety before entering a public situation. The NATs for this period are obscure in the patient's account. The therapist pursues the scenario anticipating that specific NATs will become evident as the situational account unfolds. As anxiety increased in the account of the situation, this is used to signal questioning of thought content. At this juncture the patient reports secondary cognitions pertaining to the desire to leave the situation. In order to determine the NATs behind the secondary (escape/avoidance) cognitions the therapist asks whether anything bad could happen. This produces the NAT, 'My legs would give way, and I'd collapse'. The therapist asks for a belief rating of the NAT—a high rating can signify the importance of the thought in anxiety, and the rating should be tracked through the reattribution process as a marker of treatment effectiveness.

When negative automatic thoughts are not immediately evident, elicitation of the types of emotion experienced in situations and a description of emotional symptoms can prime negative automatic thoughts and make them more amenable to introspection.

The use of specific sequences of questions in the recounting of recent emotional episodes is the basis for constructing idiosyncratic vicious circle formulations as in the conceptualisation and treatment of panic disorder, to be discussed in Chapter 5. However, in some instances, particularly when avoidance is extensive, an individual is unable to remember and report a recent anxious situation. In these circumstances, other techniques like those discussed below may be used to elicit negative automatic thoughts.

*Affect shifts*

An affect shift is a change in emotion. Changes should be monitored during the course of a treatment session and are indicative of the activation of negative automatic thoughts. When an affect shift is detected by the therapist, the presence of emotion is acknowledged first, this may then be followed by asking the patient to describe the feeling experienced (this can be used to intensify awareness of the affective experience), and then attempts are made to elicit the content of thought associated with the emotion. The following extract illustrates the use of an affect shift to elicit salient negative automatic thoughts.

P:  I can't explain the feeling, it's like everything has changed around me.
T:  When you say things have changed around you, what is that like?
P:  It's as if everything is unreal, as if I'm drifting away.
T:  As if you're drifting away? Is it like you are detached from things around you?
P:  Yes. It's like being in an unreal world, it's scary. I've got it now just talking about it. (Patient places his hand over his eyes and shakes his head.)
T:  It looks as if you're feeling a little anxious right now.
P:  Oh God, I feel panicky, I don't want it to be like this.
T:  What thoughts are going through your mind right now?
P:  It's terrible, I think I'm just going mad or something.
T:  That's a frightening thing to think. How much do you believe that you are going mad right now?

Changes in affect can occur during discussion of symptoms and emotion, and also occur in the context of exposure experiments and induction of symptoms. In these circumstances questions can be used to elicit the content of thought. In some cases the therapist is able to direct the line of conversation in such a way that affect shifts are more likely. Unfortunately, there may be a tendency for some patients to direct the course of conversation in the opposite direction in an attempt to produce sessions that are affect-free. Cognitive affective avoidance of this type is often marked by a tendency to discuss situations in fine detail combined with a seeming inability to give direct answers to the therapist's questions. It should be noted, however, that such attention to detail may be a characteristic of the individual's personality rather than situation-specific emotional avoidance.

*Dysfunctional Thoughts Records (DTRs)*

Dysfunctional thought records take different forms. The general standard form of a DTR is presented in Figure 4.0.

DYSFUNCTIONAL THOUGHTS RECORD (DTR)

| DATE | SITUATION | EMOTION | AUTOMATIC THOUGHT | ALTERNATIVE THOUGHT | OUTCOME |
|------|-----------|---------|-------------------|---------------------|---------|
| | Note situation or thought/recollection leading to unpleasant emotion | 1. Note type of emotion (sad, anxious, angry etc)<br><br>2. Rate intensity of emotion (0-100) | 1. Write automatic thought<br><br>2. Rate belief in automatic thought (0-100) | 1. What's another way of viewing the situation<br><br>2. Re-rate belief in automatic thought (0-100) | 1. Note type of emotion<br><br>2. Re-rate intensity of emotion (0-100)<br><br>3. What further action can I take |
| | | | | | |

**Figure 4.0**   Dysfunctional Thoughts Record (DTR)

DTRs are used for a number of purposes. Early in treatment they provide a means of recording negative automatic thoughts associated with emotional change. In this respect they provide information concerning the content of negative automatic thoughts and they offer a means by which the individual can develop an awareness of the links between thoughts and feelings. Thought records and diary measures also provide information on symptom patterns. The existence of patterns in symptoms can be used in some circumstances to strengthen the cognitive formulation of emotional problems, and in the case of health anxiety to falsify the patient's physical illness model. Disorder-specific DTRs should be used when negative automatic thoughts are associated with specific identifiable bodily sensations or other specific stimuli. In the treatment of panic disorder for example, a DTR might consist of additional columns for recording a range of bodily sensations and then a column for recording the negative misinterpretation of these sensations. Disorder-specific cognitive models can be used to develop DTRs that assess the salient NATs implicated by these models. In obsessive-compulsive disorder for example, in which the cognitive model specifies that the negative appraisal of intrusive thoughts is important, the DTR should consist of columns for monitoring intrusive thoughts and columns for noting the negative interpretation of the intrusive thought or NAT (see Chapter 9 for more details). The cognitive model of social phobia predicts that negative self-evaluation is as important as fear of negative evaluation by others in problem maintenance. Therefore, DTRs may consist of columns for recording negative automatic thoughts about the self and for recording negative automatic thoughts concerning other people's evaluation of the self in anxiety-provoking situations.

### Exposure tasks

Exposure is used as a means of activating fear. Patients may be exposed to analogue stressful situations or real-life situations. Access to salient NATs may be restricted when the individual's 'fear mode' is inactive. In these circumstances it is useful to activate the patients' fear in order to increase accessibility of NATs. The effect of 'fear mode' activation on NATs is evident in patient's reports of the believability of negative appraisal. For instance, social phobics believe highly that they are the centre of other people's negative attention when in social situations. However, when questioned away from the situation the level of belief is often diminished. Similarly, panic patients report strong beliefs in catastrophe during panic attacks but are able to question the validity of their belief when not panicking. Exposure exercises provide a mechanism for accessing situationally moderated NATs. Moreover, when avoidance is extensive the reversal of avoidance facilitates access to otherwise inaccessible dysfunctional appraisals. In the following therapy excerpt, the therapist accompanies an agoraphobic patient on a exposure expedition to a normally avoided shopping centre. Initial attempts to determine the content of the patient's NATs in the consulting room were unsuccessful, and it was decided to explore the thoughts elicited by exposure to a feared situation. The example illustrates the types of questions that can be used to determine primary NATs.

T: I'd like you to take a walk along this parade on your own and return back to me in 5 minutes. How do you feel about doing that?

P: I'm feeling anxious already. I'm not sure I can do that.

T: What are the anxious feelings that you have right now?

P: I feel breathless and I'm trembling inside.

T: What thoughts are you having right now?

P: I'm not having any. I just feel anxious.

T: Can you just walk a short way for me on your own? Say to the end of this parade and back.

P: I can try.

T: How do you feel right now?

P: I still feel nervous, it's not getting any better.

T: Do you think anything bad could happen if the symptoms get worse?

P: I just feel so foolish being like this.

T: When you say you feel foolish, do you mean that you might appear foolish?

P: Well, people might notice something odd about me.

T: What's the worse thing they could notice?

P: They could see me walk funny.

T: What would that look like if you walked funny?

P: Well they might see me staggering and think I was drunk or something.

T: One of your frightening thoughts seems to be that you will walk funny and everyone will notice and think that you are drunk. How much do you believe that could happen right now?

P: The way I'm feeling now I think it probably could.

T: On a scale of 0–100 per cent, how much do you believe that could happen right now?

P: About 80 per cent

T: OK, can you go ahead and do the walk right now and let's see what happens?

In this example, the patient's fears concerning negative evaluation by others became clear on exposure to a feared situation. Apart from the information presented in this excerpt, the therapist followed through with the exposure task in order to determine the patient's subtle safety behaviours used during the situation. The information gained was used in building an initial formulation of the patient's problem.

*Role-plays*

Role-plays are a useful form of exposure-based exercise in cases of social anxiety. An advantage of role-plays over real-life exposure is that the variables in some role-plays can be manipulated and controlled more efficiently than real-life social circumstances. This allows for the modulation of social factors in a way that increases fear activation and the accessibility of NATs. In social phobia, for example, the predominant fear may be of one-to-one interactions involving self-disclosure. Analogue situations of this type can be created through role-plays with the therapist. During such role-plays the patient is asked to monitor his/her level of anxiety and to signal an increase in anxiety or distress to the therapist. At this point, the role-play is halted and discussion is focused on the NAT's accompanying anxiety. Dimensions of the role-play can be manipulated in order to increase affect. For example, the therapist may move closer to the patient, may act in a more critical and less friendly way or may ask more personal questions.

*Audio-video feedback*

Audio or video recording of therapy sessions offers the advantage of collaboratively reviewing the tape with a view to determining NATs. The tape is paused at a point where the patient shows signs of an affect shift and the therapist can ask questions to determine the content of thought at that particular time. In effect, feedback is used as a means of prompting memories of negative automatic thoughts at particular instances in time. An advantage of this procedure is that it can distance the individual from situational affect which is useful when affect itself is overwhelming. This technique is also useful in situations where the patient is engaged in some form of social interaction task and it would be disruptive to probe for negative automatic thoughts in the situation. Audio and video recording is particularly prone to activate negative automatic thoughts concerned with public presentation and appearance, and it can therefore be used in conjunction with other exposure procedures to enhance self-consciousness and public performance anxiety.

*Manipulation of safety behaviours*

Since the cognitive model predicts that individuals use safety behaviours to prevent feared catastrophes, it follows that reduction or elimination of safety behaviours during exposure to fearful situations should increase the perceived likelihood of catastrophe thereby rendering negative appraisal more salient. Safety behaviours may be manipulated in two ways: they may be decreased, and they may be increased. Increasing safety behaviours in some circumstances exacerbates bodily sensations and makes misinterpretations more likely. The following extract illustrates an increased safety behaviours manipulation to elicit NATs in a panic disorder patient.

T: When you feel anxious or panicky, do you do anything to try to control the anxiety?

P: I try and take deep breaths and try to relax.

T: If you didn't control your breathing, could anything bad happen in a panic attack?

P: I'd just feel more panicky.

T: What's the worst that could happen if you panicked and didn't control your breathing?

P: Nothing. I suppose the panic would go away eventually.

T: Can I ask you to control your breathing right now, like you do in a panic attack?

P: You mean take deep breaths?

T: Yes. Show me exactly what you do when you're panicking, and practise that until I ask you to stop.

P: (Patient begins slow deep breathing.)

T: That's good, carry on like that.

P: It's making me feel a bit panicky.

T: What are you feeling right now?

P: I feel a little breathless and dizzy.

T: Can I ask you to carry on doing that some more?

P: I'd rather not really.

T: What would happen if you carried on with that?

P: I'd get to feel worse. It feels as though I can't breath.

T: What do you mean you can't breath?

P: It feels as if I could run out of air.

T: Do you think you could run out of air during a panic attack?

P: Yes, I worry that I can't breath properly and that I will be unable to catch my breath.

T: During a panic attack, how much do you believe that you will be unable to breath?

In this example, the patient's use of safety behaviours elicited bodily sensations and associated catastrophic misinterpretations of them. In some cases, merely suggesting the abandonment of safety behaviours during exposure or role-plays will enhance fear and increase the accessibility of negative predictions associated with negative automatic thoughts. For example, an obsessional patient was recently asked not to control his thoughts next time they occurred. His immediate response was 'I couldn't possibly do that, I would lose control.' Clearly this person's NATs centred on themes of loss of behavioural and/or mental control. Increased safety behaviours manipulations are closely associated with symptom induction techniques in that the procedure can be used to induce feared bodily sensations in some cases of panic, social phobia or hypochondriasis.

### Symptom induction

We have already discussed the role of exposure to situations as a means of determining the content of dysfunctional thoughts. Another type of exposure task depends on exposure to internal bodily cues. The elicitation of bodily sensations or cognitive symptoms that are the focus of preoccupation and/or misinterpretation can provide access to a wide range of cognitions concerning danger. For example, an obsessional patient recently was unwilling or unable to articulate his negative automatic thoughts about intrusive thoughts. His fear became accessible, however, when he was asked to deliberately form and hold in mind an unwanted intrusive image. The patient refused to comply with this request and the therapist asked about the worst consequences of performing the task. It became evident that the patient feared that he could cause harm to his family by having particular thoughts. Symptom induction techniques, both for the elicitation of NATs and for challenging them, are illustrated in the panic, social phobia, and generalised anxiety disorder chapters. Physical symptom induction through hyperventilation and exercise are common methods in the treatment of panic and health anxiety.

### Ask about imagery

The occurrence of imagery is easily overlooked when eliciting negative automatic thoughts. If negative thoughts are difficult to elicit, the therapist should check for the presence of negative appraisals in the form of images. Negative automatic images may be difficult for the patient to articulate in verbal form. Whenever the content of thought is elicited or questioned, the therapist should check for the occurrence of images. Spontaneous images of catastrophe can be manipulated in session in order to activate a broader range of negative appraisals. Imagery manipulation strategies can produce affect shifts.

## REATTRIBUTION METHODS

Cognitive therapy aims to modify belief at the level of negative automatic thoughts, and schemas. Durable modification of problems depends on conceptualising and changing the range of variables responsible for maintaining belief at NAT and schema levels. To this end reattribution consists of a range of interlocking strategies, the application of which is determined by the nature of individual case conceptualisations. In this section, reattribution methods are broadly divided into verbal reattribution techniques, and behavioural reattribution techniques, although this distinction is somewhat arbitrary, and both types of technique are used in unison to produce effective cognitive-behavioural change.

## Verbal reattribution

Verbal reattribution techniques rely principally on discussion, and are embedded in the socratic dialogue. Twelve techniques are briefly reviewed in this section. This is by no means an exhaustive list and therapists are encouraged to devise their own reattribution methods 'on-line' during the course of therapy sessions.

### Defining and operationalising terms

The first step in challenging negative automatic thoughts is to develop an understanding of the meaning of such appraisals to the patient. As we saw earlier, the meaning may not be immediately apparent at the surface level. Clearly, it is difficult to effectively challenge beliefs in negative automatic thoughts if their meaning is obscure. A definition of the concepts represented in negative automatic thoughts is required. For example, if a salient thought is 'I can't cope' the precise meaning of the coping concept should be elicited before any challenge of that concept is initiated. Similarly, if an individual states that his/her main fear is one of 'losing control' it is necessary to understand the meaning of this concept for the individual. In this example, what precisely is the patient fearful of losing control of, and what would loss of control look like? The fear could conceivably involve loss of behavioural control, loss of mental control, or loss of emotional control and its appraised consequences. Once the precise nature of the fear is determined verbal and behavioural reattribution can be specifically targeted at that concept. Some useful questions for operationalising terms are:

- When you say that you (can't cope, will lose control, can't stand it), what do you mean?
- If you could not (e.g. cope, etc.), what is the worst that could happen?
- What would (e.g. not coping, etc.), look like?
- If that were true, what would it mean to you?
- If that were true, what would be bad about that?
- What does (e.g. coping, being in control, etc.) consist of?
- If you could (e.g. cope, have control, etc.), how would things be different from the way they are now?

*Questioning the evidence*

Some of the most frequently used verbal reattribution techniques are based on questioning the patient's evidence in support of negative automatic thoughts, assumptions and beliefs. Often there is some form of supporting evidence. Rather than challenging belief in negative appraisals head-on it is useful to elicit and collaboratively explore the quality of patients' evidence in support of negative automatic thoughts. Reinterpretation of evidence that supports NATS or the discovery by the individual that there is little supporting evidence can loosen belief in NATS. The following questions are useful for this purpose:

- What's your evidence that (catastrophe) will happen?
- What makes you think that?
- How do you know that will happen?
- What is you reason for believing (catastrophe) will happen?

In the absence of evidence belief may be weakened. However, when evidence is given the task then becomes one of collaborative evaluation of the quality of the evidence. This can be achieved through reviewing alternative explanations for the evidence, reviewing counter-evidence, and labelling thinking errors as discussed next.

*Reviewing counter-evidence*

Questions for eliciting counter-evidence include:

- What is the evidence to suggest that (catastrophe) is not true or cannot happen?
- What is another way of looking at the problem?
- What is the evidence to support an alternative way of looking at it?
- Has the (catastrophe) happened yet? Why not?

A further line of questioning that may be used in this context is the *'worst, best, most likely* consequences scenario'. Here the patient is asked to describe the worst that could happen in a feared situation. This is followed by a description of the best that could happen, and is concluded by discussion of the most likely thing that could happen. This procedure is an effective means of *'balancing out'* catastrophic thinking and should be followed up with questions aimed at eliciting evidence in support of the most likely scenario. In the following dialogue a combination of questions and techniques are used:

T: When you say that you might act foolish, what do you mean by that?
P: People will think I'm foolish.

T:  What will happen to make people think that?

P:  I will do something foolish and draw attention to myself.

T:  What will you do?

P:  I will get my words wrong and I won't know what to say.

T:  So your negative thought is that you will get your words wrong and people will think that you are foolish?

P:  Yes. I don't want people to think that.

T:  Do you have evidence that that will happen?

P:  It's happened before when I've been anxious in situations. I don't know what to say and my mind goes blank.

T:  It's true that your mind goes blank sometimes, but what makes you think that people see you as foolish?

P:  Well, I don't know for sure.

T:  How would people react to you if they thought you were foolish?

P:  I suppose they wouldn't talk to me and they would ridicule me.

T:  Is there any evidence that people do that to you?

P:  No. Some people might, but people don't usually do that.

T:  So it sounds as if there might be some counter-evidence, some evidence that people don't think you're foolish?

P:  Yes, I suppose there is when you look at it like that.

T:  What is the evidence that people don't think you're foolish?

P:  I have a couple of good friends and I get on well with people at work.

T:  What do you mean by getting on well with people at work?

P:  Some people ask my advice about jobs they are working on.

T:  Is that evidence that they think you are foolish?

P:  No, quite the opposite.

T:  It seems that sometimes you have difficulty knowing what to say when you are anxious, but it seems that people don't think that you are foolish. If people don't think that you are foolish, what else could they think?

P:  Well, they probably don't even notice that I'm being quiet.

T:  Even if they did notice, what might they think?

P:  They might think I'm just being quiet or thoughtful or something.

T:  Thinking about it now, how much do you believe people will think you are foolish?

In this example, a combination of questions were used to define the meaning of acting foolish, to examine the patient's evidence, and to review counter-evidence. At the end of this process a more realistic appraisal was elicited. Notice how the patient produced evidence in support of the occurrence of symptoms of anxiety in social situations (i.e. mind going blank). However, there was little evidence that others thought he was foolish. This distinction is a subtle but crucial one in questioning negative automatic thoughts and predictions. The aim of verbal reattribution is not to challenge predictions concerning the occurrence of anxiety responses. The aim of reattribution must go beyond anxiety symptoms and modify belief in the appraised *consequences*, *meanings*, and *implications* of experiencing anxiety symptoms in cases where these symptoms are themselves a source for concern. For example, if an initial negative automatic thought is 'I will panic' it is meaningless to challenge the thought at this level. Instead, the therapist should determine the implications and meaning of having a panic attack (e.g. 'What is the worst that could happen if you did panic?'). Verbal reattribution should target the meaning or implication of experiencing symptoms.

### Labelling distortions

Identifying and labelling cognitive distortions or 'thinking errors' provides a means of invalidating negative automatic thoughts and beliefs. Burns (1989) has developed the *Triple Column Technique* for identifying distortions in automatic thoughts and for generating more realistic thoughts. Individuals are asked to write down automatic thoughts when they occur and rate belief in them on a scale of 0–100. The next step involves identifying distortions present in each thought such as *black and white thinking, personalising, catastrophising* and so on. The final step involves substituting a rational response for each thought followed by a rating of belief in each alternative response. The three-column technique can be used as a shorthand method of invalidating negative automatic thoughts. It relies on educating patients about different thinking errors and training them to identify thinking errors in their negative automatic thoughts. Initially, patient and therapist may review negative automatic thoughts on previously completed dysfunctional thoughts records and attempt to identify particular thinking errors during the therapy session as an educational exercise.

### Use of rational responses

An end-point of questioning the evidence and identifying thinking errors should be production of rational responses to negative automatic thoughts. Rational responses are entered on the dysfunctional thoughts record in the 'alternative thought column', or they may be written on flash-cards that individuals can carry with them. A rational response flash-card may consist of a rational self-statement on one side of the card and on the reverse side the evidence in support of the response is presented. Patients should be encouraged to generate rational responses to their negative automatic thoughts, and when this is difficult flash-cards can be used to help them challenge dysfunctional thinking. Caution should be exercised, however, since rational responses in some instances may become safety behaviours. For example, individuals fearful of intrusive thoughts may falsely assume that controlling their thinking or using rational responses averts some form of mental catastrophe. In some instances, such as performance situations, it will be helpful for individuals to use rational responses or positive self-statements to regulate their anxiety and maintain task focus. However, care should be taken with this type of usage since some self-regulatory strategies have the potential to interfere with performance, and may become additional safety behaviours. If rational responses are used as safety behaviours to prevent feared catastrophes, they may block belief change. While it is recommended that rational responses should be practised whenever necessary, the effect of this strategy, and the individual's motivation for its usage, should be closely monitored.

### Cost–benefit analysis

Cost–benefit analyses have two aims: (1) to increase patient motivation; and (2) to elicit assumptions and beliefs underlying particular behaviours or underlying the maintenance of particular cognitions. The strategy is also known as an *advantages–disadvantages* analysis. The steps in this procedure are as follows. First, an attitude, belief or behaviour that the therapist and patient wish to modify is selected. Second, a two-column table is constructed and one column is labelled 'costs' or 'disadvantages' and the other column is labelled 'benefits' or 'advantages'. In the next step, therapist and patient work collaboratively in eliciting the patient's appraised *advantages* of holding a belief or engaging in a particular behaviour. Some of the advantages elicited reflect assumptions and beliefs concerning the negative consequences of abandoning particular behaviours or attitudes. When cognitions of this type are present, challenging them may increase compliance with treatment. For example, a generalised anxiety disorder patient was ambivalent about experiments in which she was invited to suspend worrying. For her, worrying had a number of appraised advantages. In particular, she believed that if she worried about the welfare of her children they would remain healthy and safe. She also believed that worrying indicated that she was a good person and a caring mother.

The second step in the cost–benefit analysis consists of listing the *disadvantages* of engaging in the particular behaviour or holding the particular attitude. An effort should be made to generate more disadvantages than advantages. Advantages and disadvantages may also be weighted by assigning a numerical value to each one, and the total weight of disadvantages versus advantages should be compared. When the disadvantages of maintaining a behaviour or attitude outweigh the advantages, the individual should be more motivated to change. The advantages associated with continuing unhelpful behaviours or attitudes should be challenged. Alternative and less problematic ways of acquiring the advantages may be explored.

*Pie charts*

Pie charts offer a means of exploring a range of alternative explanations for events with the aim of reducing likelihood or probability estimates for catastrophic outcomes. Construction of the pie chart is implemented in a number of stages. Once a negative appraisal of an event has been elicited, and belief in the appraisal has been obtained, the first step involves generating a comprehensive list of the potential explanations for the event. For example, if a health-anxious person misinterprets headaches as a sign of a brain tumour, the therapist works with the patient in collaboratively eliciting a range of possible explanations for headaches. These may include: eye strain, migraine, muscle tension, hangover, cold and flu, dehydration, posture, stress, anxiety, and brain tumour. The second step consists of drawing out a pie diagram consisting of a circle with segments allocated to the different explanations listed. The therapist should begin with the most benign explanations for symptoms and leave the catastrophic explanation until last for inclusion in the pie diagram. Usually when a range of explanations for symptoms are taken into account, the likelihood of a catastrophic explanation is reduced. In the following example based on a social phobic case, a pie chart is used to gain a balanced perspective on the negative thought: 'My boss thinks I'm stupid.'

T: What makes you think that?
P: He seemed annoyed when I asked him for an address.
T: Does he often seem annoyed with you?
P: No, we usually work well together.
T: How much do you believe his behaviour meant he thought you were stupid?
P: I should have known where to find the address. I believe it 70 per cent.
T: I'd like to explore with you some other reasons why your boss might seem annoyed. Can you think of any?
P: He doesn't like me.
T: Do you think that's true of your boss?
P: No.
T: Can you think of any other reasons?
P: He could have been having a bad day.
T: Yes, that sounds possible. What else?
P: He might not have been feeling well.
T: Yes that's a good possibility. What else?
P: He was probably stressed.
T: OK. What else can you think of?
P: I don't know, that's about it.
T: Can you think of anything that would make you act that way?
P: Yes, feeling tired.

T: OK. What other things?

P: I can't think of any more.

T: How about too much work, being worried, getting out of the wrong side of bed?

P: Yes I suppose so.

T: Now we have a reasonable list, I'm going to draw a pie chart so that we can get a balanced perspective on these possibilities. If this circle represents all of the explanations we've listed I'd like us to assign a segment of it to each one. Starting with the first explanation. How likely do you think it was that your boss was having a bad day?

P: It's possible. I'll say 25 per cent.

T: Good. How likely is it that he was feeling unwell?

P: Ten per cent.

T: What about him feeling stressed?

P: That's a good one. Forty per cent.

T: What percentage would you give to tiredness?

P: Twenty per cent.

T: How about worry?

P: Ten per cent.

T: I don't think there's room in the circle for ten per cent. Perhaps we should put everything else in this last 5 per cent category, so that each has about one per cent.

P: OK.

T: Looking at the pie chart. See how your original interpretation takes up the smallest amount of space. Taking into account all of the possibilities how likely is it that your boss acted the way he did because he thinks you are stupid?

P: It doesn't seem very likely at all.

T: How much do you believe that now?

The completed pie chart for this example is presented in Figure 4.1.


*Education*

Information that corrects patients' faulty knowledge or lack of understanding can be used to modify belief in thoughts and schemas. This information can be presented verbally or in the form of written material ('bibliotherapy'). In presenting new information the therapist may deviate from a socratic approach and present information in a more didactic way. Education is particularly relevant in anxiety cases in which danger appraisals centre on misinterpretations of bodily sensations or mental events. In panic, for example, information about the effects of hyperventilation is presented and it is emphasised that the symptoms are normal and harmless. In cases

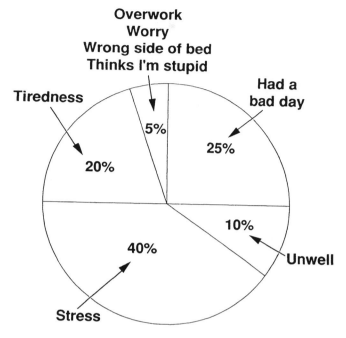

**Figure 4.1** Pie-chart for a social phobic case

involving fears of choking or suffocation the patients understanding of swallowing and breathing mechanisms, and safety reflexes such as coughing are enhanced. The presentation of new information is often preceded by an exploration of the patients existing understanding so that new information can be directed at correcting faulty understanding rather than it merely acting as a 'blanket reassurance'. Education can be a powerful means of normalising patients experience of symptoms. For example, obsessional patients should be educated about the normal occurrence of obsessions, and when appropriate research papers and similar material supporting new knowledge may be given as additional bibliotherapy.

*Continuous presentation of the model*

A clear understanding by the patient of the cognitive formulation is central in determining a framework for belief change and for understanding the use of particular treatment strategies. The formulation offers an understanding and alternative set of beliefs about presenting problems that often differ from a patient's initial understanding of the problem. In health anxiety, for example, through repeated presentation of the cognitive model a health-anxious patient begins to view his/her problem as one of worry about illness and disease as opposed to a problem of actual physical illness.

### Point and counter-point

This technique consists of patient and therapist alternating roles of presenting a negative automatic thought, or counter-arguments or counter-evidence. The therapist may begin by articulating one of the patient's key negative automatic thoughts, and asks the patient to argue against the thought. When the patient begins to find this difficult, the roles are reversed and the therapist then continues the challenge of the negative thought(s). Both therapist and patient speak in the first person (e.g. 'I think . . .') during the task when presenting NATs.

### Imagery techniques

Negative automatic thoughts occur in imagery as well as verbal form. While verbal reattribution techniques are suitable in most cases for modifying the meanings and implications that dysfunctional images contain, imagery itself can be manipulated in the exploration and challenging of meaning.

In anxiety disorders images represent potential future disasters, in which case they have a predictive quality, and/or they can represent intrusive recollections ('flashbacks') of stressful past events, as in cases of post-traumatic stress disorder. Often patients terminate images before or at their worst point since exposure to them is distressing. Initially the meaning and significance of having the image should be explored. In some cases, such as post-traumatic stress or obsessive-compulsive disorder, the image is appraised as dangerous. For example, a patient may believe it is a sign of 'mental breakdown' or 'loss of control'. Negative automatic thoughts about imagery should be elicited and *challenged* whenever necessary. Intrusive negative images are likely to be terminated at their worst point in the portrayal of events. In some cases it is useful to 'finish-out' images and take them beyond the worst point. This procedure reduces the amount of distress accompanying the image and shifts the patient out of danger processing mode. In the following example *finishing-out* was used with an obsessional washer who feared contracting disease and subsequent death. He frequently experienced an intrusive image in which he had died but was somehow trapped inside his body. The intrusive image was causing significant distress.

T: I'd like you to close your eyes and form the image right now. Try to make it as clear as you can. When you have a clear image signal to me by raising a finger on your right hand.

P: (Raises finger.)

T: OK. Can you describe to me what is happening in the image right now?

P: Yes. I'm dead and it's all dark.

T: Where are you right now?

P: I'm in a coffin, I'm underground, I've been buried.

T: OK. What's happening now?

P: Nothing, I'm trapped.

T: I'd like you to run the image on, allow time to pass in your image. A few days and weeks, and now several months. What is happening to you now?

P: I'm still trapped nothing much has changed. The winter has turned to summer but I'm not a part of it.

T: What has happened to your body in this time. Is it the same?

P: Well no. I suppose its started to decay.

T: OK. Staying with that image take the time on a few more months, so that your body decays even more. What is happening to you now?

P: That's it I'm free. I'm no longer trapped in my body because it no longer exists.

T: Staying with that image of being free. How does that make you feel now?

P: I feel better. It's OK now. I'm not going to be trapped for ever.

In this example, the therapist offers some prompting concerning how the image might change. However, in some cases merely staying with an image or simply suggesting running the image forward or backward in time is all that is required for a spontaneous modification to take place. When a more spontaneous change seems unlikely the therapist should take a more active role in manipulating the contents of the image. In the example above, the patient was asked to practise finishing out the image whenever it was activated between sessions. He found that he had to do this only a few times since the image lost its initial salience following this procedure. In this example, imagery modification changed the patient's belief that he would be trapped in his body following death.

Aside from 'finishing-out' as a means of modifying belief and the affective significance of images, basic verbal reattribution techniques such as questioning the evidence for the events portrayed, and generating counter-evidence should also be used. However, in some instances the effect of verbal reattribution seems to be a less profound experience for the individual than belief change through direct imagery manipulation. A technique of manipulation that has been used in the treatment of early traumatic memories in personality disorder involves recalling events in imagery and instructing the patient to introduce into the image modifications that counteract negative affect and threat (e.g. Layden, Newman, Freemen & Morse, 1993). For example, if the patient is a child in the memory, the instruction might be to grow older in the image and to assert control over the situation, or to have a trusted adult enter the situation and provide safety.

A strategy of prolonged exposure to traumatic images following exposure to traumatic events such as rape has been used as a component of cognitive-behavioural treatment of post-traumatic stress disorder (e.g. Foa, Rothbaum, Riggs & Murdock, 1991). A rationale for the use of repeated exposure is that it facilitates assimilation of new material in memory in a way that reduces fear activation (e.g. Foa and Kozak, 1986).

*Action plans*

Action plans consist of generating strategies for dealing more effectively with difficult situations. This can encompass selecting and practising particular skills for dealing with stressful social encounters, and generating summaries of adaptive responses for use in situations. New ways of dealing with situations may be mentally rehearsed and 'de-bugged' before implementation (*cognitive rehearsal*). A central element in relapse prevention work is the attempted forecasting of difficult situations that could arise in the future following therapy and the generation of a plan of how to deal with the situation should it arise.

## Summary of verbal reattribution

A range of the most useful and commonly used verbal strategies was presented in the first part of this chapter. These techniques are not intended to be used in isolation, but are intended for use in conjunction with each other and in conjunction with behavioural reattribution strategies. The selection and use of techniques is guided by the individual case conceptualisation. In many instances verbal reattribution offers only a preliminary step in cognitive-behavioural change, it is not an end in itself. Verbal reattribution techniques offer a means of loosening belief and presenting a foundation for attitude change. The most significant change in cognitive therapy of anxiety is usually obtained when behavioural reattribution is used. We consider the use of behavioural strategies next.

## BEHAVIOURAL REATTRIBUTION

Behavioural strategies offer the most powerful means of cognitive change in cognitive therapy. Many of the techniques used in the treatment of anxiety resemble strategies used in other treatment approaches such as behaviour therapy. In the more eclectic varieties of cognitive-behaviour therapy such strategies are often imported from other orientations and applied with little or no modification. Readers will probably have gathered that I do not favour such an approach, and the theme running throughout this book is that cognitive therapy should use techniques that are geared towards modifying the variables that maintain anxiety disorder as specified by an appropriate cognitive model. Typically this requires that procedures not originally based on a cognitive model are modified and finely tuned in order to produce optimal therapeutic effects. For example, it is common for relaxation to be used in the treatment of anxiety disorders, however an important question concerns the appropriateness of this technique in treatments that aim to maximise belief change. While relaxation is likely to modify particular types of belief, it may not modify belief in primary NATs. For example, it may increase the belief that anxiety is controllable but if a primary fear driving anxiety is that anxiety is harmful, teaching control could prevent modification of this. Returning to the concept of safety behaviours (Salkovskis, 1991; Wells et al., 1995b), discussed in Chapter 1, the provision of relaxation or distraction in some treatments could be equivalent to introducing new safety behaviours, and their attendant problems. This is not to imply that relaxation or other symptom control procedures do not have a place in anxiety treatment, just that their usage should not compromise modification of primary dysfunctional thoughts and schemas.

## Use of exposure in cognitive therapy

Broadly speaking two classes of exposure have been used in cognitive therapy of anxiety: (1) exposure to feared external stimuli, and (2) exposure to feared internal stimuli. We have seen how exposure may be used to elicit negative automatic thoughts for the purposes of assessment and case conceptualisation. However, it is predominantly used in connection with challenging belief in negative automatic thoughts and schemas. In this context exposure constitutes a component of *behavioural experiments* designed to modify belief at negative automatic thought and schema levels. This differs from its usage in behavioural treatments. Some treatment packages have used exposure to internal bodily sensations (interoceptive exposure) in the treatment of panic disorder, or have introduced anxiety control strategies such as relaxation and breathing retraining (e.g. Barlow, Craske, Cerny & Klosco, 1989). While these approaches are capable of modifying misinterpretations of bodily sensations they are based on different models of panic to the one considered in this book. Cognitive therapy of panic is effective without the provision of control techniques such as breathing re-training (Salkovskis, Clark & Hackmann, 1991).

## Behavioural experiments

Behavioural experiments have three basic aims: socialisation, reattribution, and modification of affect. Experiments are used to socialise patients in the cognitive model. Following derivation of an individual case formulation the therapist aims to 'sell' the model to the patient. Behavioural experiments offer one effective means of demonstrating the principles represented in the formulation. Examples of socialisation experiments include manipulating safety behaviours and observing the effect on bodily sensations. Safety behaviours may be increased, and decreased and the effects on anxiety, self-consciousness and performance contrasted (Wells & Clark, 1995). More specifically, when selective attention to the self is a component of problem maintenance, patients can be instructed to focus attention on bodily or mental events and observe the effects on symptom intensity, anxiety or performance. In panic cases selective attention manipulations such as focusing on particular parts of the body are used to demonstrate the effect of thinking on symptom perception. The paired associates task is another socialisation experiment used in panic. This involves the reading of symptom-catastrophe word lists (e.g. chest tight—heart attack; dizziness—fainting; breathless—suffocate; unreality—insane; palpitations—dying) and the effect of dwelling on these words on anxiety and symptoms is discussed. Specific examples of socialisation procedure are presented in subsequent chapters of this book.

Behavioural experiments are used to challenge belief at the appraisal and schema level. In this context they represent 'reality testing' procedures that offer a means of validating particular predictions derived from patients' appraisals, and schemas. This usage of behavioural experiments predominates in cognitive therapy. In this context, experiments are used to collect and assimilate data for replacement beliefs (education). In subsequent sections the precise implementation of disconfirmatory experiments is discussed. Finally, experiments may also be used to modify affective experience. In this latter context, techniques such as activity scheduling, distraction procedures, and relaxation are used to provide *temporary* relief from symptoms and interrupt unhelpful cognitive, affective and behavioural cycles that interfere with engagement in cognitive therapy. These types of experiment can be used to socialise in the model. For example, in depression treatment activity scheduling is introduced as an experiment to illustrate how modifying behaviour and distracting from negative thoughts can influence mood. The results of such a procedure can be used as supportive evidence for the cognitive formulation of depression, while at the same time the procedure may begin to challenge negative appraisals that contribute to depressive inertia.

## Disconfirmation experiments in anxiety and depression

In anxiety treatment, behavioural experiments typically involve testing predictions concerning physical, social or psychological danger. They require a combination of *exposure* to feared events plus *disconfirmatory manoeuvres* that are intended to test out belief in thoughts. An exception to this format is the survey-based experiment. The *survey technique* consists of collecting data through observation of events or by interviewing other people. For example, a health-anxious patient who misinterpreted deviations in his heart rate and believed that such deviations were 'abnormal and must be a sign of something serious', was instructed to conduct a mini-survey by asking ten colleagues or friends if they ever noticed changes in their heart rate. The therapist also asked a further five people. The results of the survey showed that four out of the ten people whom the patient asked reported that they had noticed changes. This finding significantly reduced his dysfunctional belief.

In depression treatment experiments typically involve methods to modulate mood, challenge appraisals of hopelessness, counteract depressive inertia, and challenge specific predictions. Examples include: activity scheduling, mastery and pleasure techniques, graded task assignment, and problem solving. For more information on depression the interested reader is referred to Beck, Rush, Shaw and Emery (1979).

## Designing and implementing effective experiments

Effective experiments are primarily those that modify belief in the cognitions that maintain anxiety. Four principles should be considered in designing experiments. First it is necessary to identify *Key target cognitions* that are to be challenged in the experiment. Second, key cognitions should be *operationalised* in concrete observable terms. This means vague ideas require reframing as specific tangible concepts. For example, the social phobic who states that s/he will 'look stupid' in a particular situation should be asked to describe what 'looking stupid' would actually consist of (e.g. babble uncontrollably). Similarly if a panic patient fears 'losing control' this will need operationalisation. Some appraisals and beliefs, for example 'having a heart attack; fainting; losing bladder control', have clear observable consequences and thus require less operationalisation. Third, the therapist and patient should determine which variables are to be manipulated in experiments so that thoughts can be challenged. This is achieved by examining the nature of the patient's avoidance and safety behaviours. Typically, reversing avoidance, dropping safety behaviours, or intensifying symptoms will provide a means of testing appraisals and beliefs. A *testable prediction* should be established based on the patients thought's. For example, the social phobic who thinks 'I'll babble uncontrollably', might predict that if s/he interacts with a stranger while not engaging in safety behaviours (i.e. not avoiding eye contact, and not mentally rehearsing sentences before saying them), the catastrophe will happen. By tape-recording an interaction under decreased safety behaviour conditions it is possible to disconfirm this prediction. In the case of a panic patient who leaves situations before anxiety reaches a peak because the fear is one of collapsing, a key avoidance or safety behaviour is escape. By reversing this behaviour so that the individual remains in the situation during peak anxiety the belief in collapsing can be challenged. The fourth principle to consider when designing an experiment is *rating of belief* level. Belief in appraisals should be elicited before and after execution of the experiment. Changes in belief are indicative of the effectiveness of the procedure. An experiment may have to be repeated a number of times in its original or a modified form in order to achieve maximal belief change.

Behavioural experiments in cognitive therapy of anxiety can be conceptualised as consisting of two central elements: **exposure** to a feared situation or stimulus, *plus* the execution of a **disconfirmatory manoeuvre**. The disconfirmatory manoeuvre serves to unambiguously **test** a prediction or thought, and typically involves, abandoning safety behaviours, staying with anxiety to see what really happens, or paradoxical symptom enhancement procedures.

The actual implementation of an experiment can be viewed in terms of a sequence of stages:

*Stage 1:* Focus on a key cognition and discuss the evidence supporting belief in the cognition. The elicitation of evidence can provide ideas about what should be manipulated in the experiment. At this initial stage some verbal challenging of evidence is often desirable since it serves to loosen the belief, and can enhance compliance with the subsequent experiment.

*Stage 2:* Identify situations or events that elicit anxiety, *and* identify behaviours or variables that prevent disconfirmation of belief (usually avoidance, in-situation safety, escape, or checking behaviours).

*Stage 3:* Establish a cognitive set that facilitates belief change. Basically, this consists of sharing with the patient a rationale for the experiment. A rationale should emphasise the role of behaviours in maintaining dysfunctional belief, and the need to experiment with decreasing or increasing target behaviours (and anxiety symptoms) in order to test out belief. The rationale should be able to answer the question: 'What is the aim of running this experiment?'

*Stage 4:* Expose the patient to the feared situation, stimulus, or bodily sensation, *and* have the patient implement a *disconfirmatory manoeuvre* that disconfirms belief in catastrophe during exposure. When the feared event is a bodily sensation, as in cases of panic and health anxiety, the exposure component usually involves induction of the feared bodily sensation.

*Stage 5:* Discuss the results of the experiment in terms of the case conceptualisation and use the outcome to determine similar experimental tests that can be applied to specific thoughts (beliefs) in the therapy session and for homework.

It is important to obtain belief ratings for target thoughts before and after the experiment. This can be done simply by asking the patient: 'How much on a scale of zero to one-hundred, do you believe that . . .?' If a degree of belief remains, the basis for this should be explored, and new experiments and verbal reattribution should be used to reduce the belief to zero. In some instances, when behavioural experiments are used for socialisation purposes, a rationale is often omitted. This is because expectancy effects can interfere with the outcome of the experiment. (If the experiment does not work in the way specified by a rationale, this could diminish the patients confidence in the cognitive formulation.) Thus, socialisation experiments such as the paired associates and bodily attention tasks are not usually presented with a preliminary rationale.

The behavioural experiment sequence outlined here and its basic content is summarised in Figure 4.2 some readers may find it helpful to remember the mnemonic **PETS** which stands for Prepare, Expose, Test, and Summarise in implementing a behavioural experiment.

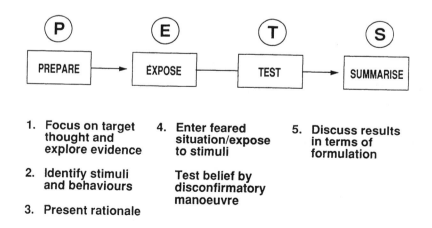

**Figure 4.2**   Summary of behavioural experiment sequence (PETS)

Cognitive therapists typically design and implement several experiments in the course of a single treatment session. Use of experiments early in treatment is advisable for accelerating cognitive-behavioural change.

## Difficulties with behavioural experiments

A number of difficulties are commonly reported by cognitive therapy trainees concerning use of behavioural experiments: inability to think of a suitable experiment; patient non-compliance with the experiment; and therapist anxiety about running experiments.

An inability to generate a suitable experiment is often the result of a vague or incomplete case conceptualisation. If this is so, more time should be devoted to generating a specific case formulation that can be used to make predictions about the mechanisms maintaining the disorder. In a related vein, it is difficult to generate experiments if the primary negative automatic thoughts or beliefs associated with anxiety are unclear. The solution is to focus efforts on eliciting primary cognitions. One of the simplest ways of generating disconfirmatory manoeuvres relies on identifying the patient behaviours that are used to prevent feared catastrophes (e.g. avoidance, safety behaviours, checking, selective attention) and manipulating these behaviours in feared situations. Apart from this tactic other experiments consist of collecting information from various sources, for example by mini-survey or observational strategies. This type of procedure should be used when fears are partially supported by a lack of knowledge about other people's experiences or a lack of knowledge about other people's reaction in the environment. These techniques are useful for 'normalising' events.

Non-compliance with experiments is not a common problem, despite the fact that experiments require exposure to feared situations and events. When non-compliance does occur this is usually the result of a lack of understanding of the reason for the experiment, or due to a strong belief that catastrophe will occur. A lack of understanding can be overcome by clear presentation or re-presentation of a rationale. If the patient is too fearful initially to comply with the experiment, gentle but firm persuasion should be used, the therapist should persist in trying to implement the experiment but not to the point where it could threaten the therapeutic relationship itself. In order to increase compliance the therapist should perform the experiment with the patient, perhaps even modelling the experiment before the patient tries it. Another strategy is to break the experiment up into more manageable 'chunks' so that a graded approach is used. For example, a panic patient may initially be asked to take only five deep breaths in a hyperventilation task, and then try ten breaths and so on, until s/he can hyperventilate for an extended time period in order to discover that catastrophe does not occur.

A therapist's own negative automatic thoughts can interfere with the use of experiments. These can range from a fear of 'making the patient worse'; 'causing a panic attack'; 'causing the patient to drop out of treatment', or actually causing a feared catastrophe. In order to overcome this problem it is necessary for the therapist to work on his/her own negative automatic thoughts. When a concern is that the patient will become distressed in the session, it is helpful to run the experiment close to the beginning of the session so that extended time can be given for discussing the implications of the experiment and for allowing emotion to subside.

## SAFETY IN TREATMENT

The patient's physical well-being must be safeguarded in treatment. Therefore, before running experiments that involve strenuous physical exercise or hyperventilation the patient's physical health must be checked, and the patient's medical doctor should be consulted for advice on whether these procedures could cause a problem. In cases where there are physical conditions such as asthma, potentially life-threatening cardiovascular complaints, pregnancy, and epilepsy, hyperventilation and vigorous exercise should not be used. As an alternative rely on situational exposure plus dropping of safety behaviours, or extended exposure to situations in order to provide disconfirmation.

## Schema-focused techniques in anxiety disorder

Much of the initial therapeutic effort in the treatment of anxiety disorders centres on challenging and modifying cognition at the level of appraisals/negative automatic thoughts. When there are concurrent problems of personality disorder a greater amount of time may need to be devoted to conceptualising and modifying underlying dysfunctional schemas concerning the self and the world. Schema-focused interventions whether they are anxiety disorder related or related to underlying personality problems should normally be introduced following symptomatic-focused interventions. More specifically, schema work should constitute a later stage of therapy following successful implementation of symptom-focused cognitive therapy. Some schemas are clearly related to presenting anxiety problems. In particular, health-anxious patients may have assumptions concerning the significance of stress and anxiety responses for physical and mental well-being. Similarly, some social phobics hold assumptions linking anxiety to social acceptability—for example: 'If I show signs of anxiety, people will think I'm foolish.' Beyond these conditional assumptions there may also be unconditional beliefs associated with anxiety disorders. Some examples of assumptions and beliefs across anxiety disorders are presented in Table 4.0.

In the remainder of this chapter techniques for eliciting and challenging assumptions and beliefs are discussed.

## ELICITING ASSUMPTIONS

Schematic content can be determined in several ways. Several questionnaires exist for eliciting schemas in personality disorders and depression

**Table 4.0**   Examples of assumptions and beliefs in five anxiety disorders

| Disorder | Assumption | Belief |
| --- | --- | --- |
| Social phobia | If I can't think of something to say, people will think I'm boring | I'm boring/inadequate |
| | If I tremble, people will notice and think I'm weird | I'm different I don't fit in |
| Generalised anxiety | If I worry, I'll be able to cope | Worrying helps me cope (I can't cope) |
| | I must control my worries or I'll cease to function | My worry is uncontrollable (I'm losing my mind) |
| Panic | If I become over-anxious my breathing could stop | I'm vulnerable (Anxiety is dangerous) |
| | If I panic it means I'm mentally weak | I'm weak (I've damaged my brain) |
| Obsessive–compulsive | If I don't check I'll never be able to relax | My emotions could overwhelm me |
| | If I think I've harmed someone, I probably have harmed them | My bad thoughts are real |
| Hypochondriasis | If I have unexpected physical symptoms, it signals serious illness | I'm going to be punished . . . (by illness) |
| | If I become ill, I'll be a worthless person | I am what I do |

such as the Schema Questionnaire (Young, 1990) and the Dysfunctional Attitude Scales (Weissman & Beck, 1978). These instruments may not be particularly relevant to cases of anxiety alone. Questionnaires do exist that appear to be more relevant to anxiety. Cartwright-Hatton and Wells (1997) developed the Meta-Cognitions Questionnaire (MCQ) to assess dimensions of assumptions and beliefs associated with intrusive worrying thoughts. This measure may be used to determine salient schemas in anxiety disorders in which intrusive thoughts predominate such as Generalised Anxiety Disorder and Obsessive-Compulsive Disorder. Wells and Hackmann (unpublished) have developed a Death Beliefs Questionnaire based on earlier work with imagery in health anxious patients. This measure covers a range of attitudes and assumptions concerning illness and death. The Social Cognitions Questionnaire developed by Wells, Stopa and Clark (unpublished) assesses a range of cognitions associated with social phobia. Some of the items on this scale represent beliefs. Where pre-existing measures of attitudes and assumptions are unavailable, therapists should construct individual rating scales for use with clients. The assumptions presented in Table 4.0 may be used as a thematic guide for this purpose.

The themes present in patients' automatic thoughts are typically indicative of similar themes that exist in underlying assumptions and beliefs. More specifically, if negative automatic thoughts concern themes of negative social self-appraisal, as in cases of social phobia, schemas should consist of rules concerning social performance and/or conditional assumptions concerning the social implication of particular events. Similarly, unconditional beliefs should represent dysfunctional constructions of the self as a social object. If negative automatic thoughts centre on catastrophic misinterpretations of bodily sensations, as is characteristic of panic or hypochondriasis, beliefs and assumptions should reflect the meaning and significance of bodily and mental events for physical and psychological well-being. Unconditional beliefs may reflect themes of physical or mental weakness or beliefs concerning the presence of damage to the body (e.g. 'I am weak'; 'My heart is damaged'). In health anxiety, general assumptions concerning biological mechanisms in the body and the way the body 'should' function may predominate (e.g. 'A healthy body should be symmetrical').

Schematic content may be determined by the vertical arrow technique (Burns, 1980). Here the meaning of an automatic thought is repeatedly questioned in order to determine the 'bottom line'. This process proceeds with the questions *'If that were to happen, what would that mean to you?'* or *'If that were true, what would be so bad about that?'*. The results of using a vertical arrow on the negative automatic thought 'What if I babble or talk funny?' is presented in Figure 4.3.

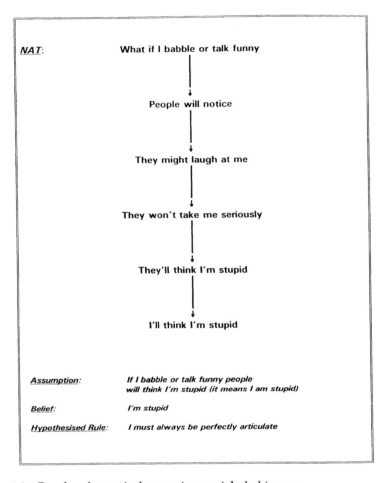

**Figure 4.3**   Results of a vertical arrow in a social phobic case

The sequence of questions used to achieve the result depicted in Figure 4.3 was as follows:

P:  What if I babble and talk funny?
T:  If you did babble and talk funny, what would be bad about that?
P:  People will notice.
T:  And if they noticed, what would that mean?
P:  They would laugh at me.
T:  What would be bad about that?
P:  They wouldn't take me seriously.
T:  What would that mean if they didn't take you seriously?

P: They'll think I'm stupid.

T: What would it mean if they thought that about you?

P: It probably means that I am stupid.

T: What would that mean if it were true?

P: It means everyone would know I'm stupid.

T: You seem to hold the assumption that if you babble or talk funny it means that people will think you're stupid or perhaps you'll believe that you are stupid. How much do you believe that?

P: Well it is a pretty stupid thing to do. It's not normal, is it?

T: So how much do you believe that babbling or talking funny means people will think you are stupid?

P: 80 per cent.

T: How much do you believe that you are stupid?

P: Well I don't normally think that I am stupid, but when I feel anxious around other people, then I believe it.

T: How much do you believe it in that situation?

P: Completely.

In this example the patient's responses are taken and reformulated as an assumption. A belief rating in the assumption and its link to anxious situations is then elicited to verify its validity. The data present in this vertical arrow can also be used to construct hypothesised rules that the patient may hold. In this example the belief was 'I am stupid'. This belief was not chronically activated but was activated by particular situations. In this example the patient's rule for social performance led to the use of a range of self-regulatory or safety behaviours such as closely monitoring her speech, carefully pronouncing words and saying little in social encounters in order to prevent the appraised catastrophes of performance failure. Typically the bottom of the vertical arrow is marked by a failure to progress to new concepts and a return to thoughts or implications represented in an earlier step of the sequence. Figure 4.4 illustrates the vertical arrow for an obsessive-compulsive patient. In this case negative automatic thoughts in the form of doubts or questioning of personal actions acted as triggers for checking rituals.

## Meta-cognition and the vertical arrow

A meta-cognitive analysis of disorders of intrusive thought (Wells, 1995) in which appraisal of thought is a central feature, such as 'worry about worry' or negative appraisal of intrusions, presents implications on the way in which the vertical arrow is executed. In particular the differentiation between Type 1 and Type 2 worries (Wells, 1995), in which Type 1 worry

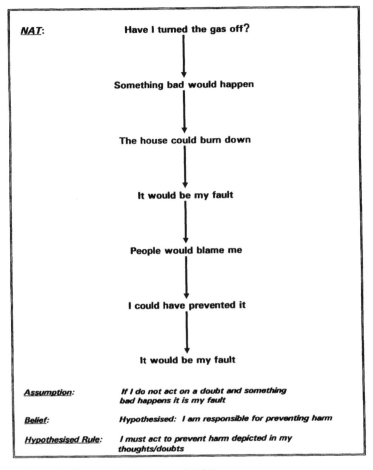

**Figure 4.4**   A vertical arrow in the case of OCD

concerns external events and non-cognitive internal stimuli, and Type 2 worry concerns cognitive events themselves, suggests two distinct implementations of the vertical arrow in cases of generalised anxiety and obsessive-compulsive disorder. It is possible to question the implications and consequences of the events depicted in an intrusive thought (Type 1 vertical arrow), and to question the implications and consequences of having the thought itself (Type 2 vertical arrow), Figure 4.4 above shows the results of a Type 1 vertical arrow and 4.5 shows the results of a Type 2 vertical arrow on an individual with checking rituals in which a checking episode was triggered by the negative automatic thought (actually an 'automatic doubt'): 'Have I turned the gas off?'

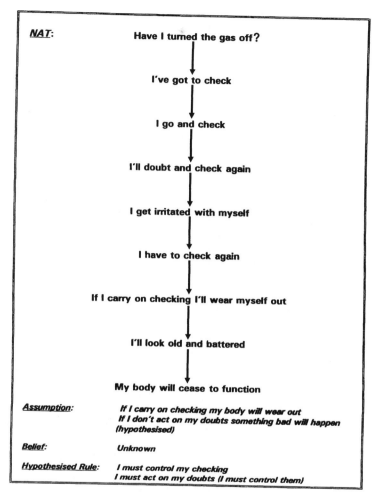

**Figure 4.5** A meta-cognitive vertical arrow in the same case of OCD

In Figure 4.4 it is apparent that questioning the negative implications represented in the thought, revealed concepts of self-blame and being blamed by others. These concepts are closely associated with the notion of responsibility in obsessive-compulsive disorder (e.g. Salkovskis, 1985). However, by using the Type 2 variant of the downward arrow, as illustrated by Figure 4.5, different underlying assumptions and beliefs were elicited. Broadly, these two usages are associated with meta-cognitive and cognitive conceptualisations of the problem. In particular, a meta-cognitive approach (Wells, 1995) implies that the vertical arrow should be focused on the implications of having particular types of thoughts, hence the initial question 'What's so bad about thinking that?'. In contrast, a more general cognitive approach questions the meaning of the catastrophe inherent in the negative automatic thought or doubt as illustrated in Figure 4.4. In general clinical practice, it is useful to implement both types of vertical arrow in the exploration of underlying schemas and meanings. The sequence of questions used to determine the vertical arrows displayed in Figures 4.4 and 4.5 are presented below.

*Figure 4.4 dialogue*

P: Have I turned the gas off?
T: *If you hadn't turned it off, what would be bad about that?*
P: Something bad would happen.
T: What would happen?
P: The house could burn down.
T: What would that mean?
P: It would be my fault.
T: What would be so bad about that?
P: People would blame me.
T: What's bad about that?
P: I could have prevented it.
T: What's bad about that?
P: It means it would be my fault.
T: What would be bad about that?
P: Nothing else, that's it. I wouldn't be able to live with myself, I'd feel so guilty.

*Figure 4.5 dialogue*

P: Have I turned the gas off?
T: *What's so bad about having that thought?*
P: I've got to check.
T: What's bad about that?
P: It means I go and check.
T: And what's bad about that?
P: I'll end up doubting and have to check again.
T: What's bad about that?
P: I get irritated with myself and feel uncomfortable.
T: And then what, what's so bad about that?
P: I have to check again.
T: And what's so bad about that?
P: If I carry on checking, I'll wear myself out.
T: And if you wear yourself out, what will that mean?

P: I'll look old and shattered.
T: What do you mean by that?
P: My body will cease to function.
T: And what's so bad about that?
P: Well no one wants that to happen, do they?
T: No, I suppose you're right, no one does.

## Imagery and schemas

Imagery techniques can be used to elicit the content of underlying schemas. The meanings of events represented in spontaneously occurring intrusive images should be questioned to determine underlying meanings. The types of image that normally occur in anxiety can be induced in the therapy session and the vertical arrow may be performed while the patient holds the image in mind. Particular bodily sensations or affect experienced in conjunction with images can be explored to determine the nature of early learning experiences that may have led to the formation of early maladaptive schemas. For example, a health-anxious patient reported the experience of an intrusive image in which he saw himself trapped in a barrel at the bottom of the sea. He was instructed to form this image in the therapy session and the nature of his feeling associated with this image was elicited. He reported feeling trapped, helpless and suffocated. When he tried to move or break free, the barrel would shrink around him and restrict his movements. When asked what the barrel image meant to him, the patient disclosed that he thought it was like being dead. From this material it was hypothesised that the patient had some dysfunctional assumptions and beliefs about death and dying. More specifically, it transpired that being dead would mean being trapped and alone for ever. It was hypothesised that such a schema would contribute to hypervigilance for bodily symptoms and misinterpretation tendencies. Accordingly the schema was modified during relapse prevention work in therapy.

## Restructuring of rules, assumptions and beliefs

Once the stages in the vertical arrow and the bottom line have been established, the predominant theme should be reformulated as an assumption, belief and/or hypothesised rule. Cognitive therapy may then proceed by challenging these assumptions and beliefs. One strategy is the restructuring of the vertical arrow itself. The vertical arrow is drawn out so that the patient may see it, and verbal and behaviour reattribution strategies are used to challenge the linkages between each level of the downward arrow represented by the arrows themselves. For example, in restructuring the links between concepts in the vertical arrow, the types of thinking errors represented by each linkage can be identified. The evidence for each linkage can be questioned. An example of restructuring the vertical arrow is presented in Figure 4.6. Alternative more realistic concepts should be generated, and behavioural experiments should be run to test out the likelihood or probability of events depicted.

Belief at the schema level should be modified in the same way as belief at the level of negative automatic thoughts and appraisals. The verbal and behavioural reattribution strategies reviewed throughout this chapter are applicable to the modification of cognition at both levels. Specific schema modification strategies have been developed and applied in the treatment of personality disorders, and the interested reader should refer to the texts by Layden et al. (1993) and Beck and Freeman (1990). Schema-focused

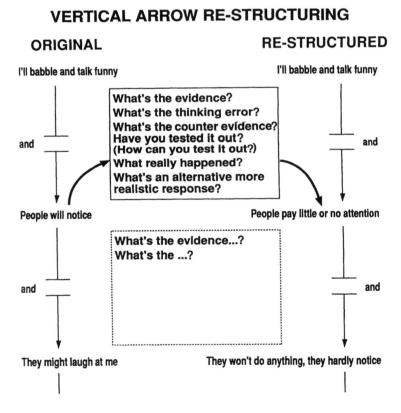

**Figure 4.6** Diagram depicting the process of restructuring the vertical arrow

interventions begin with the identification of schematic content. The next step consists of educating patients about schemas. At the most basic level, this educational process conveys the following information: *Beliefs and assumptions guide interpretations of events and influence behaviour and emotion. Some beliefs result from early learning experiences while others develop later in life, sometimes as a consequence of suffering from emotional problems such as anxiety. In order to understand vulnerability to anxiety and to reduce such vulnerability in the future, it is helpful to identify underlying beliefs and assumptions that may be relevant and to change them. These underlying assumptions and beliefs are given a name and they are usually called schemas.* The existence of schemas can be discussed in the context of more general beliefs that people have and the way in which these beliefs shape behaviour and emotions. For example, the effects of religious or political beliefs may be discussed. The next step of schema modification consists of challenging schemas directly. In this context particular emotive techniques can be used such as imaginary dialogues with parents, role plays of appropriate 'ventilation of emotions'. Cognitive techniques in addition to those discussed previously include the use of *continua* to modify dichotomous thinking, development of flashcards to contradict schemas, and repetition of rational responses.

Since schemas often consist of dichotomous concepts, continua work offers a means of introducing shades of grey in the patient's system of judgement. There are different ways of constructing continua. Typically both ends of the continuum are defined and based on these definitions other points along the continuum are operationalised with reference to other people or characteristics of people or situations. A continuum used in the treatment of a socially anxious person with the belief 'I'm boring' is presented in Figure 4.7.

The stages in collaboratively generating the continuum depicted in Figure 4.7 were as follows. First, the concept of being a boring person was defined. The characteristics that constitute a boring person were listed. Second, the opposite end of the continuum, characteristics of being interesting were listed. Third, examples of different points along the continuum were sought (these can be examples of people that the patient knows or, in this case may be generated from contributions of particular characteristics). Fourth, the patient was encouraged to locate himself on the continuum. When he did this he could see that he had most of the characteristics at the 40 per cent level and some characteristics from the 60 per cent level and so he located himself at 50 per cent. In the process of constructing the continuum, the patient conceded that he probably would not wish to be anything above 60 on the scale since people with an excess of the characteristics he considered desirable could be annoying and socially undesirable.

```
┌─────────────────────────────────────────────────────────────────┐
│                      CONTINUA WORKSHEET                          │
│                                                                 │
│  Belief:    "I'm boring"                                        │
│                                                                 │
│                                                                 │
│      0   10  20  30  40  50  60  70  80  90  100               │
│      |   L   L   L   L   L   L   L   L   L   |                 │
│    Boring                    ▲              Not boring         │
│                                                                 │
│                                                                 │
│     0 (Boring)  =   No friends, no interests, never goes out,  │
│                     ignored by everyone, is useless, never says │
│                     interesting things, has never travelled,   │
│                     has no personality of his own.             │
│                                                                 │
│       20        =   Has one or two friends, has a hobby, people │
│                     show some interest, is able to hold people in│
│                     conversation, has a viewpoint on things.   │
│                                                                 │
│       40        =   Has a group of friends, is invited out, ask │
│                     him for advice or seek his opinion, can talk│
│                     about a range of things, has a number of   │
│                     hobbies.                                    │
│                                                                 │
│       60        =   Is lively, can make people laugh, is       │
│                     intelligent can talk about current affairs, tell│
│                     stories about his experiences.  Has a group │
│                     of friends.                                 │
│                                                                 │
│       80        =   Has travelled extensively, is able to do a lot of│
│                     things, is the "life" of the party, talks about│
│                     almost anything, always has something to   │
│                     say, is attractive.                        │
│                                                                 │
│      100        =   (Same as above but more so).               │
└─────────────────────────────────────────────────────────────────┘
```

**Figure 4.7**   Results of a continua worksheet

Finally in this section, consideration should be given to the use of personal flashcards. These consist of evidence against negative schemas and answers to schemas in the form of replacement responses or beliefs. The aim of developing flashcards is to facilitate repetition of rational responses and potentiate challenging of negative schemas when they are activated. In a different use of flashcards, they may contain summaries of desirable behavioural responses that should be executed in feared situations. The behavioural responses may be tied to challenging belief at the automatic thought or schema level and serve as reminders for implementing behaviour change. As we shall see in Chapter 10, recent advances in modelling cognition in emotional disorders suggest that it should prove useful for long-term change to *rescript* patients' cognitive, attentional and behavioural responses in problematic situations (Wells & Matthews, 1994): flashcards present one way of summarising and facilitating the use of new behavioural and cognitive responses.

## CONCLUSION

In this chapter a range of cognitive therapy techniques have been reviewed. Cognitive therapy is not a technique-driven treatment. It should be driven by individual case conceptualisations that are based on a specific cognitive model. Verbal and behavioural reattribution strategies should be combined to produce optimal cognitive-behavioural change. It is recommended that behavioural reattribution experiments are used as early as possible in therapy. In this chapter, a framework for generating behavioural experiments and for their implementation was presented in detail. We have also seen how schemas may be elicited and modified. In most cases schema-work should be undertaken only after successful implementation of symptom-focused cognitive therapy. However, in some cases progress in treatment appears to be blocked, and the difficulty may arise from the presence of underlying schemas. If this is suspected, it may be necessary to conduct provisional work at the schema level before returning to symptomatic treatment in order to resolve the therapeutic impasse. Although there are a range of commonly used techniques in cognitive therapy, therapists should attempt to devise and experiment with their own cognitive and behavioural reattribution techniques. Skilled cognitive therapy consists of flexibility in moving between strategies, a seamless integration of different techniques, and an ability to generate and modify strategies 'on-line' as therapeutic requirements demand.

Chapter 5

# PANIC DISORDER

A detailed account of cognitive therapy for panic disorder is presented in this chapter. It is helpful to be familiar with the conceptualisation and treatment of panic before considering the treatment of other anxiety states, since panic is one of the simpler problems to model and offers an introduction to themes which are recurrent across other disorders. A central theme is the use of cyclical models for purposes of conceptualisation and socialisation, which illustrate the key relationships between cognition, behaviour, and affect, considered to maintain anxiety problems. In the first part of this chapter a description of panic is presented along with a brief review of the different types of panic attack. A cognitive model of panic (Clark, 1986) is then presented in detail, and the transition from model to practical case conceptualisation is discussed. The remainder of the chapter focuses on how the basic formulation can be developed, and on cognitive therapy treatment techniques. The cognitive therapy approach presented here closely follows the treatment developed by Clark et al. (1994) in the Oxford Cognitive Therapy programme and outcome trials.

## CHARACTERISTICS OF PANIC ATTACKS

Panic attacks are defined as rapid occurrences of anxiety or rapid escalations in current anxiety in which there are at least 4 of 13 somatic or cognitive symptoms (DSM-IV; APA, 1994). Four or more symptoms have to escalate or occur within a ten-minute period, to meet panic criteria. These symptoms include physical responses such as palpitations, dizziness, sweating, choking, trembling or shaking, breathlessness, depersonalisation, and cognitive symptoms such as fear of dying, suffocating, going crazy, and so on. In some instances fewer than four symptoms occur in an attack, and these are known as *limited symptom attacks* but the distinction is somewhat arbitrary. Panics can also be differentiated in a way that relates to the conditions under which they occur. More specifically, panics may be situational (cued) or spontaneous (uncued). Spontaneous panics occur unexpectedly, while situational panics occur in situations that almost always cause anxiety. In order for an individual to meet criteria for panic disorder in accordance with DSM-IV (APA, 1994), the presence of recurrent, unexpected panic attacks followed by at least one month of persistent concern about having another panic attack or a significant behavioural change related to the attack is required. At some time during the problem there should have been at least two spontaneous panic attacks (which did not occur in anticipation of, or on exposure to, a situation which invariably caused anxiety). In addition it is important to establish that organic factors are not maintaining the problem. Organic factors which should be ruled out include: caffeine or amphetamine intoxication, and hyperthyroidism. Panic attacks occur in disorders other than panic disorder; for example, a social phobic or claustrophobic may panic on exposure to the feared situation.

Panic attacks can be nocturnal in which case an individual may wake from sleep in a state of intense anxiety. Panic commonly occurs in conjunction with agoraphobia, although not all agoraphobics have panic attacks or meet criteria for panic disorder. Agoraphobic avoidance develops in cases of panic disorder when individuals avoid situations in which they fear they might have another panic attack. The avoidance can lead to a highly restricted lifestyle in more severe cases. Panic disorder with agoraphobia is diagnosed when a person who meets diagnostic criteria for panic disorder is also agoraphobic. Agoraphobia is defined in DSM-IV as: 'Anxiety about being in places or situations from which escape might be difficult (or embarrassing) or in which help may not be available in the event of having an unexpected or situationally predisposed panic attack' (p. 396).

## COGNITIVE MODEL OF PANIC

There are several cognitive models of the development and maintenance of panic disorder and agoraphobia (e.g. Goldstein & Chambless, 1978; Beck, Emery & Greenberg, 1985; Clark, 1986). The approaches of Clark (1986) and Beck and associates (1985) are based on the principle that panic patients fear the experience of certain bodily or mental events. Goldstein and Chambless (1978) offer a more learning theory based account of this 'fear of fear' concept. Their approach is analogous to the concept of interoceptive conditioning (Razran, 1961) in which bodily sensations become conditioned stimuli for the conditioned response of panic. However, Goldstein and Chambless (1978) add more cognitive elements to this concept. They assert that, having suffered one or more panic attacks, patients become 'hyperalert' for bodily sensations and interpret these as a sign of oncoming panic. Since these feared stimuli are carried around with the patient there is a generalisation of fear and external situations themselves become anxiety provoking, thus contributing to agoraphobia. The interoceptive conditioning approach has led to the development of treatments that attempt to extinguish fear of fear by strategies such as systematic exposure to internal sensations (e.g. Griez & van den Hout, 1986).

The model of panic proposed by Clark (1986) is one of the most useful for the cognitive conceptualisation and treatment of the disorder. The model has many overlapping features with the generic cognitive theory of anxiety proposed by Beck et al. (1985), and it deals specifically with the cognitive factors involved in the aetiology and maintenance of panic. More specifically, Clark's (1986, 1988) model proposes that a certain sequence of events leads to panic attacks. This sequence is circular and the model has become known as the 'vicious circle model' of panic. However, vicious circles are useful for conceptualising anxiety disorders in general, although the precise pattern of cyclical relationships and the elements within cycles differs between disorders. In Clark's model, panic attacks result from the 'catastrophic misinterpretation' of bodily or mental events. These events are misinterpreted as a sign of an immediate impending disaster, such as the sign of having a heart attack, of collapsing, suffocating, or going crazy. For example, physical sensations such as dizziness may be interpreted as a sign of fainting, and speeded heart rate as a sign of a heart attack. Mental events such as difficulty concentrating or the experience of racing thoughts can also be misinterpreted, often as a sign of a mental or social catastrophe such as losing control of one's mind or behaviour. According to the model the sensations that are misinterpreted are mainly those associated with anxiety, but other non-anxiety sensations may also be misinterpreted. Non-anxiety sensations include feelings of shakiness or lightheadedness caused by low blood sugar, the sensations associated with postural changes in blood pressure, effects of alcohol withdrawal, tiredness, and so on. Many normal bodily sensations or deviations in physiological activity can become the target of misinterpretation. The vicious circle that culminates in a panic attack consists of a sequence of thoughts, emotions, and sensations which can begin with any of these elements. The basic model is presented in Figure 5.0.

In this model any internal or external stimulus which is appraised as threatening produces a state of anxiety and bodily symptoms associated with that state. If these symptoms are interpreted in a catastrophic way a further

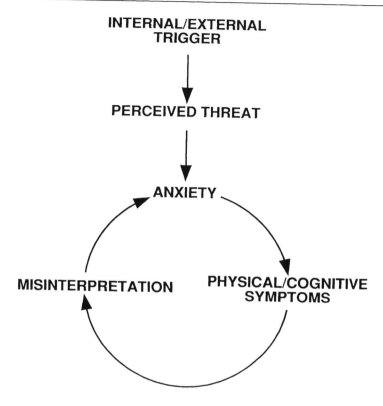

**Figure 5.0**   Clark's cognitive model of panic (adapted from Clark, 1986)

elevation in anxiety occurs and the individual becomes trapped in a vicious circle that culminates in a panic attack. Once panic attacks have occurred at least three other factors contribute to the maintenance of the problem: (1) selective attention to bodily events; (2) in-situation safety behaviours; (3) avoidance (e.g. Clark, 1988; Salkovskis, 1991; Wells, 1990).

*Selective attention* to bodily events and increased bodily focus can contribute to a lowered threshold for perceiving sensations and may also be involved in increasing the subjective intensity of these events. As a result the patient is more likely to activate the cycle of misinterpretation. Panic patients develop situational *safety behaviours* aimed at preventing feared catastrophes. These responses prevent disconfirmation of belief in catastrophe and can intensify bodily symptoms. For example, patients who misinterpret feelings of weakness in the legs as a sign of imminent collapse may sit down, hold onto or lean on something, crouch down, put themselves on the floor, or tense the muscles in their legs in order to prevent collapse. The symptom intensification effect of safety behaviours is most evident in panickers who misinterpret breathlessness or shallow breathing as a sign of suffocating, and take deep breaths, or try to control breathing in order to avert the feared catastrophe. These control behaviours can lead to symptoms of hyperventilation: dizziness, dissociation, heightened breathlessness, etc. In summary, safety behaviours maintain panic in two ways. First, they prevent disconfirmation of the patient's belief in misinterpretations, since the non-occurrence of the feared catastrophe can be falsely attributed to the use of the safety behaviour rather than correctly attributed to the fact that anxiety does not cause physical catastrophes such as collapsing. Second, certain safety behaviours directly exacerbate physical and cognitive symptoms which can make catastrophe more believable. Finally, *avoidance* is a maintaining factor in panic. Avoidance of anxiety-provoking situations, such as crowded shops, or activities such as exercise restrict the panicker's opportunity to

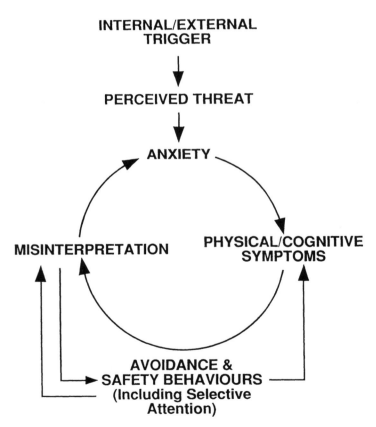

**Figure 5.1**  Cognitive model of panic with maintenance cycles added

experience anxiety and to discover that it does not lead to catastrophe. These maintaining factors should be fully explored and included in idiosyncratic case conceptualisations. Figure 5.1 presents the basic model with these additional maintenance cycles incorporated.

## FROM COGNITIVE MODEL TO CASE CONCEPTUALISATION

The model presented in Figure 5.1 is directly translatable into an individual conceptualisation of panic attacks. The cognitive therapist has this model in mind when conducting the cognitive-behavioural assessment interview. In the next section specific assessment issues pertaining to the derivation of the panic model are considered.

### Assessment

Cognitive-behavioural assessment in panic is aimed at eliciting idiosyncratic data for construction of a vicious circle model. The main information sought concerns: (1) the nature of catastrophic misinterpretations (content and belief levels); (2) detailed descriptions of the main feared sensations; and (3) the nature of safety and avoidance behaviours. One of the main outcome measures in the treatment of panic should be a measure of panic frequency and intensity, although measures of general anxiety (the Beck Anxiety Inventory) and of avoidance should also be used on a regular basis. Recommended measures are reviewed in Chapter 2. Panic frequency data can be collected in the form of a daily panic diary (see Figure 5.2 for an example of such a diary). Sessional use of the Panic Rating Scale presented at the back of this book is recommended for tracking change in symptoms, target safety behaviours and misinterpretations.

In the first few treatment sessions the conceptualisation may consist only of the primary vicious circle and the other contributory influences of safety behaviours may be omitted for simplicity and to facilitate patient understanding. However, whenever possible a full model of the symptomatic problem should be derived in the first session. Any conceptualisation of vulnerability factors (general beliefs and assumptions) and their inclusion in a more detailed cognitive conceptualisation should normally be postponed until a reliable cessation of panics is achieved.

## DERIVING THE VICIOUS CIRCLE

The construction of the panic circle depends on identifying the sequence of events involved in *specific* panic attacks. Difficulty in the identification of

Panic Diary

| Date | Situation | Main bodily/mental sensations (e.g. dizziness, mind-racing, breathless, palpitations) | Negative thought (misinterpretation) | Answer to negative thought | Total number of panic attacks |
|------|-----------|------|------|------|------|
| MON | | | | | |
| TUES | | | | | |
| WED | | | | | |
| THURS | | | | | |
| FRI | | | | | |
| SAT | | | | | |
| SUN | | | | | |

*Instructions:*   *When you feel panicky make a note of the situation in which panic occurred (e.g. driving in a car) in the Situation column. Write down your main bodily sensation in the Main bodily sensation column. Write down the frightening negative thoughts that you had during your attack in the Negative thought column. Under the Answer to negative thought heading, write in your answer or rational response to your negative thought, this may be a verbal answer or a particular behaviour. Make a note of the total number of panic attacks you have each day in the Number of panic attacks column.*

**Figure 5.2**   Example of a panic diary

misinterpretations and sequence involved arises from several sources: focusing on panic in a general abstract way; the presence of high degrees of
patient avoidance behaviour leading to inaccessibility of 'hot cognitions';
and a failure to slowly 'track' the course of attacks. Difficulties are minimised by identifying a specific and recent panic attack, and analysing it in

detail as if it had occurred in 'slow motion'. The vicious circle contains three basic elements: emotional reactions; bodily sensations; and negative thoughts about sensations (misinterpretations). These elements are linked in a sequence which follows a particular pattern which can begin with any one of the elements but always follows the same circular sequence:

sensations → thought → emotion → sensations → thought → emotion, etc.

As illustrated in Figure 5.0, the vicious circle closes following the misinterpretation of bodily sensations associated with anxiety. The stem that leads to anxiety (apprehension) at the apex of the vicious circle can vary in length, and may consist of a chain of thoughts, sensations, or emotions other than anxiety such as anger or excitement. When constructing the panic circle it is most convenient to locate anxiety at the bottom of the stem so that it becomes the start of the circle. With anxiety in this location it is more convenient for closing the circle. An example of an idiosyncratic panic circle derived from a 26-year-old male panicker is displayed in Figure 5.3.

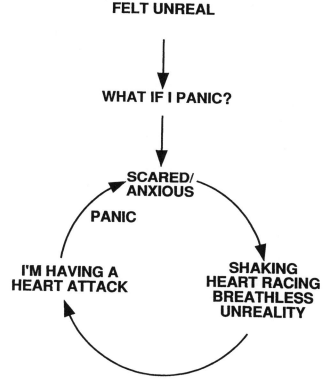

**Figure 5.3**   An idiosyncratic panic cycle

The therapist–patient socratic dialogue used to elicit the information for this conceptualisation was as follows:

T: When was your most recent panic attack?
P: I had one yesterday, in the morning. It was quite a bad one.
T: I'd like to ask you some questions about that attack. Is it clear in your mind?
P: Yes, I think so.
T: Was it a typical attack?
P: Yes it was fairly typical, but not as bad as some I've had in the past.
T: OK. Let's focus on that attack so that we can begin to find out exactly what happened. Where were you and what were you doing just before the attack started?
P: I was at work talking to a customer on the telephone, and then it just suddenly hit me.
T: It sounds as if it occurred very quickly. What was the very first thing that you noticed as the panic started to develop. Did you have a body sensation or a thought?
P: I felt unreal, as if I wasn't really part of what was going on.
T: When you noticed that feeling of unreality what thoughts went through your mind?
P: I thought, oh no, what if I panic?
T: When you had that thought how did it make you feel?
P: I felt that I didn't want to panic in that situation.
T: I really mean how did you feel emotionally when you had the thought?
P: I was scared in case it developed into a full panic.
T: So you felt scared and anxious.
P: Yes, I thought it was going to be a bad one, I felt I just wanted to get out of the situation.
T: OK. Let's continue to examine slowly what happened in that attack. You said you felt scared, what sensations did you notice when you felt scared?
P: I started to feel shaky, and my heart was racing.
T: Did you notice any other sensations. What happened to the unreal feeling for example?
P: Oh, it got much worse, and I felt breathless.
T: When you had all of those sensations; feeling shaky, heart racing, unreal and breathlessness, what thought went through your mind?
P: I knew I was panicking and couldn't control it.
T: Did you think anything bad could happen when you had all of those symptoms?
P: Yes, I thought that was it, that I could die.
T: How did you think you could die?

P: I thought I was having a heart attack.

T: What happened to your anxiety when you had that thought? (The response to this question closes the panic circle.)

P: It got worse, I felt really panicky.

T: In that panic attack, how much did you believe you were having a heart attack when the symptoms were bad—on a scale of zero to one hundred: zero being no belief and one hundred being convinced the thought was true?

P: Oh, I was pretty sure, about 80 per cent.

The standard sequence of questioning illustrated above allowed the therapist and patient to identify the components of the panic cycle. In this case the trigger was feeling unreal, the quick negative automatic thought in the vicious circle stem was 'What if I panic?'. This led to the emotional response of anxiety and then to associated sensations (heart racing, etc.), and then the catastrophic misinterpretation (I'm having a heart attack) which culminated in further anxiety and panic. This sequence is illustrated in Figure 5.3. Note that panic is actually labelled on the vicious circle, so that it is clear to patients. In this example the therapist elicited the patient's belief in the misinterpretation during the panic attack. Belief ratings are essential, since therapy is focused on directly challenging and eliminating belief in misinterpretations. Changes in the level of these ratings are therefore an essential guide in determining the effectiveness of interventions used in cognitive therapy.

## DEVELOPING THE BASIC CONCEPTUALISATION : INCORPORATING SAFETY BEHAVIOURS AND AVOIDANCE

Once the basic panic circle has been constructed, the next stage is the identification and inclusion of behaviours. Avoidance behaviours may be clearly apparent from the outset, particularly if agoraphobia is a problem. However, more subtle forms of avoidance and safety behaviours may be less apparent, and they should be carefully explored. Examples of subtle avoidance include avoidance of strenuous activity or exercise, avoidance of being alone, avoidance of medical information and so on. In most instances asking the question *'Are there any situations that you are avoiding because of your anxiety?'* is sufficient to elicit some avoidance behaviours. This should be followed by other questions probing for detailed information about avoidance in an attempt to develop a comprehensive list of feared and avoided situations associated with panic. Self-report inventories such as the Marks and Mathews (1979) Fear Questionnaire and the Panic Rating Scale (Chapter 2) are aids to identifying avoided situations.

The identification and analysis of safety behaviours proceeds with questions designed to access the behaviours which the patient believes have prevented feared catastrophes from happening during anxiety/panic attacks. These behaviours can be elicited with questions about panic attacks in general, but the best strategy is the use of questions which probe safety behaviours in specific attacks already conceptualised. An example, of a dialogue used to elicit safety behaviours in the panic case presented previously follows:

T: If we look at the vicious circle (points it out on the marker board). When you felt anxious and believed you were about to have a heart attack, did you do anything to save yourself? To prevent a heart attack?

P: I just tried to relax and slow my heart down.

T: What did you do to try and relax and slow your heart down?

P: I told myself to relax and tried to breathe deeply and more slowly.

T: Can you show me how you breathed?

P: I just took deep breaths, to try and slow things down.

T: So you took deep breaths to try and relax. Did you do anything else?

P: I sometimes breathe in and out of a paper bag, but I couldn't on that occasion.

T: It sounds as if you've developed a few tricks for controlling your anxiety. How much do you believe that if you hadn't used these control strategies during this panic attack that something bad would have happened, like having a heart attack?

P: I think I probably could have had a heart attack or maybe collapsed.

T: So how much do you believe that controlling your breathing has prevented a heart attack or collapsing, on a scale of 0–100?

P: Oh, probably about 60 per cent.

Behavioural responses should be included in the initial panic cycle as a secondary positive feedback loop. The full formulation for this particular patient, which includes the behavioural loop, is presented in Figure 5.4.

The behavioural loop should be drawn as originating from the misinterpretation, and generates two potentially positive feedback influences: one is an exacerbation of bodily sensations, and the second denotes the prevention of disconfirmation of belief in misinterpretation. When the model has been presented in this form behavioural experiments should be used to illustrate the symptom intensification linkage, and metaphors can be used to illustrate the blocked disconfirmation linkage. Examples of these socialisation procedures are presented later in this chapter.

For purposes of clinical reference, examples of misinterpretations and safety/avoidance behaviours for a sample of seven patients treated by the author with a primary diagnosis of panic disorder with no to moderate agoraphobic avoidance (DSM-IV; APA, 1994) are presented in Table 5.0

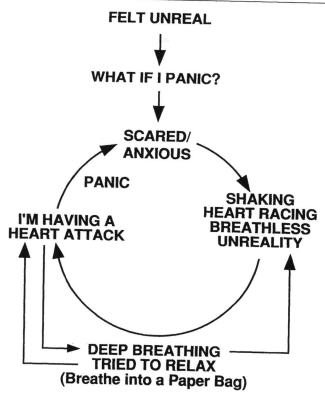

**Figure 5.4**   A full idiosyncratic panic cycle

## SOCIALISATION

Socialisation begins with building and presenting the panic cycle. This should be done for several panic attacks (to show that all panics fit the sequence). At this stage it is important to determine the patient's reaction to the model, and to this end questions like the following should be used:

- Does this seem to fit with your experience of panic (if not why not)?
- Is there anything in the model which you feel is not right or you don't understand?

The aim of socialisation is to offer an explanation of panic attacks as caused by the catastrophic misinterpretation of bodily sensations. These two variables can be linked by explaining that belief in catastrophe leads to an 'adrenalin rush' which exacerbates anxiety. The arrows in the model which

**Table 5.0** Examples of main sensations, misinterpretations and safety behaviours for seven panic patients

| Sensation(s) | Misinterpretation | Safety behaviour/avoidance |
|---|---|---|
| Palpitations Chest tightness | Heart attack Dying | Relax Slow down heart rate Sit down, avoid exercise Avoid physical exertion |
| Unreality (dissociation) | Loss of control Madness | Keep control of mind Check memory Try to control thoughts Look for exits |
| Breathlessness | Suffocate | Take deep breaths Sit by open windows Go into open air Suck menthol sweets |
| Throat tightness | Choking | Carry bottle of water Try to clear throat |
| Dizzyness | Fainting Collapsing | Control breathing Sit down Hold on to partner Avoid going out alone |
| Blurred vision | Blindness Stroke | Check vision Wear sunglasses Take aspirin Avoid stress |
| Jelly legs | Falling Collapsing | Leave situations Stiffen legs while standing Walk close to walls Wear flat shoes |

occur after appraisals are usefully described as adrenalin surges. Where possible, behavioural experiments should be used to gain evidence in support of the model and illustrate linkages between its components.

## Sample socialisation experiments

*The paired associates task*

This task (Clark et al., 1988) aims to illustrate the effect of thinking on anxiety and associated bodily sensations by testing the supposition that thinking about physical catastrophes can elicit or heighten bodily sensations and/or anxiety. The task is presented without an explanation of its aims, since a rationale can interfere with the impact of the task. The patient is asked to dwell on pairs of words and think of their meaning while reading them aloud. A period of about 5–8 seconds should be allowed for dwelling on each word pair, which are presented in list format. The words used for constructing the pairs consist of common anxiety sensations partnered with physical calamities typical of the content of panic misinterpretations. For example, the following word pairs would be repeated on the list:

| Breathlessness | — Suffocate |
| Dizziness | — Fainting |
| Chest tight | — Heart attack |
| Numbness | — Stroke |
| Palpitations | — Heart attack |
| Unreality | — Insane |
| Weakness | — Collapsing |

After performing the task for a few minutes, the patient should be asked if he/she noticed anything while reading the words. Occasionally the task invokes high anxiety, but most often a more subtle increase in anxiety or awareness of bodily sensations is reported. The patient should then be asked what sense he/she makes of this result in terms of the model, and in terms of the impact of their thinking. The task does not work with all patients. When it fails, closure of the exercise can be achieved by explaining that it was a test to see what the patient's general reaction was to reading unpleasant material, and the fact that there was little reaction is fine.

*Body-focus task*

A different demonstration of the effect of 'thinking', or more specifically the effect of selective attention on symptom perception, can be achieved with self-focused attention manipulations. The task serves to show that attentional strategies can increase awareness of bodily sensations which are normally present, and that it can exaggerate perceived symptom intensity. Patients are asked to focus attention on sensations in particular parts of the body such as the feet, or sensations in the fingertips. After a couple of minutes monitoring they are asked to report what is noticed. The procedure is normally used in conjunction with questions which facilitate the framing of the results of the task in terms of the panic model. Typical questions include the following:

- Were you aware of the sensations before you focused on that part of your body?
- What happened to the sensations when you focused on them?
- If focusing your thoughts on your body leads you to notice sensations that you were not previously aware of, how might that contribute to the vicious circle?

A variant of the self-focus task involves visual fixation on parts of the body, such as staring at the back of one's left or right hand, and noticing what happens to perception, such as perception of size, clearness of the image, and extent to which the hand seems part of the individual. If there is evidence to suggest that a patient engages in this type of self-monitoring as a safety/checking behaviour this is likely to be a useful socialisation task since self-monitoring can exaggerate feared responses such as distortions in perception of size and feelings of unreality.

### Increased safety behaviours tests

Safety behaviours can be manipulated in-session to demonstrate the role of behaviours in maintaining and intensifying sensations, and as an introduction to the concept of such behaviours preventing disconfirmation. For example, if a panicker uses deep controlled breathing to avert an appraised catastrophe such as suffocating, deliberate controlled deep breathing can be employed to illustrate the effect of this behaviour on sensations. A range of sensations can be produced by more vigorous over-breathing including: dizziness, palpitations, feelings of faintness, depersonalisation, blurred vision, feelings of weakness, etc. While it should be acknowledged that the patient probably does not breathe in such a vigorous way when panicking, it should be stressed that the exercise is intended to illustrate what can happen, and that even small changes in sensations produced by smaller changes in breathing tend to be more perceptible during panic attacks when fears are activated.

The effective use of increased safety behaviours tests relies on the detailed exploration of the actual behaviours used by the individual when anxious, and the selection of those which are likely to be involved in symptom intensification and thus can be used to illustrate the model.

### Metaphors and allegories as socialisation

The effect of safety behaviours in preventing disconfirmation of belief can be illustrated with metaphors and allegories. Two examples are given below:

1. In South America there are a tribe of people who believe they are the guardians of the world. In order to keep the world spinning and humankind existing they have to conduct a special ceremony each year. They fear in case something should prevent them from doing this. They believe that if they did not perform their ceremony the world would end. How can they discover that their belief is false?

In the same way, how can you discover that your world will not end in a panic attack? (Probe: Can you discover that nothing bad will happen so long as you use safety behaviours?)

2. Some people believe in vampires, and so they become very anxious when it's time to sleep at night. In order to keep safe they sleep with cloves of garlic around their neck. Of course no one has seen a vampire and so the garlic must be working. How can these people discover that there are no vampires?

Both of these scenarios present the importance of abandoning safety behaviours in challenging belief in negative appraisals. In addition to abandoning safety, it is helpful for patients to push symptoms during an attack to unambiguously prove that catastrophe does not occur. We return to this principle later.

## REATTRIBUTION STRATEGIES

Socialisation is a prerequisite to the more direct forms of reattribution strategies. One of its central functions is to provide a *cognitive set* which facilitates the processing of disconfirmatory experiences. The central aim of cognitive therapy for panic disorder is the reduction of belief in misinterpretations, and the elimination of avoidance. This is dependent on strategies that break the feedback cycles which block disconfirmation, and strategies that directly challenge belief.

### The evolution of treatment strategies in panic

Earlier cognitive-behaviour treatment of panic used symptom control strategies such as controlled breathing exercises during panic attacks. The use of control strategies such as breathing exercises or relaxation is contra-indicated by the safety behaviours analysis in panic disorder. These strategies could contribute to the panicker's armoury of responses which prevent disconfirmation of belief in catastrophe. In contrast to using anxiety/symptom control procedures such as slow controlled breathing, more appropriate tasks are symptom provocation procedures designed to test predictions based on patients' beliefs. However, this does not mean that control strategies never have a place in treatment. In some instances, such as physical illness complications, symptom provocation is inadvisable and it is helpful to have a range of back-up treatment procedures.

## BEHAVIOURAL EXPERIMENTS

Many of the behavioural experiments used in the treatment of panic involve the active induction of panic sensations in order to challenge belief in misinterpretations. So-called 'panic inductions' are therefore the cornerstone of behavioural reattribution experiments in this disorder, and are typically among the first experiments employed in treatment.

## Guidelines for effective symptom induction experiments

Effective symptom induction or *panic provocation* tests are normally those that produce sensations which *closely* resemble the sensations which are normally misinterpreted during panic attacks. Failure to achieve a close match has a tendency to reduce the power of the provocation task in producing belief-change (reattribution). The therapist should have a good knowledge of the patient's feared sensations, and the precise idiosyncratic misinterpretations associated with them (plus belief level) before designing and implementing an induction experiment. These experiments are targeted at modifying the patient's belief, and a mere induction of symptoms is usually insufficient for this to occur. Thus, experiments are usually presented in conjunction with a clear rationale and a *disconfirmatory manoeuvre* as discussed in Chapter 4. The rationale should be based on a shared conceptualisation. The rationale serves both to provide a cognitive set for the effective processing of disconfirmatory experiences, and it also increases patient compliance with the task. Compliance is rarely a problem, although in many instances some gentle persuasion is necessary. Compliance may be enhanced if the therapist first models the induction procedure and executes the procedure in parallel with the patient.

In order to assess the efficacy of the induction, patient belief in a specific feared catastrophe (misinterpretation) should be rated before and after the experiment. If some belief remains the reason for this should be questioned. The induction may have to be repeated several times, perhaps more vigorously in order to maximise disconfirmation. In the event of minimal or no belief change a number of factors should be explored which can contribute to the reduced effectiveness of the procedure. First, the patient may have used in-situation safety behaviours during the task which have prevented full disconfirmation. Close observation of behaviour during induction often reveals the use of particular safety behaviours, such as suddenly disengaging from the task, holding onto or leaning on things, sitting down, taking deep breaths (or not taking deep enough breaths during forced hyperventilation), tensing muscles, and so on. These responses should be eliminated during induction, and several inductions may have to be repeated before this is fully achieved. The second interfering factor can be a poor match between induced symptoms and the symptoms normally misinterpreted during panic attacks. For best results a good match should be achieved for disconfirmation to occur. The third factor which modulates the degree of anxiety and belief activation during induction, and can therefore affect experimental impact, is the presence of *rescue factors* built into the environment. For example, fear may not be fully activated by bodily sensations in the presence of the therapist or in the clinic setting if the patient appraises the therapist or setting as the best source of emergency help in the event of catastrophe. Situations like this draw on the therapist's creative problem solving in designing induction experiments that exclude perceived rescue factors. A solution is to ask the patient to perform the induction while alone in the consulting room, or conducting the procedure away from the clinic setting altogether.

It is useful to recognise that induction experiments not only elicit anxiety in patients but can also be a source of anxiety for therapists. There may be a reluctance to push patients in symptom inductions. This is often based on faulty assumptions held by the therapist. There may be a fear that the patient will panic and the therapist will not be able to handle the situation, or the therapist may believe that a person can actually faint in a panic attack. It is important that therapists identify and challenge their own unhelpful assumptions. Some common examples of therapist thoughts/assumptions are:

- I must always make my patient feel better rather than worse.
- If I ask my patient to do this he/she will get mad at me.
- If I ask my patient to do this he/she will drop out of treatment.
- If I make my patient panic I won't be able to cope.
- What if my patient does lose control?

In the next section specific examples of behavioural experiments commonly used in the treatment of panic are presented. The general rules for the conduct of behavioural experiments outlined in Chapter 4 should be used in conjunction with these procedures.

## Hyperventilation provocation task

The hyperventilation task is one of the most common induction procedures since it is often effective in provoking a wide range of panicogenic sensations. It offers a particularly powerful means of inducing sensations of dizziness, faintness, dissociation, visual changes, feeling hot, speeded heart rate and paradoxical breathlessness. The task is therefore useful for challenging beliefs in misinterpretations of these types of symptoms. The task is most often practised with the patient in a standing position and is followed by various disconfirmatory manoeuvres, such as a prolongation of hyperventilation to push symptoms in order to discover that catastrophes do not occur, or walking in a straight line, standing on one leg, or hopping on one leg to challenge beliefs about loss of balance or collapsing. The induction may be immediately followed by, or used in parallel with, other disconfirmatory manoeuvres. For example, a panic patient reported a panic attack in which he misinterpreted being dazzled by sunlight as a sign that he was going blind; this led to feelings of dizziness and unreality which served to reinforce his belief. An in-session disconfirmatory experiment involved staring at a bright light while hyperventilating (to produce subsidiary visual anomalies and unreality). The patient had a 40 per cent belief that the exercise would lead to blindness before the task if he stared at the light for longer than a few minutes. The experiment consisted of staring at the light and hyperventilating for four minutes (longer than the time he predicted for blindness to occur) and was followed by a text-reading task (an additional disconfirmatory manoeuvre to show that his vision still functioned). Following the experiment the patient's belief fell to zero.

The reversal of particular safety behaviours during hyperventilation serves as a further source of disconfirmation in certain cases. More specifically, if the main fear concerns 'going crazy' during panic, and safety behaviours consist of keeping control of one's mind, hyperventilation can be combined with attempts to lose control by thinking 'crazy thoughts'. Similarly, in cases where fears of loss of behavioural control predominate, loss of behavioural control can be attempted (e.g. rushing around the room making bizarre gestures, and shouting) following hyperventilation.

There are a number of common myths concerning hyperventilation. Some medical practitioners suggest that panickers control their breathing or use the paper-bag technique in order to prevent hyperventilation. This approach reinforces the views that hyperventilation can lead to catastrophe such as fainting. The cognitive therapist must counteract the false beliefs that patients have acquired. Prolonged forced hyperventilation gives rise to a range of bodily symptoms but these subside as hyperventilation continues (van den Hout, de Jong, Zanderberger & Merckelbach, 1990). In rare instances it may produce muscular spasm. Fainting does not result from panic or hyperventilation. In some cases of blood injury phobia, individuals exposed to medical procedures, blood, etc., may faint. In these individuals an initial increase in heart rate and blood pressure is followed by a sudden drop in blood pressure when exposed to a feared situation. In contrast, in panic and other anxiety disorders blood pressure is elevated during exposure to feared situations. Since it is a drop in blood pressure that causes fainting, patients are less likely to faint in a panic attack. (The problem of blood injury phobia is treatable by training patients to use *applied tension* to increase blood pressure during exposure: Ost & Sterner, 1987.) Forced hyperventilation should not be used when particular medical conditions are present (cardiac problems, asthma, high blood pressure, pregnancy). The therapist must check with the patient's doctor to determine if there are any health reasons why the patient should not be asked to engage in *vigorous* hyperventilation or exercise.

## Physical exercise tasks

Physical exercise tasks are indicated in cases where strenuous activity is avoided, and are useful strategies for challenging cardiac concerns and concerns about physical robustness and strength. Typical exercise tasks include jogging, walking quickly up and down steps, skipping with a rope and so on. These strategies may be combined with other strategies to emphasise particular symptoms; for example, if the main panicogenic symptoms are speeded heart rate and sweating, the exercise may be conducted in a particularly hot environment, or with the patient wearing a coat, in order to push symptoms and thus disconfirm beliefs.

## Chest pain strategies

In some cases the sensations that are misinterpreted consist of chest tightness or chest pain. There are several ways of inducing different types of chest discomfort. Discomfort can be induced by asking patients to completely fill their lungs with air, and then breathe around full lungs without letting all of the air out. After practising this technique for a few minutes chest discomfort is likely. Another strategy involves taking a deep breath and pushing a finger between the ribs around the heart region and slightly to the side of the sternum. This pushes against the delicate intercostal muscles between the ribs and tends to produce a sharper type of stabbing pain. Chest pain procedures are perhaps best employed as behavioural experiments which can be used in conjunction with education about the causes of bodily sensations in panic. In some cases, for example, chest sensations can be attributable to certain safety behaviours such as overuse of thoracic musculature due to controlled deep breathing, or the repeated palpation of the chest wall in an attempt to reassure oneself that the pain is muscular rather than of cardiac origin. An example is the use of such exercises to illustrate that the chest is full of many delicate muscles which can become tense when anxious and can give rise to chest pain which is not indicative of a heart attack.

## Strategies for inducing visual disturbances

Visual grids can be used to produce a range of visual anomalies. Visual grids consist of narrowly spaced lines, usually printed in black ink on a highly contrasting white background. Patients are asked to stare at the centre of the grid and report their visual 'sensations'. As with all of the strategies reported here, the grid test can be used as an aid to education about normal visual responses, and it can also be used to test specific beliefs about particular symptoms. In a recent case, a panic patient misinterpreted slight visual disturbance as an indication that he was 'going blind'. A visual grid successfully induced the types of sensations that he misinterpreted, and it became clear through questioning that he believed that if he made the sensations worse he would lose his sight. In order to test this prediction the patient was asked to stare at the grid for an extended period of time to determine if the catastrophe occurred. His belief fell from 50 per cent to zero by doing this, and he took the grid home so that he could push the symptoms next time he felt panicky.

Eye fixation and staring exercises can also produce unusual vision effects. An analysis of the patient's safety behaviours in response to particular fears about sight often suggests particular amplifications of safety behaviours that can be used to elicit feared sensations. For example, repeatedly closing and opening one's eyes in an attempt to focus on different objects, or perhaps staring at print on a page of text could be used to induce blurred vision.

## Dissociative experiences

Feelings of unreality or disconnectedness can often be produced with visual exercises like those suggested previously. Hyperventilation can be a powerful inducer of this type of feeling. However, it is also worth experimenting with induced day-dreaming combined with eye fixation, and also with induction of relaxed states in order to produce these effects.

## 'Acting as if' experiments

Primary concerns about the social consequences of events such as collapsing or fainting can be modified by acting out the catastrophe (e.g. faking a collapse) in public situations. The therapist may have to model this first before the patient is prepared to carry out the procedure. The aim is to test belief concerning the negative reaction of others.

# VERBAL REATTRIBUTION TECHNIQUES

General verbal techniques, as discussed in Chapter 4, should be applied in cases of panic disorder although their application can become more complicated in cases where agoraphobic avoidance is severe and specific cognitions seem less accessible. Appropriate modification of belief in misinterpretations through verbal techniques depends upon a *precise* understanding of both the nature of the feared catastrophe and the idiosyncratic evidence on which the misinterpretation is based. In some cases questioning the evidence for a particular misinterpretation will lead the patient to concede that there is no evidence. However, in some instances the patient will offer evidence of various types. Evidence should be subject to a *detailed* analysis which in itself is likely to suggest alternative appraisals, both to the patient and the therapist. Detailed analysis is crucial in panic cases where the patient reports that feared catastrophes have actually happened as a result of anxiety. In some cases, for example, patients claim to have collapsed, that is, their legs gave way or they 'fainted' during an attack of anxiety. However, detailed questioning usually reveals that on believing that a catastrophe was likely the patient actually flopped into a chair, crouched down or sat on the floor, and that these were voluntary behaviours designed to minimise social or physical harm to the self. In these cases there was no loss of consciousness, or non-deliberate physical collapse. Only through careful detailed analysis can the patient discover that these were safety responses. Panic and anxiety symptoms can then be contrasted with actual symptoms of fainting and collapse (see symptom contrast technique, p. 128), in order to produce reattribution.

## Questioning the evidence

Standard questions should be used to facilitate the patient's evaluation of evidence for specific misinterpretations. This form of reattribution may be used prior to behavioural experiments which are themselves intended to reinforce the reattribution, or may be used after an experiment to consolidate new information and elaborate disconfirmatory experiences. Examples of useful questions are:

- How do you know that panic will cause (catastrophe)?
- You've had lots of panics. Why haven't you (catastrophe) yet? (This question can elicit safety behaviour.)
- What makes you think that anxiety can cause (catastrophe)?
- What's the mechanism that would allow anxiety to do that to you?
- Do you know what causes (catastrophe)? Do you think anxiety is part of that mechanism?

In the process of challenging the patient's evidence the concept of thinking errors can be introduced. In panic disorder the main errors are *catastrophising* and *arbitrary inference*. In addition it is useful to acknowledge the diminished ability to *reality test* which commonly occurs during a panic attack. While panickers can readily challenge belief in misinterpretations using verbal techniques when not in a panic attack, this ability is markedly reduced during an attack. Some patients refer to this in terms of their seeming to be two sides to their mind, a rational side and an irrational side, the latter of which seems to 'take over' during panic. The acknowledgement of this phenomenon can be used to reinforce the necessity for conducting behavioural experiments *when anxious* to directly challenge fear, and to emphasise that rational responding is not intended to be used to control panics (since this would be the provision of another safety behaviour). Once the patient has learned to identify thinking errors, these should be labelled when misinterpretations occur as a short-hand means of challenging belief in misinterpretations. However, in isolation these verbal techniques are a poor substitute for disconfirmatory experiments.

## The panic cognitions diary

The panic diary is a central source of data on the efficacy of treatment in reducing panic frequency and intensity (Figure 5.2). It is also crucial for the identification of misinterpretations and for logging verbal and behavioural 'answers' to them. The diary increases patients' awareness of negative misinterpretations, which offers evidence for the model, and permits the identification of misinterpretations which may not have been identified at interview or by questionnaire. The panic diary may differ from diaries used in other disorders in a number of ways. The diaries used by Clark and colleagues in the treatment of panic (e.g. Clark, 1989, p. 64) consist of additional columns for checking a range of bodily sensations, for stating the main sensation, and the negative misinterpretation, as well as the standard columns for describing the situation and the rational response.

Panic diaries should be completed by patients on a daily basis for homework. In this format the diary presents additional information on main feared bodily sensations which can be a guide to selecting induction experiments. Patterns in the occurrence of panic attacks (i.e. day or time patterns) can also emerge from the daily diary. An identification of patterns can be used to challenge beliefs about organic pathology when these exist, and used for identifying factors which may give rise to panic triggers. For example, if panic is often triggered by feelings of dizziness, and this symptom seems to occur mid-morning, this may be indicative of low blood-sugar levels, or withdrawal from alcohol as potential triggers. Such possibilities should be investigated by asking appropriate questions. In the first couple of weeks of treatment patients are usually asked only to complete the first columns of the diary up to and including the column identifying misinterpretations. The 'answer to negative thought' column is completed when disconfirmatory evidence has been gained through behavioural and verbal techniques. It can be particularly effective to use the responses column of the diary to log the use of behavioural experiments such as dropping safety behaviours or pushing symptoms during panics. A tracking of belief level before and after these responses is powerful for reinforcing the cognitive model and the aims of treatment. It is also a marker for problems in the effective challenging of beliefs, the causes of which should be explored and modified.

## Education and exploring counter-evidence

Belief in negative appraisals of symptoms can be challenged and alternative appraisals can be strengthened by eliciting and exploring counter-evidence, and by presenting new incompatible information. These techniques should be backed up with behavioural demonstrations to increase their power, and wherever possible guided discovery should be used. Strategies of this type are useful in modifying general assumptions that panickers often hold concerning the negative consequences of anxiety. In particular, the panicker may assume that intense anxiety can kill, cause insanity, lead to fainting, heart attacks and so on. Counter-evidence can be collected based on the patient's own disconfirmatory experiences or by reviewing other scenarios not relevant to the self, through education, and via behavioural techniques like those already reviewed. In the following section, examples of educational manoeuvres used in the treatment of panic are presented. These procedures are intended for use as part of an integrated cognitive therapy package which utilises guided discovery and behavioural experiments to test out new information.

## Selected educational scenarios in panic

*Misinterpretation: I'll faint during a panic attack. Anxiety will make me collapse*

T: One of your fears is that during a panic you will collapse. What do you mean by collapse?
P: I feel dizzy and like I'm going to faint or collapse.
T: When you say collapse what do you mean?

P: That I'll actual pass-out if the panic gets really bad.

T: Have you ever passed out?

P: No it's never happened but I've been close to it a time or two.

T: So you're concerned that in a bad panic you could pass-out, but it hasn't actually happened yet. You've had lots of bad panics in the past, yet you've not actually passed out yet, how do you explain that?

P: Well I don't know I'm just waiting for the time when it does happen.

T: Do you know what causes people to pass-out?

P: I'm not really sure. Is it lack of air?

T: Well you could suffocate due to lack of air, but that's different. What typically causes fainting?

P: I don't know. Anxiety can cause it.

T: Well, the thing that causes fainting is a drop in blood pressure. When it is very low then fainting occurs. What do you think happens to your blood pressure when you're anxious?

P: It goes up I suppose.

T: Yes that's right. How do you know it goes up?

P: I can feel it, everything seems to be going faster.

T: Yes, what happens to your heart rate when you're anxious?

P: It speeds up.

T: And if you increase the rate at which a pump like the heart works in a sealed system, what happens to the pressure?

P: It increases.

T: That's right, your blood pressure increases when you're anxious, so you're even less likely to faint. It just isn't going to happen. Next time you feel anxious you can do an experiment to prove that you won't faint. You could push the symptoms by trying the overbreathing we've talked about, or you could try taking your pulse next time you're anxious to prove that your heart rate has increased, and compare it with what it is when you're relaxed.

*Misinterpretation: I'll stop breathing/suffocate; run out of air*

T: What makes you think you'll stop breathing in a panic attack?

P: I feel breathless and I get a tight feeling around my chest.

T: Do you do anything to make sure you don't suffocate?

P: Yes, I'm often conscious of my breathing and I try to take deep breaths and keep it under control.

T: What would happen if you didn't do that?

P: I'm afraid that it might stop.

T: It sounds as if you believe that you have to be conscious of breathing otherwise it might fail.

P: Yes.

T: What about when you're asleep. Are you consciously controlling your breathing then?

P: No, I'm not aware of it.

T: So what does that tell you about your breathing?

P: That it can look after itself?

T: Yes that's right. Breathing is normally automatic and it goes on without you having to think about it or do anything about it. It's controlled automatically by the brain. The brains control is very powerful and it will take control even when you try to stop your breathing. However, you can also control your breathing voluntarily. But when people try to control activities which are normally automatic it can make them seem difficult. For example, running up a flight of stairs is automatic and you don't have to think about your movements. But if you focus on every footstep what's likely to happen?

P: I'd probably trip or something.

T: That's right. The activity would seem much harder and you might trip-up. If you focus on your breathing and try to control it, it also begins to seem harder, but of course you can't really disrupt it permanently because your brain is always ready to take over automatic control. Let's do an experiment right now to show that you cannot stop yourself from breathing. (Implementation of breath-holding exercise and irregular breathing exercise.)

*Misinterpretation: I'll have a heart attack*

P: When I'm panicking it's terrible I can feel my heart pounding, it's so bad I think it could burst through my chest.

T: What thoughts go through your mind when your heart is pounding like that?

P: Well I'll tell you what I think, It's so bad that I think I'm going to have a heart attack. It can't be good for your heart beating like that.

T: So you're concerned that anxiety can damage your heart or cause a heart attack.

P: Yes, it must do some damage. You hear of people dropping down dead from heart attacks caused by stress.

T: Do you think more people have stress in their lives than die of heart attacks?

P: Yes I suppose so.

T: How can that be if stress causes heart attacks?

P: Well I suppose it doesn't always cause problems. Maybe it does only in some people.

T: Yes, that's right; stress can cause some problems in some people. It tends to be people who have something wrong with their hearts in the first place. But stress is not necessarily the same as sudden anxiety or panic. When you panic your body releases adrenalin which causes the heart to speed up and your body to work faster. It's a way of preparing you to deal better with danger. If adrenalin damaged the heart or body, how would people have evolved from dangerous primitive times. Wouldn't we all have been wiped out?

P: Yes I suppose so.

T: So maybe panic itself doesn't cause heart attacks, there has to be something physically wrong for that to happen. When people have had heart attacks they are often given an injection of adrenalin directly into the heart in order to help start it again. Do you think they would do that if it damaged the heart even more?

P: No I'm sure they wouldn't.

T: So how much do you now believe that anxiety and panic will damage your heart?

*Misinterpretation: I'm going blind*

T: What are the sensations that make you think you are going blind?

P: My vision goes blurred and now I've noticed specks floating in my eyes.

T: Have you had your eyes tested?

P: Yes, I'm a little short sighted and should wear glasses, but I don't like wearing them because they make my eyes feel strange.

T: When do you notice your eyes are blurred?

P: When I'm driving or when I look at something for a long time.

T: Do you find that you are staring at things at these times?

P: Yes, I stare at things because I can't see clearly and also I'm checking-out my eyesight to see if it's OK.

T: Let's do an experiment right now to see what happens when you stare at something. Stare at the writing on this paper. What do you notice?

P: Yes, it begins to look blurred, that's how it is when I think there's something wrong with my eyes.

T: It seems as if the blurring you get is a combination of being short sighted, and this may be made worse by staring at things. When most people stare in this way it leads to noticeable changes in vision, and that's quite normal. Now what about those things floating in your eyes? They are called floaters, do you know what they are?

P: No, but I'm worried that they will get bigger and then I won't be able to see any more.

T: Let me draw you a picture of the eye and then you can see what they are (shows cross section of eye). The eye is filled with fluid, that's what enables it to keep its shape. Like most liquids—even water if you look at it closely—it contains small particles. What you can see are the small particles which are floating in the fluid of your eye. It is quite normal to have them and at least it tells us that you do have fluid in your eye like you're supposed to. If you look out of the window and blink a few times whilst moving your eyes around you'll notice the floaters floating about in your eye, you'll probably be able to see the different shapes and sizes they are. The more you focus on them the more of them you see, it doesn't mean they are getting worse. For homework what about asking other people to notice their floaters, to prove that they're normal?

*Misinterpretation: I'm having a stroke*

T: Do you know what causes a stroke?
P: Well I thought it was when the brain stopped working.
T: How can your brain stop working?
P: Well stress can cause a stroke can't it? It must damage you.
T: If stress can damage your brain why is it that after all of your panic attacks your brain isn't damaged?
P: Well if it goes on like this it could happen.
T: So it seems as if one of your worries is that anxiety might cause a stroke. A stroke is caused when part of the brain is starved of oxygen carried by the blood. Then part of the brain can die. Blood can be blocked off when the small arteries become constricted or blocked. Do you think anxiety causes that to happen?
P: Well I don't suppose so, but where does it come from?
T: A stroke is caused by a blood clot. But anxiety doesn't cause that. So anxiety, no matter how intense would not cause a stroke. Let me check that you've understood the difference between anxiety and a stroke. Why doesn't anxiety cause strokes?

*Misinterpretation: I'm losing control/going crazy*

T: When you say that in a panic you're afraid of losing control and going crazy what do you mean by that?
P: I'd just lose it and act like a mad person.
T: What would that be like? For example, what would it look like if you lost it in that way?
P: I'd just lose control and rush around screaming.
T: Do you get an image of that in your mind when you're panicking?
P: Yes, I can see myself rushing about screaming and hitting things, and everybody thinks I'm crazy.
T: What is it that makes you think that panic can send you crazy?
P: My mind starts racing, I can't concentrate on anything and everything seems like a dream.

T: When you say 'like a dream' do things seem unreal as if you're not a part of what's going on?

P: Yes, it's a really weird feeling, I can't explain it.

T: That feeling often seems strange, but it's a common symptom of anxiety and it's called derealisation. It's not a sign that you're going crazy, it's just a symptom of anxiety and is harmless. It's also common for someone's mind to race when they feel anxious. Anxiety is designed to help you defend yourself from harm, that wouldn't work very well if it sent you crazy. When your thinking speeds up it's a sign that your mind is working more quickly so that you can detect threats more easily and work out escape routes and so on. It doesn't mean that you will lose control of your behaviour. Think about people under great anxiety like motor-racing drivers at the start of a race, or people involved in accidents, do they go crazy?

P: No they don't. But I've rushed out of situations before when I've been panicking.

T: It sounds as if you think that rushing out means you've lost control of your behaviour.

P: It's not normal is it?

T: Well you are a normal person. Many people have panic attacks at some time in their life, and you probably have had a good reason for leaving situations. What were you afraid would happen if you stayed in situations where you felt panicky?

P: I thought I would go crazy.

T: It seems as if you are confusing your decision to leave with losing control. Your decision seems a sensible one to me if you believed such a bad thing would happen if you stayed. Does that sound like the behaviour of a crazy person to you?

P: No it seems quite sensible.

T: Have there been times when you were afraid of going crazy but were unable to leave the situation?

P: Yes, when I'm at work I can't just rush off and leave a customer.

T: It sounds to me then as if you can control what you do, and leaving the situation is based on your conscious decision. What do you think?

P: Yes, I suppose you're right, I'd never really looked at it that way before.

T: Let us do some experiments to see if we can test out your belief that you will go crazy.

In the educational scenarios above, guided discovery is employed as much as possible and new information is presented which is specifically targeted at the patient's misunderstanding. The procedure begins with exploration and definition of a specific fear, this type of breakdown is essential for understanding the patient's view of reality and suggests ways in which knowledge is faulty, and at which point the most effective educational correction may be made. Educational procedures are a small but important part of the overall cognitive restructuring strategies used in treatment, and they should be integrated with the techniques of questioning the evidence for misinterpretations and behavioural experiments. Initial questioning of the evidence not only elicits important idiosyncratic information but also 'loosens-up' the patient's thinking in preparation for the assimilation of new information.

## Counter-evidence

In exploring the counter-evidence for catastrophic misinterpretations in panic, the occasions on which panic has not led to catastrophe can be highlighted. Counter-evidence should be listed; this evidence can be gained from discussion of general issues, and of results of experiments, as well as other personal experience. Table 5.1 shows an evidence/counter-evidence worksheet for a panic patient's cardiac misinterpretations.

**Table 5.1** Evidence/counter-evidence worksheet of a panic patient with cardiac concerns

| *Misinterpretation*: Panic will cause me to have a heart attack | |
|---|---|
| *Evidence* | *Counter-evidence* |
| Read about people dying of stress | I've never heard of anyone dying of panic |
| Anxiety affects my heart | Stress is only a problem if there's something seriously wrong with heart |
| There's an old saying that you can die of fright | People under intense stress (e.g. soldiers on battlefields) don't die of stress |
| I get tingling in my fingers and chest pain when I panic | Anxiety and panic associated with adrenalin release. Adrenalin is administered to start hearts not stop them |
| | Anxiety is a survival mechanism. It does not harm people |
| Anxiety increases blood pressure and high blood pressure is bad for the heart | I've pushed my heart when anxious and nothing went wrong |
| | Panic caused temporary increases in blood pressure like exercise. And exercise is good for the heart. It's only when blood pressure is constantly too high that it's a problem |

We saw earlier how in some instances patients claim that catastrophe has actually happened, such as collapsing or fainting. Some safety behaviours, such as putting oneself on the floor, can be misconstrued by the patient as evidence that the catastrophe has occurred (i.e. collapsing). This type of evidence should be reframed in the context of the safety behaviours analysis as a strategy used by the individual to prevent catastrophe.

### Symptom contrast technique

The symptom contrast technique is useful in instances where an individual has experienced events such as fainting or vomiting which have subsequently become the themes of misinterpretations of anxiety. The technique relies on the provision of a discriminative context for appraisal which challenges the patient's restricted interpretation of symptoms (e.g. the view that 'dizziness' means fainting). The procedure consists of listing in detail the symptoms which accompanied the event and compares these with the symptoms of panic so that a pattern of the presence and absence of particular symptoms across the two states can be assessed. The subjective experience of fainting is usually quite different from the subjective experience of anxiety symptoms which are misinterpreted as a sign of fainting. The contrast for a particular panic patient is set out in Table 5.2.

**Table 5.2**   A symptoms contrast table for fainting versus panic

| Symptoms of fainting | Symptoms of panic |
| --- | --- |
| Everything goes black | ✗ |
| Felt sleepy | ✗ |
| Things slowed down | ✗ |
| Felt warm | ✓ |
| ✗ | Things seem fuzzy and brighter |
| ✗ | Weakness in legs |
| ✗ | Heart racing |
| ✗ | Dry mouth |

The contrast should be written out on paper or on a marker board, to facilitate patient processing of the material. The dialogue used to elicit the contrast presented in Table 5.2 was as follows:

T: I'm going to draw two columns on the board. In the left-hand column I'd like us to list all the symptoms you experienced when you fainted, and in the right-hand column the symptoms associated with panic. When you fainted what was that like?

P: I was ill with flu and I was on my way to the bathroom and I just came over all faint.

T: Did you feel anxious at that time?

P: No, I wasn't anxious.

T: When you felt faint what was that like? What were the feelings that you had?

P: Everything seemed to go black, and I felt sleepy.

T: Any other sensations that you noticed?

P: Yes it was as if everything had slowed down, and I felt warm.

T: OK. Let me write down these sensations under the fainting column. Now let's take each of these sensations in turn and see if you have them when you're panicking. First of all do things seem to go black?

P: No, not at all. But I do feel light-headed.

T: OK. So we'll put a cross next to that in the panic column. And we'll come back to the light-headed feeling in a minute. Do you feel sleepy when you're panicking?

P: Oh no, the opposite if anything. I can't relax.

T: OK. So we'll cross that in the panic column. What about feeling slowed down when anxious?

P: No I never feel slowed down, everything seems to be moving much faster.

T: OK. So we can cross that one off the panic experience. What about feeling warm?

P: Yes, I do get hot when I'm having a panic attack.

T: Is it the same type of hot feeling as when you fainted?

P: Yes similar.

T: So we'll put a tick next to that in the panic column. OK. Let's look at the feelings you get when panicking that lead you to think you will faint. What are they?

P: I feel light-headed and my legs feel weak.

T: What do you mean by light-headed?

P: Things seem fuzzy around me and brighter somehow.

T: That sounds like the opposite of fainting, didn't things seem black then?

P: Yes, you're right. It's not the same.

T: OK. So I'll cross that under the fainting heading. What about the feeling of weakness in your legs—did you get that when you fainted?

P: No I didn't notice that.

T: What else do you notice when you're panicking?

P: My heart races and my mouth goes dry.

T: Did you notice either of those when you fainted?

P: No, not at all.

T: So we now have a picture of the symptoms associated with fainting and those with panic. Do they look like the same ones to you?

P: No they're actually very different. I can see what your getting at.

### The survey technique

In panic disorder the experience of particular symptoms can be normalised by survey methods. The patient is asked to question other people, usually relatives and friends, to determine whether they also experience specific symptoms. The precise questions that patients ask should be determined beforehand in the therapy session.

## DEALING WITH AVOIDANCE

The degree of agoraphobic avoidance in panic varies. An essential dimension of treatment is the elimination of avoidance when this is present. A regular check on the degree of avoidance is therefore necessary. The reversal of avoidance should be a priority. This is accomplished through exposure experiments directed at challenging negative beliefs concerning symptoms that are situationally activated. Exposure should be combined with decreased safety-behaviour manipulations or paradoxical symptom induction strategies in challenging specific catastrophic predictions. While hierarchies of anxiety-provoking situations are not necessary in the cognitive use of exposure, it can be useful to break exposure tasks down into more manageable units in order to facilitate compliance.

## RELAPSE PREVENTION

The last two to three sessions of cognitive therapy should be increasingly devoted to relapse prevention work. Since the cognitive model predicts that residual belief in misinterpretations constitutes a vulnerability to future anxiety and panic, belief level should be checked and remaining beliefs modified before the end of treatment. Self-report measures such as the Agoraphobic Cognitions Questionnaire (Chambless, Caputo, Bright & Gallagher, 1978) and items of the Panic Rating Scale are capable of highlighting residual beliefs. These beliefs should be modified with combinations of verbal and behavioural procedures outlined previously. In addition to the elimination of residual belief, remaining avoidance, and safety behaviours should also be reversed. Central components of relapse prevention are: development of the *Therapy blueprint*; presenting a reframe for possible future anxiety; and scheduling a limited number of booster sessions. These are considered in turn.

## Therapy blueprint

The blueprint for panic consists of a written summary of everything that the patient has learned during treatment about the causes of panic, the maintaining factors, and the ways of overcoming the problem. It should consist of an example of a vicious circle, an account of the role of safety-behaviours and avoidance, a detailed account of techniques for challenging belief in misinterpretation, and summaries of counter-evidence.

## Reframe and booster sessions

Asking patients to rate how distressing they would find a future panic attack (0–100) presents a guide to the remaining problem level. If this is high the reasons need to be investigated and challenged. The possible (but unlikely) event of future panics should be reframed as an opportunity to practise the techniques used in treatment in order to challenge remaining beliefs. The experience of panic in the future should be viewed, not as a relapse, but as an opportunity to strengthen cognitive therapy skills. Two or three booster sessions should be scheduled at intervals of 2–3 months in order to ensure that gains are maintained.

## EXAMPLE TREATMENT OUTLINE

*Session 1*

(a) Map out panic circle for a recent attack.
(b) Socialise using circle and socialisation procedures.
(c) Identify range of misinterpretations and beliefs, plus safety behaviours.
(d) Homework : Fill out panic diary with misinterpretations. Listen to tape of therapy session.

*Session 2*

(a) Map out circle for recent panic recorded in diary.
(b) Focus on key beliefs and use behavioural and verbal reattribution.

(c)  Introduce concept of safety behaviours.
(d)  Homework : Continue diary. Experiment by dropping safety behaviours. Listen to tape of therapy session.

*Sessions 3–7*

(a)  Continue to map out circles for panics, including safety behaviours. Focus on key beliefs.
(b)  In-session induction experiments to challenge different beliefs.
(c)  Verbal reattribution and generation of rational responses based on this and on behavioural experiments.
(d)  Homework : Specific exposure experiments plus dropping of safety behaviours and pushing symptoms. Continue panic diary and include rational responses. Listen to tape of therapy session and write a summary.

*Sessions 8–12*

(a)  Challenge remaining beliefs.
(b)  Identify and eliminate remaining safety behaviours and avoidance.
(c)  Relapse prevention.
(d)  Homework : Continue pushing symptoms. Go in search of a panic to test fears. Work on blueprint.

*Note*. Use sessional responses on the Panic Rating Scale (PRS) to guide the focus of treatment sessions.

Chapter 6

# HYPOCHONDRIASIS: HEALTH ANXIETY

Hypochondriasis is classified in DSM-IV as a somatoform disorder not an anxiety disorder. Notwithstanding this, hypochondriasis can be usefully viewed as a problem concerned with *anxiety* about health, and has overlapping features with anxiety disorders such as panic, at least on a cognitive-behavioural conceptual level, hence its inclusion in this book. The treatment approach described here is based on that of Salkovskis (1989) and Warwick, Clark, Cobb and Salkovskis (1996).

The central defining features of this disorder are: belief that one has, or fear of developing, a serious disease which is based on the misinterpretation of bodily signs or symptoms. An appropriate medical evaluation does not identify a medical condition that fully justifies the person's concerns about disease or physical signs or symptoms. In hypochondriasis the belief is not of delusional intensity. That is, 'the person can acknowledge the possibility that he or she may be exaggerating the extent of the feared disease, or that there may be no disease at all' (DSM-IV, APA, 1994, p. 463). The preoccupation should cause significant distress or impairment, and the problem should be of at least 6 months' duration to warrant DSM-IV diagnosis. The preoccupation should not be better accounted for by Generalised Anxiety Disorder, Obsessive Compulsive Disorder, panic disorder, major depression or another somatoform disorder. These unwarranted fears are not allayed by medical reassurance. Some hypochondriacs frequently seek reassurance from their GP while others, because of a general fear of illness-related material, tend to avoid contact with the medical profession and with medical information. Reassurance seeking may be extensive and constitute—'doctor shopping'.

Hypochondriasis may occur in conjunction with panic attacks, and illness concern tends to fluctuate in severity over a time course of days or months. Acute phases of the disorder may be punctuated by periods of relatively low levels of distress and health concern. Health-anxious patients tend to respond to medical reassurance with an immediate reduction in distress and worry; however, the effect of reassurance tends to be transient, typically lasting for a few hours to a few days.

## A COGNITIVE MODEL OF HYPOCHONDRIASIS

The main tenant of the cognitive model is that the disorder results from, and is maintained by, the misinterpretation of normal bodily signs and symptoms as a sign of serious organic pathology. This is similar to the process which is central in the cognitive model of panic. However, the misinterpretations in panic tend to differ from those in health anxiety in a fundamental way that reflects the patient's perceived time course of the appraised catastrophe. More specifically, panickers tend to believe that the catastrophe is immediately impending during a panic attack while health-anxious individuals believe that the catastrophe (e.g. death or painful suffering) will occur at some time in the more distant future. When the catastrophe is appraised as immediate, panic attacks may be more likely to occur.

Salkovskis and Warwick are leading proponents of the misinterpretation model of health-anxiety (Salkovskis, 1989; Warwick & Salkovskis, 1989, 1990). In their model individuals are considered to develop hypochondriasis when critical incidents activate dysfunctional assumptions concerning health. These assumptions may form early or later in life but are modified through ongoing experience.

The critical incident may be the experience of unexpected physical symptoms, noticing previously unnoticed bodily signs, the death of a relative or exposure to illness-related information. Once activated these beliefs lead to the misinterpretation of bodily sensations/signs as evidence of serious physical pathology. These misinterpretations occur as negative automatic thoughts, which may involve vivid negative images. In health anxiety these images typically consist of parts of the body 'giving-out' or functioning improperly. For example, patients report images of the heart quivering, the lungs only partially inflating, the brain haemorrhaging, and cancer 'taking over' the body. In consequence, a number of related mechanisms are activated which are involved in the maintenance of health preoccupation and

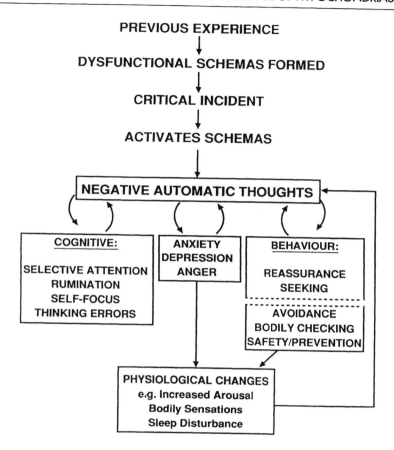

**Figure 6.0**  A cognitive model of health anxiety (adapted from Salkovskis, 1989; Warwick & Salkovskis, 1990)

anxiety. Four categories of maintenance mechanism are distinguished; cognitive, affective, behavioural, and physiological. A cognitive model of hypochondriasis based on Warwick and Salkovskis (1989) depicting a relationship between these mechanisms is presented in Figure 6.0.

## Cognitive factors

Selective attention processes in health anxiety may resemble those found in panic disorder. For example, there is typically an increased focusing on internal bodily processes such as heart rate, gastro-intestinal activity, swallowing, breathing and so on. In addition, some health-anxious patients focus on the outwardly observable aspects of their bodies and are hypervigilant for signs such as asymmetry of the body, bumps and blemishes on the skin, hair loss or irregular hair growth, and pupil size. Preoccupation with products expelled from the body such as the colour of one's saliva, faeces and urine may also be present. In these latter cases patients are often checking for noticeable changes in functioning such as the presence of blood colorations. Aside from selective attention to the body, attentional bias for external negative illness-related information is also common. This may take the form of increased sensitivity to particular types of information during clinical consultation and enhanced awareness of external illness information presented in the media. Rumination in the form of worry or mental 'problem solving' is a common feature in some cases. Worry about health may be a manifestation of a hypervigilant strategy adopted by the individual so that early signs of illness may be detected, or may be a superstitious strategy intended to ward off dangers of positive thinking (Wells & Hackmann, 1993). Continued rumination about health maintains bodily awareness and contributes to affective symptoms (e.g. sleep disturbance), factors that can contribute to misinterpretation.

Common cognitive distortions (thinking errors) in health anxiety are: discounting of alternative non-serious explanations of symptoms, selective abstraction, and catastrophising. A tendency to discount medical feedback and the results of investigations that fail to find illness may result from particular beliefs, such as: 'It is possible with the appropriate tests to know with *certainty* that one is not ill.' Selective abstraction is a distortion that operates in clinical consultations, it consists of placing undue emphasis on, and taking out of context minor bits of information. For example, the health-conscious patient may be given feedback that his/her blood pressure is 'within the normal range and should be checked again at a later date'. The idea of repeating the check may be taken out of context and used to infer that there is something seriously wrong that needs monitoring. Catastrophising involves overinflating the significant of signs and symptoms and is often accompanied by a failure to consider benign explanations for them.

## Affect/physiological changes

The affective response which accompanies misinterpretations is typically anxiety (although depression is often a secondary feature of longstanding health preoccupation). Autonomic symptoms of anxiety are commonly misinterpreted symptoms in health anxiety. Changes in bodily processes such as bowel function, heart rate, and change in sleep patterns resulting from arousal may be misinterpreted.

## Behavioural responses

Several behavioural factors contribute to the maintenance of misinterpretations in health anxiety: checking, avoidance, safety behaviours, reassurance seeking.

Repeated checking of the body such as palpation of the abdomen to check for discomfort, or self-examination such as checking for rectal bleeding, or repeated checking for breast or testicular lumps can lead to soreness and tissue trauma. Discomfort resulting from checking behaviours is likely to be misinterpreted as further evidence of serious physical illness. Even in the absence of physical damage, bodily checking maintains awareness of the body so that normal and benign symptoms are more easily noticed—a perceptual change that can be falsely interpreted as evidence of worsening symptomatology rather than of increased attention. Other examples of bodily checking contributing to physiological changes include repeatedly taking deep breaths to check that the lungs are functioning properly, which can produce muscular strain and chest discomfort; forced swallowing to check for feared anomalies in the throat, which typically makes swallowing seem more difficult; and checking one's pulse, which increases awareness of its natural variability.

Avoidance behaviour takes several forms. Avoidance may be of certain activities such as strenuous physical exertion, or avoidance of situations which activate health rumination and anxiety such as exposure to media material about illness. In some instances the health-anxious patients will try not to think about illness by attempting to control their thoughts or by distraction. Avoidance of 'risky' behaviours such as physical exertion prevents exposure to disconfirmatory experiences, and avoidance behaviours maintain preoccupation with concepts of illness. Attempts to suppress thoughts may be problematic because that leads to a paradoxical increment in unwanted thoughts (see Chapter 8).

A third type of behaviour tied to problem maintenance is the patient's use of safety behaviours. Specific safety behaviours in health anxiety are intended to reduce the risk of illness in the future. In particular, these are 'preventative' behaviours. For example, a patient with cardiac concerns may take an aspirin each day, or vitamin supplements are used on a daily basis when there is no medical reason to do so. In moderation these particular behaviours may not produce problematic bodily responses, however they serve to maintain preoccupation with illness and health concepts, and are capable of maintaining beliefs such as one's body is weak and needs all the assistance available to remain healthy. Other precautionary responses, such as extensive resting, can be problematic because they contribute to loss of physical fitness and body strength. These symptoms may then be taken as further evidence of serious illness. Some safety behaviours consist of adopting particular bodily postures or controlling bodily responses such as swallowing or breathing. These behaviours maintain bodily-focused attention and intensify symptoms.

Repeated reassurance seeking is the fourth behaviour to be considered in the conceptual analysis of factors responsible for maintaining dysfunctional belief at the misinterpretation and schema levels. Reassurance can be sought in different ways; reassurance seeking behaviours are often subtle and may involve asking a partner or family members about symptoms, or it may involve persistently mentioning and describing symptoms to others. Reassurance seeking may consist of visits to the doctor and requests for investigations and tests. Reassurance seeking can manifest itself in the form of studying medical articles and books in an attempt to self-diagnose and rule-out serious illnesses.

A number of problems exist with reassurance seeking. One of the more salient problems is that conflicting or inconsistent information is given about symptoms, and after repeated presentations to medical professionals patients may feel that they are not being 'taken seriously'. These factors are capable of strengthening a patient's desire for further investigations and contribute to the development of negative beliefs about medical competency so that failure to find a physical cause of symptoms provides little comfort.

## Summary of model and new directions

In summary, the cognitive model of health anxiety maintains that misinterpretation of bodily signs and symptoms and the physiological/affective, cognitive, and behavioural factors (checking, reassurance seeking, avoidance and safety) associated with them are involved in the aetiology and maintenance of the disorder. The model asserts that individuals misinterpret symptoms partly because of the assumptions and beliefs that are held about the meaning of bodily events. Recent work by Wells and Hackmann (1993) has explored in detail images and associated beliefs in health-anxious and panic patients. For some individuals illness has extremely negative and sinister implications. In these cases there is a strong fear of death and images and beliefs that death will be an experience of external distress or punishment. In other cases there is an inherent concept that following death there will be a continuation of awareness, but this is an awareness of the things that have been left behind. In other cases a key belief is that illness will lead to a change in ability to work or function, and when this is an important determinant of self-esteem there is a predicted diminution in self-concept. Beliefs about death and spiritual concepts ('meta-physical' beliefs) may interact with more general negative beliefs about the self in contributing to a fear of illness, and of death.

## GENERAL TREATMENT ISSUES

There are two general issues that should be considered in implementing effective cognitive therapy for health anxiety. The first deals with the precise *aim* of treatment for this disorder. The second, with engagement of patients in treatment.

The primary aim of treatment is *not only* to challenge the patient's belief that he/she is seriously ill. The aim of cognitive therapy is to offer the patient an alternative and hopefully more credible explanation of the problem. Therapy focuses on collecting evidence for an alternative psychological model which should present a conceptual shift away from the disease model held by the patient. In practise effective treatment involves a combination of directly challenging disease conviction and building an alternative model. In cases involving feared 'mechanical' failures of the body such as cardiac failures, breathing failures and so on, it is possible to devise experiments (like those in panic) to directly challenge belief by trying to make the failure happen. However, when misinterpretations concern diseases, such as cancer, that have a more general effect on the body, experiments mainly focus on collecting evidence for the cognitive model. More specifically, experiments cannot focus on making the catastrophe happen, but focus on demonstrating the effects of selective attention, rumination, bodily checking, etc.

### Engagement in treatment

Engagement of health-anxious patients in treatment can be difficult and is hindered by negative patient expectations and attitudes towards health professionals. These attitudes may be based on past deteriorating doctor–patient relationships. In addition, problems can arise from a patient's seemingly insatiable appetite for listing and describing signs and symptoms in minute detail, and a general preoccupation with physical symptoms at the expense of a concern with psychological factors. Attendance for cognitive therapy is not a guarantee that health-anxious patients are considering psychological explanations of their problem, and can merely reflect an attempt to show that the psychological approach does not work and, therefore, 'there must be something seriously physically wrong'.

Given this sort of profile it is not surprising that many clinicians initially find some health-anxious patients difficult to engage in treatment. However, steps can be taken to diminish the problem. Engagement in treatment can be facilitated by using the following routine, or similar combination of these methods:

1. Present cognitive therapy as a 'nothing to lose' opportunity to discover what the problem may be. This is presented by reviewing the strategies used by the patient so far in attempting to sort out his/her problems. The fact that the patient's existing approach (usually repeated medical consultations) has been unfruitful should be highlighted. The therapist should then suggest.that a psychological approach may be worth while, but even if it is not, at least the patient will have tried a different perspective and may then be considered more favourably by other professionals when they resume the medical approach. In this framework the psychological approach is presented as a 'no-lose' experiment.
2. Challenge erroneous patient assumptions concerning the psychological perspective. Some patients assume that the psychological approach views symptoms as 'all in the mind' or 'imagined'. The therapist should emphasise that symptoms are real, not imagined, but may have causes other than serious physical illness.
3. Discuss the collaborative nature of treatment and the importance of both patient *and* therapist entering treatment with an 'open mind' about the problem, in search of possible answers.
4. Construct a basic conceptualisation based on the model and begin socialisation.
5. Design and implement behavioural experiments in the *first* treatment session which illustrate elements of the model and alternative explanations. Discuss any temporary ameliorative effect of medical reassurance on symptoms as support for the model (see example below).
6. Shift the patient from focusing on signs and symptoms to identifying and articulating emotions and thoughts (misinterpretations) associated with focusing/dwelling on symptoms.

*Example of the 'no-lose' engagement dialogue*

T: It sounds as if you've had worries about your health for a long time. What have you done about it?
P: I've been to see the doctor a few times and he sent me for an ECG, and he's done blood tests, and they all seem normal.
T: Do you think that your visits to the GP and the tests have helped at all?
P: Well it puts my mind at rest, but only for a while and then I notice something in my chest and it starts again.
T: What you have just said might be very important for understanding your problem. You said that visits to the doctor 'put your mind at rest', and

then things seem better for a while. What does that tell you about your problem?

P: I don't know, I wouldn't worry if I didn't have the chest pain.

T: Would reassurance take the problem away if it had a physical cause?

P: No, I don't suppose so.

T: So what does that suggest about the problem?

P: That it has to do with what I'm worrying about.

T: That's right. Maybe a big part of your problem has something to do with worry and preoccupation with health rather than a serious illness.

P: Well I'm not sure, I will have to think about that. I don't get anxious or worried unless I notice the chest pain first.

T: The way I see it is that you have tried the medical option and it hasn't got you very far. What about giving the psychological approach a chance, just for twelve sessions? There is nothing to lose and you can only gain by it.

P: But I'm not sure it's going to help.

T: You can benefit no matter how it turns out. If it does work then that's great. If it doesn't at least you have given it a try and maybe your GP will be more motivated to explore other possibilities with you, having ruled out this one. What do you think?

P: I suppose you're right, I don't have anything to lose, do I?


## FROM COGNITIVE MODEL TO CASE CONCEPTUALISATION

Although Figure 6.0 can be translated into an idiosyncratic case conceptualisation with little modification, simpler forms of the conceptualisation may be presented initially. When panic attacks are present, the first conceptualisation should take the form of the standard vicious circle model of panic (see Figure 5.1, p. 102). An initial formulation of panic offers a convenient way into the cognitive model, and panic attacks should be targeted for treatment before dealing with more chronic health concerns. Successful treatment of panic offers a means of socialising in the psychological model. Since the first stages of treatment focus on symptomatic relief (i.e. reduction in anxious health preoccupation) it is unnecessary to include predisposing beliefs in the conceptualisation at this stage. The central variables are negative misinterpretations and the cycles of maintaining factors as depicted in the idiosyncratic conceptualisation of Figure 6.1.

The construction of the conceptualisation is based on reviewing in detail recent health-anxious episodes, which may be exacerbations of general background health preoccupation. An illustrative excerpt of a therapeutic dialogue used in eliciting material for the conceptualisation in Figure 6.1 is

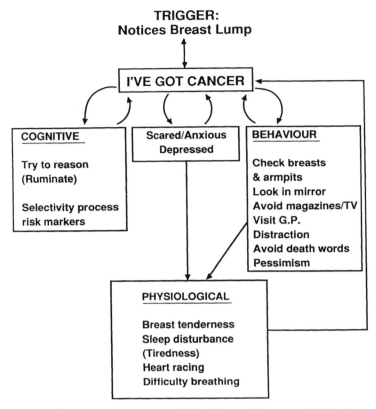

**TRIGGER:**
**Notices Breast Lump**

**I'VE GOT CANCER**

**COGNITIVE**

Try to reason
(Ruminate)

Selectivity process
risk markers

Scared/Anxious
Depressed

**BEHAVIOUR**

Check breasts
& armpits
Look in mirror
Avoid magazines/TV
Visit G.P.
Distraction
Avoid death words
Pessimism

**PHYSIOLOGICAL**

Breast tenderness
Sleep disturbance
(Tiredness)
Heart racing
Difficulty breathing

**Figure 6.1** An idiosyncratic symptomatic health-anxiety conceptualisation

given below. In this dialogue the therapist explores the cognitive, behavioural and affective factors associated with the maintenance of health preoccupation and disease conviction. In the example presented, note that there are a number of points which could have resulted in departures from the therapeutic goal of building a basic symptomatic conceptualisation. However, the therapist remained as focused as possible and flagged important themes for later exploration:

T: I'd like to find out more about what happens when you get worried about your health. Have you been worried this week?

P: I'm worried every week, it never seems to go away.

T: What have you been concerned about?

P: It's always cancer. I've noticed a new lump under my arm and I think I've got it.

T: How much do you believe that you have cancer, 0–100 per cent?

P: About 60 per cent now, but when I'm in a state about it I'm convinced it's cancer.

T: What happens to put you into a state about it?

P: If I notice a new lump under my arm or in my breast, that can start me off. There's been a lot written in magazines recently about breast cancer. Some magazines have listed the risk factors, and I have quite a few of them.

T: OK, let me see if I've got this right. It seems that noticing a lump, reading or hearing about cancer can start you worrying. It sounds like you're checking your body looking for signs, is that right?

P: Yes. I check my breasts and under my arms to see if anything is developing.

T: How often do you check?

P: It varies. At least once a day, usually after I've showered, but sometimes I check more often like five or six times a day.

T: Do you check any other parts of your body?

P: I sometimes look in the mirror to see if my face has changed, to see if I look old.

T: What would that mean if you noticed a change?

P: That might mean that I've got cancer.

T: When you check what do you notice?

P: It sometimes feels tender.

T: You've mentioned checking, and I think that's important. Do you do anything else such as avoid certain things?

P: Well, I don't watch medical programmes or those hospital dramas, and if I see something in a magazine I'll skip over it.

T: OK. Let me make a note of that. What about asking for reassurance or talking to people about your symptoms?

P: I've been to the doctor a few times. I think she's fed up with me. She said the lump I had was unlikely to be serious, and to leave it a few months.

T: OK. What about telling other people?

P: I tell my husband about it, but he's just sick of hearing about it.

T: So it sounds as if other people are not responding as well as you would like.

P: They don't seem to care. It's like being alone with all this. Sometimes I think I'm the only one and I'm going to die. (Begins to cry.)

T: (The therapist is faced with a decision at this stage. Either to explore the affect shift and explore cognitions about dying, or to continue with building the symptomatic formulation. Since this is the first treatment session the latter course is chosen, although the potential relevance of death cognitions is flagged for future work.) OK, just take your time, I can see that some of these thoughts are upsetting you. I'd like to come back to your thoughts of death later, because they could be important. If we could come back to looking at what happens when you're worried about cancer, does the way in which you think change at those times?

P:  Well I can't get it out of my head. I try and reason with myself and think it through but it doesn't help. The more I think about it the worse it gets.

T:  So it sounds as if you spend a lot of time trying to sort it out. Do you ever try not to think about it?

P:  Yes, I try to distract myself by keeping busy.

T:  Do you ever do superstitious things, like not think positive thoughts or do things in certain ways to keep safe?

P:  Well, I won't let anyone mention death, like the children. And if I see a magpie or something like that I cross my fingers otherwise it's bad luck. Also I don't like to be too optimistic because that could be tempting fate.

T:  OK. I'm getting a fuller picture now of the different branches to the problem. I want to focus on the way you feel emotionally when you're worried. What's that like?

P:  I feel scared and then depressed because I can't cope with this any more.

T:  When you feel scared do you get physical sensations?

P:  Yes, my heart races, and I have difficulty breathing.

T:  What about sensations when you feel sad?

P:  I feel tired and like it can't go on like this.

T:  OK. I've written down the things you've said and I've pulled it together in a way that could explain what's going on. It's like a number of vicious circles (shows patient formulation: Figure 6.1).

A significant feature of this patient's problem was rumination as well as the usual checking and avoidance. An early component of the intervention was the exploration of beliefs concerning rumination to determine whether it had any appraised protective function. Anti-ruminative strategies were implemented early in treatment to demonstrate that reducing rumination about the cause of symptoms reduced health preoccupation.


## SOCIALISATION

Treatment success is largely dependent on patients accepting a psychological explanation of their problem. This is most problematic in cases of strong physical disease conviction. Careful consideration must therefore be given to socialising health-anxious patients. The early use of behavioural experiments, in the first few sessions, can be a powerful aid to socialisation. Many of the procedures outlined in Chapter 5 can be adapted for use in health-anxiety treatment. If panic attacks are part of the health-anxiety scenario, it is helpful to begin by conceptualising and socialising with the panic model and treating discrete attacks before moving onto background health fears. In this way, the response of panics to treatment can be used as evidence for the conceptualisation.

## Sample socialisation experiments

Treatment relies on building a credible alternative model of the presenting problem which is then adopted by the patient in preference to a physical illness model. On one level the whole treatment process can be viewed as extended and detailed socialisation. Five particular socialisation procedures are discussed below.

### Tracking symptom patterns

By tracking the occurrence of symptoms such as dizziness, palpitations, and chest tightness, patterns in their occurrence may become apparent. The existence of symptom patterns can be used to challenge belief in disease-based explanations. For example, if symptoms such as dizziness occur most often in the mid-morning and during working days, this pattern is used to question the validity of a disease explanation: 'If you have a serious disease why does it affect you most at certain times? Is there anything about these times that could account for your symptoms?' A discussion of variables that could account for the patterns should be undertaken. Possible causes include: alcohol withdrawal, low blood sugar, or increased stress at a particular time of day. Symptoms can be tracked on modified DTRs or on blank activity schedules. For this strategy to be effective daily recording should be undertaken.

### Reviewing the impact of reassurance

In cases where reassurance seeking has been evident the impact of verbal reassurance or medical test results on worry and symptoms should be reviewed. Typically, reassurance alleviates symptoms and worry and the effect can be used to reinforce a psychological explanation of the problem (i.e. 'If reassurance relieves your symptoms what does that tell you about their cause?'). Questions like the following may be used in this context:

- What happens to your symptoms when the doctor tells you that they are not serious?
- If reassurance makes you feel better, would that work if you are seriously ill? Is reassurance a cure for . . . (e.g. cancer, heart disease)?
- Would a serious illness respond to reassurance in this way?
- How do you think the reassurance works?

● What does that tell you about your problem?

*The 'intelligent disease' metaphor*

Both the identification of symptom patterns and a review of modulating influences such as reassurance effects can be used in conjunction with the *intelligent disease* metaphor. Here, the discovery of symptom patterns or response to reassurance is used to suggest that the illness or disease can 'think for itself' (e.g. How would a brain tumour know when it was being reassured?'). If symptom patterns are not evident from monitoring, or reassurance effects are absent, another strategy is a discussion of factors that exacerbate the patients symptom's. If at first this is unclear, the presence of avoidance is often a marker for exacerbatory stimuli. For example, an individual may avoid watching medical television programmes or reading illness-relevant media material because this material increases symptoms. Such responses can be used as evidence for a psychological exploration of the patient's problem (e.g. how would reading material about illness make symptoms of a brain tumour worse?)

*Selective attention experiments*

The use of self-focused selective-attention experiments was outlined in the previous chapter on panic. Similar experiments are effective socialisation strategies in the treatment of health anxiety. Prescriptive self-focusing strategies lead patients to notice normal bodily sensations (e.g. tightness of shoes on the feet, tingling in fingertips etc.) which they have normally not noticed. These procedures can also increase symptom intensity. The impact of these procedures can be discussed as analogous to the effect of bodily checking when this is prevalent. The primary supposition is that selective self-attention intensifies awareness of normal bodily signs and symptoms which are usually present, but new or intensified awareness can be confused as the occurrence of a new *serious* symptom. (Note: Re-attribution experiments also involve attentional manipulations such as attending to observable symptom-signs in other people. For example, a patient who misinterprets bald patches in beard growth as a sign of skin cancer could be asked to observe other peoples' beard growth to determine whether this is an abnormal feature and likely to be a sign of danger.)

*Education*

The role of misinterpretation and the behavioural concomitants of misinterpretation in the maintenance of health anxiety should be presented in detail with reference to the patient's case conceptualisation (e.g. Figure 6.1).

Chapter 5 presents details on the use of education, and metaphor which can be adapted for use in the health-anxiety context.

## REATTRIBUTION STRATEGIES

Cognitive restructuring in health anxiety gives equal emphasis to building an alternative understanding of the patient's problem, and to challenging particular beliefs. In some instances a misinterpretation is not readily amenable to challenges. For example, if patients strongly believe that they have a serious illness but do not know what it is, or believe that the illness is latent (e.g. AIDS), and negative test results are unreliable, direct verbal and behavioural challenges of belief are likely to be unproductive. More generally, reattribution techniques that consist of providing an explanation for each of a patient's various symptoms are also likely to be inefficient for long-term belief change. This type of approach tends to lapse into repeated reassurance giving, and the patient is likely to present with a weekly list of symptoms to be explained. Cognitive therapy for health anxiety depends on shifting the patient's emphasis of appraisal away from focusing merely on symptoms to focusing on *thoughts* and *behaviours* associated with symptoms. When direct belief challenges can be used they are useful for an initial 'loosening' of the patient's belief, which can then be followed by the collecting of evidence for an alternative model. Moreover, in cases where cardiac and respiratory concerns predominate, or generally where specific short-term catastrophic predictions can be made based on the patient's belief, direct disconfirmation through experiment is easier to accomplish.

## BEHAVIOURAL EXPERIMENTS

### Testing patient predictions

Direct belief challenges can be used when there are specific predictions based on the patient's illness conviction. When a patient believes, for example, that there is something seriously wrong with his/her heart, predictions can be made concerning the conditions under which the problem would manifest itself and lead to catastrophe. For example, vigorous exercise tasks could be employed to test this belief. As in the case of panic treatment, an analysis of the nature of avoidance and safety behaviours will usually suggest particular experiments which can be used to test predictions. These experiments will typically involve reversing avoidance and safety responses. An example of the implementation of a direct-challenge experiment in the case of a 34-year-old male health-anxious patient with a two-year history of belief in suffering from a serious muscle-wasting disease is presented below:

T: Is there anything you're avoiding right now in case it makes your problem worse?

P: I don't play football any more, and I'm trying to take it easy at home. If I exert myself for long I just get tired and my legs feel weak.

T: Do you do anything to make things better?

P: I just try and rest more.

T: How would that help with a muscle-wasting disease?

P: If I don't use the muscles as much they won't get so tired, and I won't damage them.

T: If you do have a muscle-wasting disease, and you over-tax the muscles, what's the worst that could happen?

P: They will just get weaker and then my legs will give-way altogether.

T: Okay, it sounds as if the main evidence that makes you think you have a wasting disease is a feeling of weakness and tiredness. What I would like us to do right now is test out exactly how weak your legs are, to see if you collapse if you use the muscles vigorously. How does that sound?

P: Well I know what you are saying. I probably won't collapse but it will make them feel worse.

T: They may feel worse, but perhaps there is a difference between *feeling weak* and actually *being weak*. Let's put it to the test. How much do you believe your leg muscles are weak right now because of disease?

P: Not very much, 30 per cent.
(At this juncture therapist and patient go outside to do some jogging and muscle-taxing by exercise.)

T: Okay, how are the muscles feeling now?

P: Terrible, they are really weak. I can't do any more.

T: I would like you to push the muscles even more; it's important to find out if there is anything wrong. Sprint to that tree and back, really push the muscles this time.
(Patient sprints to tree and back.)

T: Okay, now stand on one leg, let's really see if the muscles are weak. That's good . . . Now whilst standing on one leg, bend that leg and straighten it a few times. That's good. Carry on . . . Okay, how much do you now believe your muscles are weak?

P: Well obviously they're not, I don't believe it at all.

T: How bad is the weak feeling right now?

P: Actually it is not that bad.

T: Good. How much do you believe you have a muscle-wasting disease now?

P: Oh less, about 10 per cent.

T: What's keeping the 10 per cent belief going?

P: Well, I still feel tired and I still get the feeling of weakness.

T: Let's go inside and we will look at other possible explanations for those symptoms. I think they are maintained by the way your are behaving right now rather than caused by disease. (A profitable discussion about safety behaviours, and the effect of over-resting in increasing tiredness and depleting muscle strength followed. This was presented in conjunction with homework experiments involving an exercise programme to demonstrate how reversing safety behaviours could ameliorate symptoms and thus facilitated building the alternative model.)

## Survey method

The survey method involves observing other people, and questioning others about their symptom experiences. An aim of the technique is to challenge illness conviction by 'normalising' the experience of misinterpreted signs and symptoms. An example of the use of this procedure is its usage to challenge belief that irregularities in heart beat *must* be a sign of a serious heart defect. In this scenario, patient and therapist each interview five people to determine the frequency of perceived irregularities in people with no history of heart problems. Typically, a significant percentage of people interviewed report deviations in heart rate.

## Paradoxical procedures

Paradoxical procedures are used to gain evidence for aspects of the cognitive model and thereby reinforce the psychological explanation of the problem. Instructing patients to increase bodily checking or increase rumination about health can be a powerful means of demonstrating the effect of checking behaviour and rumination in increasing symptom awareness and producing changes in affect (refer to the section on rumination interventions for further discussion).

## Medical consultation during cognitive therapy

Every endeavour should be made to ensure that patients do not have physical illnesses that account for their problem prior to conceptualising and treating hypochondriasis. The therapist may decide to ask the patient to suspend efforts to obtain further medical testing during the course of cognitive therapy. This is more difficult when tests are already planned, or the patient refuses to abandon testing. In these circumstances further tests can be set up as behavioural experiments to determine how symptoms respond to reassurance, and thereby gain evidence for the psychological model. In addition, predictions can be made concerning the way in which the patient will interpret test results if they are negative. In this way, the effects of appraisal and biased thinking in problem maintenance can be demonstrated.

## Reducing reassurance seeking

The role of reassurance seeking in the maintenance of health fears should be discussed as an integral part of treatment. Reassurance may be more or less problematic across individual cases. An initial step in reducing reassurance seeking is the discussion of problems caused by this behaviour: reassurance via medical tests and consultations can lead to conflicting explanations of symptoms provided by health experts. This in turn fuels beliefs that doctors are incompetent and there could be something seriously wrong which has not been detected yet. In addition, repeated investigations increase the likelihood that something will be found to be different from normal, but this does not mean that it is the cause of the patient's presenting symptoms, although it can become yet another factor to worry about.

When the problems with reassurance seeking have been established, the patient should be instructed to postpone or ban the activity. An *advantage/ disadvantage* analysis of *repeated* reassurance seeking may be used to strengthen motivation for abandoning the behaviour when disadvantages outweigh advantages. The results of the advantages component of the analysis should be used to focus techniques on challenging the usefulness of *repeated* reassurance seeking in meeting the advantages listed. Alternative, less problematic health-care behaviours can then be explored as substitutes. This is best accomplished in conjunction with developing a plan for future medical consultation.

## Developing a plan for medical consultation

Once the problems associated with reassurance seeking have been established, therapy involves determining a plan for more appropriate medical consultation. The implementation of such a plan can be used as a behavioural experiment in which the effects of a change in consultation strategy on anxiety and health preoccupation can be observed. Changes involve the introduction of delays in consultation in which health-anxious patients are encouraged not to check signs and symptoms repeatedly and not to seek immediate consultation, but instead to make a note of the symptom in a diary one week ahead of the present time, and decide to check for its presence after the week has elapsed. If patients are still concerned after that time they may then decide to seek consultation. Asking patients to make a note of their symptom is a means of counteracting the patients' fears that they may forget about the symptoms and therefore expose themselves to great risk.

In conjunction with delay procedures, a *decision blueprint* for evaluating when to seek medical help can be produced in treatment. The blueprint should emphasise the role of important factors in the decision process such as previous consultation with the same symptoms, previous diagnosis and symptom persistence.

## Self-monitoring

We saw in the section on socialisation how monitoring of symptoms can lead to the discovery of symptom patterns. The monitoring of other variables such as stress levels, caffeine intake, alcohol use, food intake, sleep quality, and rest periods in conjunction with symptom monitoring can lead to the identification of potential triggers for symptoms. Manipulations of these triggers can be used to challenge illness conviction.

## VERBAL REATTRIBUTION TECHNIQUES

A proportion of health-anxious patients frequently seek health reassurance from their therapists during the course of therapy sessions. This leads the patient to question the therapist about the possible cause of new or old symptoms, and in its extreme form the health-anxious person may attempt to present detailed listings of sensations and symptoms. The more this occurs the less opportunity there is to guide the patient to examine and test out alternative explanations for themselves. This problem should be managed by identifying and challenging the assumptions that lead patients to use therapy sessions in this particular way. Often, assumptions centre on the idea that the therapist must know *all* of the details about symptoms in order to assess their cause, or are based on the theme that health professionals are usually inclined to miss important details, and therefore details of symptoms must be repeatedly presented if appropriate treatment is to be given.

One of the most frequent problems encountered by cognitive therapists in treating health anxiety is *therapeutic drift*. Here, the focus of sessions shifts away from working on negative appraisals and assumptions to the discussion of patient's individual signs and symptoms. It is easy to be contaminated by the patient's need to find an explanation for all signs and symptoms and thereby lose the focus on cognition and behaviour which is conceptualised as maintaining *health preoccupation*. By keeping the cognitive model in mind this problem can be minimised. However, when drift is occurring the problem should be corrected by eliciting the patient's thoughts and the meanings of thoughts which occur during health-anxious episodes i.e. in response to triggers for health anxiety (which may include noticing particular signs or symptoms).

## The health-anxiety thoughts record

It is useful to modify the standard automatic thoughts record for use in health anxiety. In this instance the record comprises an additional column for logging triggers of health anxiety. Potential triggers include: noticing symptoms, reading or hearing news items, thoughts. A note of the situation in which health anxiety occurs is also included. The identification of triggers can be used as evidence for a psychological explanation of the problem, serving a similar function to that of the symptom record. Columns for recording negative thoughts about health and for responses to these thoughts are a standard part of the record. An example of a health-anxiety thoughts record is presented in Figure 6.2.

In the 'response to thought' section of the record, behavioural responses which have been learned in therapy as well as the usual verbal rational responses should be included, as both represent ways of answering thoughts. Typical behavioural responses are experiments such as dropping safety behaviours, pushing symptoms, or exposure to feared stimuli to test out the validity of negative thoughts. Belief in negative thoughts should be re-rated on the record following these responses. A clear aim in treatment is strengthening belief in rational responses (alternative thoughts) while reducing belief in negative thoughts (appraisals of serious physical illness). Progress in this endeavour can be monitored with the thoughts record.

## Pie charts

One of the characteristics of health-anxious thought is an overestimation of serious (life-threatening) causes of signs and symptoms. One technique for dealing with this is the pie chart. Here the therapist and patient work collaboratively in listing all of the possible causes of a particular symptom that the patient is concerned about, with their particular catastrophic concern at the bottom of the list. The more causes that are generated the better. Having generated the list a pie chart is drawn out in which each segment in the pie

| Date | Situation | Trigger for Health Anxiety | Emotion | Negative Thought (rate belief 0-100) | Response to Thought (include rational response rate belief 0-100) | Outcome (re-rate belief in negative thought) |
|------|-----------|----------------------------|---------|--------------------------------------|------------------------------------------------------------------|----------------------------------------------|
|      |           |                            |         |                                      |                                                                  |                                              |

**Note:** When you become concerned about your health, make a note of the situation where this occurred. Make a note of the "trigger" for your concern, this may be noticing a symptom, have a thought, or hearing about illness. Note your emotional response. Write down your main negative thought. In the "Response" column make a note of what you did in response to the thought and write a rational response (your therapist will guide you in responding differently in treatment). In the "Outcome" column, re-rate your belief in the negative thought, and make a note of anything that you found helpful.

**Figure 6.2**   Example of a health-anxiety thought record

corresponds to one of the listed causes. The size of each segment is determined by the patient's estimation of the percentage of cases in which each cause explains the symptom. A good outcome from this procedure is that the pie becomes filled, or almost filled, before inclusion of the patient's feared explanation (cause) for symptoms. This result is then discussed in terms of the nature of the patient's explanations for symptoms. More specifically, it is demonstrated that the interpretations made by the patient do not consider a range of causes for symptoms and that his/her thinking is restricted. The patient can practise drawing pie charts for other explanations of symptoms for homework and these can be used to assist the answering of thoughts on the thoughts record. (For a detailed example of constructing a pie chart, refer to Chapter 4.)

## Inverted pyramid

A technique closely related to the pie chart is the inverted step pyramid. The technique is intended to demonstrate a tendency to catastrophise, and to challenge overperceptions of likelihood/risk. This technique involves asking the patient to estimate the number of people that have a particular symptom at a given time, how many of those for whom the symptom persists, how many consult their doctor, how many are told they need tests and so on. A dialogue used in achieving the inverted pyramid for a 37-year-old woman with brain tumour concerns is presented below (the results are presented in Figure 6.3):

T: How confident are you that your headaches are a sign of a life-threatening brain tumour?

P: About 60 per cent.

T: OK. Let's look at that thought. What I'm going to ask you to do is to estimate how many people in Manchester wake up in the morning and they have a headache. How many would you say roughly?

P: What, in percentages you mean?

T: No, give me a total number, like 3,000 or something. Whatever you think.

P: Well I don't know how many people live in Manchester. But say 2,000 have a headache.

T: OK. How many of those people still have the headache by this evening?

P: Probably about 1,000.

T: How many still have the headache tomorrow morning when they wake up?

P: About 300.

T: How many people still have the headache after three days?

P: Probably about 50.

T: How many of those people go to the doctor and the doctor sends them for further tests?

P: 20 of them.

T: So 20 are sent for tests. How many are told that the problem is serious?

P: 3 of them.

T: How many are told that it's a brain tumour?

P: One person

T: How many are not successfully treated?

P: Well, I suppose a few people.

T: If we stay with proportions of this one person, you see we are into fractions. Do you see how when you get a headache you jump to the conclusion that you are that very small percentage? Perhaps you can use this technique next time you jump to the worst conclusion in order to challenge your thought. How sure are you now that your headaches are a life-threatening brain tumour?

## Thinking errors

In the context of discussing the pie chart and pyramid procedures we have touched on the subject of thinking errors. These methods offer means of

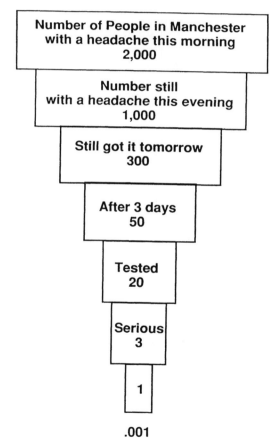

**Figure 6.3**   Results of an inverted-pyramid procedure

challenging dichotomous thinking, and catastrophising. Patients may be taught to identify and label the full range of errors as a technique for challenging thoughts. Common errors that occur in health anxiety are: catastrophising, dichotomous thinking, and selective abstraction. Selective abstraction is relevant to the processing of material discussed in the therapy session and in patient consultations with other health professionals such as general practitioners.

## Answering thoughts and imagery modification

The labelling of thinking errors can be used as an initial step in challenging the validity of negative symptom appraisals and in generating answers to thoughts. Standard questioning of evidence and generation of rational responses may be implemented. During episodes of severe health rumination some patients report difficulty in challenging misinterpretations. Flashcards, which can be an aid to questioning thoughts, may carry specific questions to be directed at challenging thoughts or rational responses which have been derived earlier in treatment.

In some instances misinterpretations occur in the form of images. For example, there may be images of blood vessels bursting, of a bruised and quivering heart, of parts of the body riddled with cancer and so on. In these instances standard verbal questioning may be less efficient and imagery manipulation procedures prove useful in providing evidence for an alternative model. For example, the therapist aims to demonstrate the role of imaging on anxiety and self-preoccupation. The procedure is most effective when the image is naturally accompanied by elevated anxiety. In rare cases it is possible to exacerbate and ameliorate particular symptoms by imagery manipulations.

Patients typically block or suppress their images before they reach the worst point. In some instances there are superstitious beliefs associated with the image—for example, the belief that images predict the future or tempt fate—in other cases the image and concepts represented in it are avoided because of a fear of being overwhelmed with worry following the image. If images are suppressed a two-stage approach to cognitive modification is available. The first stage consists of presenting a basic model of how suppression maintains the emotional salience of the image by blocking opportunities to critically evaluate the true significance of the image and its meanings. Second, the content of the image can be challenged by questioning the evidence and by presenting corrective information. This corrective information may then be incorporated in the image to modify the ending and its emotional salience and the patient encouraged to let images run to a new conclusion should they occur spontaneously.

## The 'dual model' strategy

The 'dual model' technique offers a means of assimilating alternative explanations for signs and symptoms while at the same time building supporting evidence for a psychological explanation of the presenting problem. In this technique, illustrated in Table 6.0, two columns are constructed; one is labelled 'Evidence that my problem is a (serious physical illness)' and the other labelled 'Evidence that my problem is: belief that I have (a serious physical illness)'. The material presented in Table 6.0 was generated collaboratively during one treatment session. It is easier to complete this task following several sessions by which time evidence from a variety of behavioural experiments and monitoring tasks is available for inclusion in the 'dual model'. Belief ratings in specific serious illnesses taken before and after the technique are indicative of effectiveness. The strategy can be used as a cumulative log of results of subsequent verbal and behavioural reattribution manoeuvres in treatment. In addition to listing evidence supporting the psychological model, the illness column should contain a list of *reframes* or reinterpretations of the evidence supporting the illness model.

## Dealing with rumination and worry

Some cases of health anxiety are characterised by prolonged periods of rumination concerning symptoms and health. For example, the health-

**Table 6.0**  Results of a 'dual model strategy' for a health-anxious patient

| EVIDENCE THAT MY PROBLEM IS: | |
| --- | --- |
| *A serious heart problem* | *Belief that I have a heart problem* |
| Recurrent chest discomfort | Focusing on my symptoms makes them worse |
| Heart misses beats | |
| Breathlessness | When I'm worried my heart rate changes |
| High blood pressure | Reassurance makes the symptoms go away |
| *Reframe* | |
| 1. There are lots of reasons for chest discomfort: muscle tension; body checking; controlling my breathing | I've pushed my heart by running and nothing happened |
| 2. Most heart beats change rhythm from moment to moment | It I stop checking my pulse and chest I feel better |
| 3. It's normal to become breathless due to physical exertion if you're unfit | My blood pressure is still within the normal range. It's higher when I'm anxious, but that's harmless |
| 4. My blood pressure is high when I'm anxious but it's chronically elevated blood pressure that's a problem. I don't have that | |

anxious individual may spend extended periods of time reviewing possible alternative causes of their symptoms, or thinking about the personal implications of illness and death. These worry activities may be motivated by particular beliefs. For example, patients may believe that if they are too casual and do not worry about their health this will lead to catastrophe. Or perhaps, by thinking negatively they avoid some form of punishment from God. Conversely, thinking positively may be thought of as tempting fate and therefore carries with it dangerous implications. Beliefs concerning advantages of worry include themes that it maintains vigilance such that problems can be readily detected before they become serious. In these instances cognitive therapy is focused on elucidating beliefs underlying the use of worry and rumination by patients (Wells, 1995; Wells & Hackmann, 1993). Some of these beliefs can be operationalised and tested using the experimental method. A patient who believes, for example, that thinking positive thoughts about health will lead to a catastrophe can be asked to think in such a way to determine if the catastrophe occurs. Clearly this type of manoeuvre is only useful when the precise nature of the catastrophe and the timescale of a potential disaster can be specified in advance. A timescale of one to two weeks is typically manageable but there are inherent difficulties with testing timescales of several months' duration.

The beliefs associated with rumination should be modified through verbal reattribution strategies consisting of questioning the evidence for beliefs, and in particular exploring the patients' proposed mechanisms which would account for the causal effects of worry on events. The following vignette illustrates the use of socratic questioning to explore and challenge mechanisms linking thoughts to events:

T: You said that if you allow yourself to think positive thoughts about your health then something bad might happen.

P: Yes, well it's bad to be too optimistic because that could be tempting fate.

T: And what would happen if you tempted fate?

P: Well, I could get ill.

T: So by thinking positive thoughts, that would cause you to get ill? How would thinking positively do that?

P: I don't know. I know it probably sounds stupid but maybe God would punish me for being too positive.

T: So God would cause it to happen? Does that sound like the type of God that religion and the bible talk about? A God that punishes people for being positive and happy?

P: Well that's what the nuns used to tell us at school. They used to say it was bad to be too happy.

T: Does this fit with the more widely accepted image of God?

P: Well it doesn't really fit with what people generally think.

T: That's right it doesn't really fit with the image of God that we tend to be given. One other thing concerns me about the belief. You seem to be implying that by thinking in a certain way you have the power to control what God does. Do you really think that you are that powerful?

P: (Laughs) Of course not. I don't really think that.

T: OK. So when you look at it carefully, how much do you believe that thinking in certain ways will protect you from God?

P: Well when you begin to question it I can see that it's just stupid. It doesn't make sense for God to be like that anyway.

T: So what about following this up with an experiment? Perhaps not worrying for a week and instead having a time period each day when you tell yourself that you are perfectly physically well and fit to see what happens to your mood and also to see if anything bad happens . . . (therapist proceeds to construct an experiment to test a *specific* patient prediction about thinking positively).

Another line of questioning in treatment focuses on determining the advantages and disadvantages of worrying. The aim here is to show how other non-ruminative styles of thinking can have the advantages of worry (e.g. motivates the person to seek help) while at the same time avoiding the disadvantages (e.g. does not interfere with one's ability to see things in a balanced way).

Other strategies for dealing with worry are reviewed in detail in the GAD chapter (Chapter 8), and these may be modified for use with rumination problems in health anxiety.

## Modifying assumptions and beliefs

Different types of belief in health anxiety are capable of contributing to misinterpretation tendencies. We have seen how some of these beliefs have superstitious themes of punishment by God through premature death or illness. There are also themes concerning costs of illness such that a family would not cope without the patient and that illness will involve loss of self-respect and the respect of others. Some meta-physical beliefs contain themes to do with existence after death, which is typically seen as involving a state of continued but negative consciousness such as being aware of the unhappiness and grief of the people left behind, or being aware of one's own grief and loneliness at being separated from loved ones (e.g. Wells & Hackmann, 1993).

Some beliefs concern themes of damage to the body or reflect assumptions concerning bodily characteristics. For example, a health-anxious patient may believe that both sides of his/her body should be symmetrical, that any sign of change in the body with ageing is a sign of something seriously wrong, or believe that stress and anxiety can damage the body. In some instances beliefs about body damage or weakening are associated with particular activities in which the patient has engaged in the past, such as unprotected sex, drug use, or minor surgery.

The remainder of this section focuses on modification of meta-physical belief as these can seem particularly challenging. Discussion strategies for modifying other types of belief are the same as strategies used for modifying negative interpretations. Many of the meta-physical beliefs are not amenable to challenge through behavioural experiments; however, they may be modified through a combination of *dissonance induction* and *education* within a socratic framework. Examples of each of these strategies follow.

*Modification of superstitious beliefs through dissonance*

Dissonance techniques aim to activate patients' pre-existing beliefs and use this material to generate contradictions of dysfunctional negative beliefs.

T: So you think that allowing yourself to believe that you are well will tempt fate and God will punish you. How much do you believe that?

P: 40 per cent.

T: Do you believe that you are a powerful person?

P: No not really.

T: But it seems that you believe that you are controlling God by your own thoughts. Would you say anyone who can do that is powerful, more powerful than God?

P: You're right, its a blasphemous thing to think. I don't really believe that.

T: Are you just saying that so that God doesn't punish you?

P: No, when I think about it I know it sounds ridiculous.

T: I know from our earlier discussions that you're quite religious. What sort of person do you think God is?

P: Kind and caring, and forgiving. I don't believe in the fire and brimstone God that some preach about.

T: There seems to be some contradiction in what you believe. On the one hand you think God will strike you down for thinking positive things about your health and on the other hand you think he is kind and caring. Does that make sense?

P: No, I suppose it doesn't when you look at it logically.

T: Now that you have looked at it in this way, how much do you now believe that God will punish you for thinking positively about your health?

P: I realise that it doesn't make any sense, I don't believe it.

This scenario was followed by a homework assignment in which the patient tempted fate every day for a period of a week to determine if bad things happened to her health. Not only did nothing bad happen, by substituting positive thinking for her normal negative rumination periods she also noticed an elevation in mood.

*Modification of fear of dying by socratic questioning and education*

Two examples of modifying different fears of dying are presented in this section. The therapist initially explores the idiosyncratic meaning of the event for the patient before attempting modification. This initial stage provides both a *mental* set for the patient to understand the nature of the fear, and also provides a range of *entry points* for reattribution. The therapist is then left to choose the best or identify the only entry point. Implicit in both of these cases of fear is the concept that the individual maintains some awareness of events after death. While this notion is implicit in many patients' fears, the health-anxious patient is often unaware that their fear is founded on such an assumption. Merely drawing attention to this fact can produce dissonance in patients who don't believe in a continued existence after death, and is therefore helpful in challenging the fear structure.

*Example 1*

T: What are you afraid will happen when you die?

P: I don't know, I try not to think about it.

T: Is there anything horrible about it? What's the worst that could happen when you die?

P: It's what happens afterwards, to your body.

T: What does happen?

P: When you're buried the worms and insects get into your coffin and eat your body. It's horrible.

T: If that were true what would be so bad about it?

P: I don't know, it would just be horrible.

T: Its not a nice thing to think now, but would it be so horrible when you're dead?

P: Yes, I think it would.

T: It sounds as if you think you might be aware of it happening even when you're dead. Is that right?

P: I'm afraid that I might be able to feel the insects or know what's going on.

T: An important aspect of this fear is your belief that you continue to exist in some form when you have died. What would be the point of continuing to be aware of your dead body when you no longer have use for it?

P: There is no point, but it might happen.

T: It seems unlikely to me that it would happen. In any event what makes you think that insects will eat your body?

P: Well I thought that's what happened.

T: A body decomposes quite quickly. It would have done so a long time before the coffin rotted and let any insects in. Also you should consider that worms are vegetarians and wouldn't want to eat you anyway.

P: What makes a body decompose?

T: The bacteria inside the body and in the air trapped with it are responsible. How much does death bother you now?

*Example 2*

T: The thought of dying seems to bother you. What is it that you are most concerned about?

P: It's a terrible thing. What a waste, it doesn't make any sense.

T: Is that what bothers you, the fact that it doesn't make much sense?

P: No, that's not the worst. It's leaving people and the things that I enjoy behind that upsets me.

T: What is it about leaving those things that upsets you?

P: I don't really know. It's not being able to enjoy them any more and missing people that I care about.

T: Do you believe that some part of you survives your death?

P: No not really, only in the memories of the people you've left behind. I don't believe in Heaven or anything like that.

T: So where are you when you are aware of the things that you've left behind after death?

P: I don't know, I don't suppose I'm anywhere.

T: But you seem to be saying that you have awareness of the things you've left behind, so you must be somewhere. Your memories and consciousness must be continuing after your death otherwise you wouldn't be aware of anything.

P: Well maybe I do believe that something continues then.

T: It seems so. You have the belief that following death you will be aware of unpleasant things. What about the pleasant things that you could be aware of?

P: I can't think of any, it would be lonely and I'd have a sense of loss.

T: Would you be the only person in the place that you go to?

P: No, probably not.

T: Perhaps you would meet friends and family who have gone before you. And what would happen when your children die?

P: Yes, I could be with them again. I see what you mean. I wonder where these ideas I have about death come from.

T: So it seems as if you've not really thought it through before. Perhaps you can think more about the potential positive experiences of continued consciousness after death between now and the next session. Of course, if there is no consciousness, is there anything to be concerned about?

P: Whichever way it goes it seems unlikely that I would be lonely.

## IMAGERY TECHNIQUES

Mental images play a role in health anxiety as a form of misinterpretation. Modification of images is therefore important, and this can be executed on a variety of levels. First, the events portrayed in images can be modified at the negative automatic thought level; second, the meaning of having images can be altered; and, third, images can be used to gain access to beliefs and manipulated to change belief. The type of modification adopted is determined by the nature of the image and its hypothesised role in the maintenance of health anxiety. For example, if an image is interpreted as a sign that there is something seriously wrong then this interpretation should be challenged. In contrast, if the image is suppressed before its worst point the content should be allowed to run the full course so that the meaning of the event or the events portrayed can be modified. New endings can be practised for catastrophic images. For example, in Chapter 4 we saw how a health-anxious patient reported a recurrent image of being dead and trapped in his dead body. When the image occurred he normally distracted himself from it, thus perpetuating the concept of being trapped after his death. In therapy he was encouraged to allow time to elapse in the image such that his body decayed at which point he became spontaneously freed from his imprisonment. Subsequently he was less troubled by the image and concepts of dying. Apart from 'finishing-out' images over time, alternative endings may have to be scripted. For example, a patient who repeatedly saw herself in a coffin at her funeral surrounded by weeping relatives introduced a humorous ending in which she imaged sitting up in the coffin, and climbing out of it while announcing that it had all been a joke.

In some instances images are a powerful means of evoking feared bodily sensations. The therapeutic strategy of eliciting normally spontaneous affect-laden images is a means of illustrating the effect of thinking on bodily responses. This information can be used to support a psychological explanation of symptoms and the sensations can be used to trace early events that may have contributed to the development of misinterpretation tendencies. In this latter context, the patient should be asked to recall the earliest memory of experiencing the type of affect and bodily responses present while imaging. An exploration of the events in the person's life and the meanings attached to those events can provide valuable information for understanding the origins of particular feelings and idiosyncratic meanings in the present.

## DEALING WITH HEALTH-RISK BEHAVIOUR

It is somewhat of a paradox, that while some health-anxious patients are concerned about their physical health, they continue with potentially damaging behaviours such as smoking or excess alcohol use. Moreover, engaging in these behaviours may be taken as evidence that illness and premature death are more likely. In these cases one of the goals of therapy may be reduction or elimination of the risky behaviour. For example, patients can be helped to quit smoking, motivational techniques may be useful for this purpose and aids to quitting such as nicotine patches and stimulus control applications are helpful. Changes of lifestyle such as reducing alcohol intake, stopping smoking, and the introduction of an exercise routine, offer a valuable means of *redefining* the self as a fitter and healthier individual, and can help to displace schemas of physical vulnerability.

## CONCLUSIONS

The cognitive approach to health anxiety overlaps with the approach to panic disorder. However, there a several points of divergence in the theory and treatment of these disorders which have been highlighted in this chapter. The aim of treatment for these disorders is a common one: the elimination of belief in catastrophic misinterpretations of symptoms. This is achieved by adherence to an idiosyncratic conceptualisation based on models of the disorders, and by the modification of cognitive and behavioural responses responsible for the maintenance of dysfunctional belief. In the case of health anxiety we have seen that illness and death are particularly salient and the patient associates them with certain types of cost. An aim of treatment therefore is the decatastrophisation of the meaning of these events for the individual. In some instances this requires the exploration of deeper meanings such as those pertaining to self-worth and personal identity. For example, some health-anxious patients see themselves as more vulnerable to ill health or premature death. Vulnerability may be linked with beliefs about bodily weakness, or illness and death can be understood in terms of beliefs about characterological defects and punishment.

## EXAMPLE TREATMENT OUTLINE

*Session 1*

1. Review recent health anxiety episodes and construct conceptualisation.
2. Discuss role of behaviour in problem maintenance.

3. Socialisation experiments (e.g. selective attention; decreased bodily checking).
4. Homework : monitor symptoms on activity schedule.

### Session 2

1. Go over model and share with patient.
2. Review homework—look for symptom patterns (identify triggers).
3. Explore evidence for main disease conviction and look at alternative explanation.
4. Introduce behavioural experiment to socialise/begin challenging misinterpretations; e.g.
   - Drop specific safety behaviours.
   - Push symptoms.
5. Homework:
   (a) Monitor triggers and thoughts on thought record.
   (b) Use controlled worry periods (Chapter 8) to limit rumination.
   (c) Ban bodily checking.

### Session 3

1. Check homework—discuss results in terms of model.
2. Explore role of reassurance and ban it.
3. Verbal reattribution and continue behavioural experiments.
4. Homework:
   (a) Introduce rational responding on thoughts record.
   (b) Continue checking ban.
   (c) Ban reassurance seeking.

### Sessions 4–8

1. Continue building alternative model.
2. Reframe evidence for misinterpretations (dual model strategy).
3. Continue verbal reattribution, e.g. pie-charts, inverted pyramid, label thinking errors.
4. Behavioural experiments—reverse avoidance, drop safety, push symptoms.
5. Homework.

### Sessions 9–14

1. Continue challenging misinterpretations.
2. Explore assumptions and beliefs.

3. Modify dysfunctional belief.
4. Homework.

*Sessions 15–16*

1. Check for residual beliefs and behaviours and modify if present.
2. Relapse prevention: develop therapy blueprint.
3. Schedule booster sessions.
4. Anticipate problems and rehearse coping strategies.

*Note.* Use sessional responses on the Health Anxiety Rating Scale (HARS) to guide the focus of treatment sessions.

# Chapter 7

# SOCIAL PHOBIA

Social phobia is a common problem. A central characteristic of social phobia is the fear of negative evaluation, which the social phobic anticipates will result from some form of failed performance. Performance is used here in its broadest sense, and includes the execution of emotional control skills, the performance of everyday tasks in which one is subject to the scrutiny of others such as eating in public, signing one's name or speaking to a stranger or a group. The social phobic believes that he/she will behave in an unacceptable way and this will lead to rejection and loss of self worth. The concept of fear of negative evaluation has been central in cognitive formulations of the disorder. However, the concept of negative self-evaluation is also central in the aetiology and maintenance of social anxiety (Clark & Wells, 1995; Wells & Clark, 1997). Although self-preoccupation is relevant to understanding the development of emotional disorders in general (Wells & Matthews, 1994), it has been a focus of a number of attempts to model the key cognitive components of social anxiety.

Hartman (1983, 1986) proposed a cognitive model of social anxiety in which socially anxious individuals are seen as preoccupied with their thoughts about physiological arousal, ongoing performance, and other people's perceptions of them. This type of appraisal is seen as leading to an escalation of anxiety and reduces the extent to which a socially anxious individual can experience others. As such, social performance may be compromised. Hartman (1983) emphasises the role of self-evaluation generally, in the problem of social phobia. Clark and Wells (1995) have advanced a cognitive model of social phobia that integrates features of other models and is based on the model of emotional disorder presented by Wells and Matthews (1994). This chapter is based on the Clark and Wells (1995) model, and the treatment derived from it (Wells & Clark, 1995).

## THE NATURE OF SOCIAL PHOBIA

Social phobia is defined in DSM-IV as a 'marked and persistent fear of social or performance situations in which embarrassment may occur' (p. 411). For the diagnosis to be made the social or performance situation must almost always provoke immediate anxiety on exposure to the situation and the fear must interfere significantly with the person's daily routine, occupational functioning or social life, or the person must be markedly distressed about having the disturbance. The social situation is normally avoided or it is sometimes endured with a sense of dread. Panic attacks may occur on exposure to, or on anticipation of, exposure to the phobic situation. In the feared situation people with social phobia are concerned about embarrassment and fear that others will judge them to be anxious, weak, crazy or stupid. There may be fear of eating in public because of concerns that others will see their trembling hands, or there may be great anxiety on conversing with others because of fear of appearing inarticulate or of showing anxiety such as blushing. In DSM-III-R and DSM-IV a generalised subtype of social phobia can be specified when the fears are related to most social situations, these individuals are more likely to show deficits in social skills and have more severe life impairment. A diagnosis of social phobia should not be given when the symptoms that are the focus of concern are the result of a medical condition, or when they are associated with another emotional disorder, for example concern about eating in front of others in anorexia nervosa.

## A COGNITIVE MODEL OF SOCIAL PHOBIA

The role of negative self-appraisal processes in social phobia is developed in the cognitive model advanced by Clark and Wells (1995) and Wells and Clark (1997). This model accounts for the persistence of social phobia with reference to a number of cognitive-behavioural mechanisms. Central to the model is the view that social phobics seldom encounter situations that are capable of providing unambiguous disconfirmation of their fears. Even when social phobics regularly encounter their feared situations, their processing priorities, coping behaviours, and the nature of normal interpersonal transactions conspire to impede reduction in negative beliefs. Several vicious circles are therefore responsible for maintaining the problem. The model is presented in Figure 7.0.

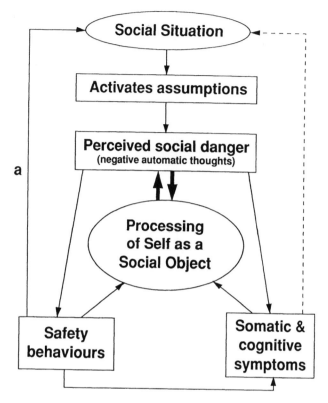

**Figure 7.0**   A cognitive model of social phobia

The central feature of social phobia is a strong desire to convey a favourable impression of oneself to others, and this is accompanied by marked insecurity about one's ability to do so. On entering social situations social phobics appraise the situation as dangerous. They believe that they are in danger of acting in an inept and unacceptable fashion and that such behaviour will have catastrophic consequences in terms of loss of status, rejection and humiliation by others. The fear of loss of status not only concerns the view held by others, but also concerns the socially anxious person's perception of the self. These danger appraisals activate an 'anxiety programme' which consists of physiological, cognitive, affective and behavioural changes which, in the evolutionary past, were probably effective in reducing objective danger in primitive environments. However, in modern environments these anxiety symptoms are further sources of perceived danger since they are appraised as threatening the persons self-presentation skills and self-concept. This leads to an escalation of anxiety and a maintenance of the problem. Social phobics become preoccupied with their somatic responses, their negative thoughts concerning evaluation by others, and thoughts of negative self-evaluation. This preoccupation or heightened processing of the social self depletes attention to external aspects of the social situation in a way that makes social performance more difficult, and reduces awareness of objective interpersonal information. For example, social phobics may believe that they are the centre of attention or that people are bored with them in social situations but they are prone to pay little attention to other people in order to check this out. Social phobics focus on a *self-generated* perception of their performance in social situations and then mistakenly assume that this accurately reflects the way others perceive them. In order to prevent social catastrophe safety behaviours are used (e.g. Wells et al., 1995b) unfortunately these act in perpetuating belief in negative interpretations and anxiety. First, some of the safety behaviours used by social phobics when anxious exacerbate symptoms (e.g. holding a cup too tightly to reduce tremor can impede normal movements), or interfere with performance (e.g. mentally rehearsing what to say before saying it impairs concentration on conversation). Second, some of the coping or safety behaviours adopted can result in the social phobic appearing less warm and friendly to others, and thus safety behaviours have the effect of contaminating the social situation (line marked 'a' in Figure 7.0). Third, the non-occurrence of catastrophes in social situations can be mistakenly attributed to use of the safety behaviours rather than to the fact that appraisals are distorted.

A novel aspect of this approach is the model's emphasis on the role of social self-processing which guides behaviour. This is essentially an impression of how the social phobic thinks he/she appears to others. The content of this impression contributes to the degree of danger appraised in social encounters. Implicit in the model is the notion that individuals are normally motivated to maintain a positive and stable public self-image. However, because of the mechanisms outlined, the social phobic's concept is unstable and prone to fluctuation. Two other mechanisms contribute to this instability and heightened self-focus in social phobia: anticipatory processing, and post-event processing.

## Anticipatory and post-event processing

In anticipation of problematic social encounters the social phobic tends to ruminate about the situation. This rumination may involve planning and rehearsing conversation and behaviour, and the content of the rumination is typically negative. It is at the anticipatory phase that the negative public self-concept is activated and the stability of the social self-concept is initially threatened. On leaving the social situation, exposure to the negative aspects of the encounter does not end. Social phobics are prone to mull-over aspects of the situation and their own behaviour. The problem with this *post-mortem* is that it does not provide any additional information that can be used to challenge negative beliefs. More specifically, because the social phobic was self-focused in the social situation, the most memorable aspect of the encounter is an image of the self or a felt-sense which is typically negative. The post-mortem contributes to an overemphasis on negative aspects of the encounter; a type of selective abstraction that prolongs negative affect. These thinking processes contribute to the maintenance of negative appraisals and beliefs.

## Processing of the social self

When the social phobic enters an anxiety-provoking social situation there is a shift of attention towards processing the self. This self-relevant processing is often from an *observer perspective* (Wells, Clark & Ahmad, 1995a). That is, social phobics see themselves as if from another person's perspective. This often occurs as an image of the way the social phobic believes they look to others or as a felt sense. The impression of the observable self is derived from interoceptive information—that is, from bodily sensations, feelings and observation of one's own performance. This internal information often presents an inaccurate picture of the way social phobics actually appear to others. For example, if a social phobic feels shaky there may be an image of looking like 'a jibbering wreck', or if the phobic feels hot and is sweating, there may be an image of rivers of sweat running from the face.

## Assumptions and beliefs

*When symptoms happen: the meaning of failed performance*

Unlike panic disorder in which the catastrophe does not occur, social phobia is a disorder in which negative feared events can happen. For example, people do stare, one can be rejected, humiliated, and found to be uninteresting.

However, the principal problem is not that these events do happen, since they happen to non-social phobics as well, but it is the meaning of these events for the individual, and the heightened perception of the likelihood of negative outcomes that presents the problem. We have seen how social phobia in the present model is associated with distorted self-perception which is a central target for treatment. However, social phobia is also characterised by distorted 'other-perception'. For example, the social phobic believes that *everyone* will notice them and judge them negatively, which will lead to rejection. It is necessary to trace the meaning and implication of specific fears so that the nature of danger inherent in social phobic appraisals can be identified. Such an analysis elicits a string of meanings or predictions that are amenable to modification in cognitive therapy. Initial negative automatic thoughts (e.g. 'I'll tremble or shake'; 'I'll get my words wrong') do not provide explicit meanings, and are difficult to challenge since they represent a self-commentary on one's own symptoms that are likely to be factual. Cognitive therapy should focus on modifying the distorted self-image concerning how these responses look, and on challenging beliefs concerning the consequences of showing symptoms or of 'failed performance'.

In the Clark and Wells (1995) model dysfunctional beliefs and assumptions render the individual vulnerable to the range of cognitive and behavioural factors that maintain social phobia. Three types of information are conceptualised at the schema level: (1) core self-beliefs (e.g. 'I'm boring'; 'I'm weird'); (2) conditional assumptions (e.g. 'If I show I'm anxious people will think I'm incompetent'; 'If I get my words wrong people will think I'm foolish'); (3) rigid rules for social performance (e.g. 'I must always sound fluent and intelligent'; 'I must not show signs of anxiety'). The pattern of onset of social phobia may be linked to the particular types of schema that exist (Wells & Clark, 1997). For example, individuals who have rigid rules for social performance may function with minimal anxiety throughout life until they encounter an event that leads to an important failure in meeting these standards. Following a critical incident of this type, social situations are perceived as more dangerous and carry with them, the potential of further 'failures'. In contrast, pre-existing early dysfunctional conditional assumptions, which may be learned through interactions with family and the peer group, and unconditional negative beliefs, may underlie more long-standing problems of social anxiety.

## Summary of the model

In summary, the cognitive model of social phobia proposes the following sequence of events when a social phobic enters a feared social situation: The situation activates assumptions concerning potential performance failure and the implications of showing anxiety symptoms. This leads to a perception of social danger which is evident as anticipatory worry or negative automatic thoughts. Examples of negative automatic thoughts are presented in Table 7.0.

**Table 7.0**  Examples of negative automatic thoughts, self-processing, and safety behaviours across five social phobics

| Negative automatic thoughts | Self-processing | Safety behaviours |
|---|---|---|
| 1. I don't know what to say. People will think I'm stupid | Self-conscious: Image of self as a plain, unintelligent 'bimbo' | Avoid eye contact, don't draw attention to self, say little, let partner do the talking, plan what to say, pretend to be interested in something |
| 2. I'll shake and lose control. Everyone will notice me | Self-conscious: 'The shaking feels so bad so it must look bad.' Image of self-losing control | Avoid cups and saucers, grip objects tightly, move slowly, tense arm muscles, take deep breaths, try to relate, avoid looking at people, hold cups with both hands, rest elbows on table |
| 3. What if I get anxious? People will notice and not take me seriously | Self-conscious: Image of self as a bright red jibbering wreck with hands and arms 'jingling' about | Grip hands together, stiffen arms and legs, look away, ask questions, cover face with hair, wear extra make-up |
| 4. What if I sweat? They will think I'm abnormal | Self-conscious: Image of beads of sweat on forehead and top lip and hair looking soaked | Wear T-shirt under shirt, keep jacket on, use extra deodorant, wear light colours, hold handkerchief, keep arms next to body, wear cool clothes |
| 5. I'll babble and get my words wrong. People will think I'm stupid | Self-conscious: Is aware of own voice and hears self as timid, weak and pathetic | Monitor speech, try to pronounce words properly, rehearse sentences mentally before saying them, speak quickly, ask questions, say little about self |

Negative automatic thoughts are associated with anxiety activation which is manifested in the form of somatic and cognitive symptoms. These symptoms are themselves subject to negative appraisal and may be interpreted as evidence of failure and social humiliation. Appraisals of danger are accompanied by a shift in attention in which the social phobic engages in detailed self-observation and monitoring of sensations, images and a 'felt-sense' (examples of self-processing are given in Table 7.0). This interoceptive information is used to make inferences about how the social phobic appears to others and how others are evaluating them.

In an attempt to conceal or avert social catastrophe safety behaviours are used (see Table 7.0) but these serve to maintain the problem. Safety behaviours contribute to:

- Heightened self-focus
- Prevention of disconfirmation
- Feared symptoms (e.g. sweating, mental blanks, trembling)
- Drawing attention to the self
- Contamination of the social situation (e.g. make the phobic appear aloof and unfriendly).

In some instances the feared social situation is avoided altogether. This is a problem because it removes opportunities for disconfirming negative appraisals and beliefs. Anticipatory processing in the form of worry and post-event worry (the post-mortem) contribute to problem maintenance by priming negative self-processing prior to social encounters, and by maintaining preoccupation with feelings and the distorted self-image after social encounters.

## FROM COGNITIVE MODEL TO CASE CONCEPTUALISATION

Figure 7.0 should be used as a template for building an individualised case conceptualisation. Initially the items in the lower part of the model incorporating feedback loops are conceptualised and the inclusion of assumptions is postponed until later in treatment. Essentially, the initial formulation represents the factors thought to be responsible for maintaining 'in-situation' dysfunctional self-processing and situational danger appraisals. The conceptualisation depends on eliciting the nature of safety behaviours and avoidance, the cognitive-somatic symptoms of anxiety, and the nature of self-processing. The situational shift to self-processing is marked by intensified self-consciousness. A modification of the model depicted in Figure 7.0 for case conceptualisation purposes, consists of including the term anxiety with cognitive/somatic responses, and includes the term self-consciousness with self-processing. Socially phobic individuals are better able to relate to these terms and therefore the model becomes more amenable to them. An idiosyncratic case conceptualisation of a 40-year-old female social phobic with a fear of writing and drinking in public is displayed in Figure 7.1.

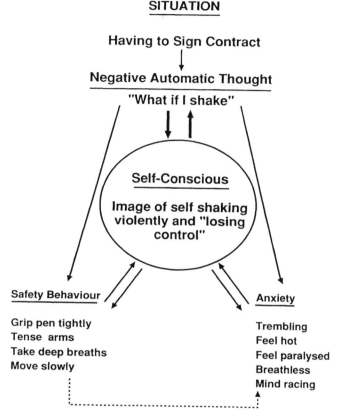

**Figure 7.1**   An idiosyncratic social phobia case conceptualisation

## Eliciting information for conceptualisation

There are two basic approaches to eliciting data for conceptualisation: reviewing several recent episodes of social anxiety; or using direct questioning during or following exposure to a real or analogue situation. In some cases, specifically where there is marked avoidance of social situations, it is not possible to review a recent social anxiety episode in the detail required for conceptualisation. If this is the case, an analogue social phobic situation should be constructed in the therapy session. Depending on the nature of the patient's fear this will typically involve introducing objects and/or other people into the consultation. For example, this involves drinking water from cups and saucers, talking in front of a small group, making conversation with a stranger, or talking to someone in authority. It may be necessary to expose to a real-life feared situation if the situation is so specific that it cannot be effectively duplicated in the treatment setting.

## Collecting data for formulation

With the basic model in mind, treatment proceeds by eliciting the data necessary for constructing a cross-sectional situational model linking negative automatic thoughts, safety behaviours, anxiety symptoms, and the contents of self-focused attention (self-consciousness). Thus, four types of information are required initially: (1) main negative automatic thoughts; (2) safety behaviours; (3) anxiety symptoms; and (4) contents of self-consciousness.

### Negative automatic thoughts

Negative automatic thoughts occurring in anticipation of exposure to feared situations, and automatic thoughts occurring in-situation should be elicited. Typically, thoughts occurring at both intervals reflect similar themes. While automatic thoughts may be readily accessible in the patient's account of social anxiety episodes in response to questions such as 'What negative thoughts went through your mind when you entered the situation?', it is helpful to focus questions on the time of occurrence of anxiety or problematic symptoms: 'When you noticed yourself feeling hot, what thoughts went through your mind?' This serves to focus the interview on relevant automatic thoughts, and assists the patient in disclosing thoughts about symptoms which he/she might otherwise be embarrassed to mention. The following dialogue illustrates a review of a recent situation and elicitation of negative automatic thoughts:

T: When was the last time you felt uncomfortable and anxious in a social situation?
P: On Tuesday. I was out with my partner and a group of his friends.
T: I'm going to ask you some questions about your feelings and thoughts in that situation. Is it clear in your memory?
P: Yes, I think so.
T: Just before you went out were you feeling anxious?
P: Yes. I didn't really want to go, but I didn't want to let my partner down.
T: What were your anxious thoughts?
P: I was worried that I might not be able to join in and I'd be quiet all night.
T: So the thoughts were something like, 'What if I can't think of anything to say?' Is that right?

P: Yes. They'd think I was boring and wonder what my partner saw in me.
T: When you entered the situation how did you feel?
P: I felt anxious, I tried to look interested but I didn't say much.
T: When you felt anxious in the situation what thoughts went through your mind?
P: I thought, I've got nothing to say. Even if I do think of something it will sound stupid.

In the example presented above negative automatic thoughts for a recent anxiety episode centred on themes of not knowing what to say in situation, and sounding stupid, as a consequence being viewed as boring. In this example the meaning or implication of the automatic thought 'What if I can't think of anything to say' becomes clear in the course of therapist questioning. The meaning of automatic thoughts is not always apparent. In particular, when thoughts represent commentaries on symptoms—for example, 'What if I sweat'; 'I'm shaking'; 'What if I blush'; 'My voice is quivering'—it is necessary to explore the meaning of these symptom experiences. The cognitive model suggests that two types of meaning are relevant to problem maintenance. The first refers to the meaning and significance that other people might attach to symptoms, and the second relates to the individual's own appraisal of the significance of symptoms such as overestimations of conspicuousness and self-concept implications. Thus, in eliciting negative automatic thoughts the meaning of such thoughts should be clearly identified. It is the *meaning* or *implication* of negative automatic thoughts or symptom experiences that are the focus of reattribution, not the statement of the symptom experience itself.

### Anxiety symptoms

Symptoms of anxiety in social phobia are maintained by negative appraisals, and symptoms are often a focus of negative appraisals. Anxiety symptoms can be divided into physiological responses and cognitive responses. In social phobia the symptoms that tend to be most problematic are those which may be observable to others, such as blushing, shaking, sweating, muscle spasm, babbling, quivering voice, crying, and mind going blank.
In constructing the idiosyncratic conceptualisation the therapist should determine the nature of anxiety symptoms and determine the extent to which appraisal of symptoms contributes to negative automatic thought and dysfunctional self-processing. To this end questions like the following should be used:

• Which symptoms bother you most?
• When you felt anxious in the situation what symptoms did you notice?

- How conspicuous do you think the symptoms are?
- If people did notice your symptoms what would that mean?

*Eliciting contents of self-processing*

At the heart of the cross-sectional conceptualisation is the social phobic's processing of the self as a social object. The content of self-processing can be determined through at least three channels: (1) exploring the contents of heightened self-consciousness; (2) questioning the social phobic's appraised level of conspicuousness of symptoms; (3) determining if safety behaviours are linked to a particular self-perception.

The initial marker for self-processing in patient accounts of situations is a report of increased self-consciousness. The therapist should specifically ask about the point in time at which the patient became highly self-conscious. The main questions then are:

- When you were self-conscious, what were you most conscious of?
- What aspect of yourself were you most aware of?
- Did you have an impression of how you looked in the situation?

Often symptoms of anxiety are the focus of self-consciousness. Therefore questioning the subjective impression of the self for periods when symptoms are intense should be undertaken:

- When you felt anxious, what symptoms were you most aware of?
- Did you have an impression of how apparent your symptoms were to others?
- How do you think you appeared?
- If I could have seen you at that time—what would I see?

The content of self-processing is also accessible through a safety-behaviours channel. In particular, when safety behaviours are attempts to conceal symptoms or appraised personal shortcomings they are typically associated with a negative public impression of the self. For example, the social phobic who hides his/her face is likely to have an exaggerated impression of the anxious features that need to be hidden. Two questions are useful in the safety-behaviours channel: the first explores self-processing associated with implementing safety behaviours, and the second explores self-processing in the hypothetical absence of safety behaviours:

- When you try to conceal your symptoms, what's your impression of how you look to others?

- If you didn't engage in your safety behaviours when you felt anxious, how would you look to others?

### Ask about imagery

The precise nature of a public self-impression should be determined. The impression often occurs as an image from the 'observer' perspective. If this is the case, the social phobic should be encouraged to regenerate a recent negative observer image and describe the image of the self in detail. In questioning the nature of the self-impression it is important to specifically ask:

- Did you have an image of the way you thought you looked when you were in the situation? Describe the image.
- Can you construct an image of how you think you looked at the time? Describe what you see.

### Identifying safety behaviours

Safety behaviours in social phobia can be overt or covert. Examples of safety behaviours are presented in Table 7.0. Overt safety behaviours are often observable and can be seen during exposure tests.

If safety behaviours have been used for a long time period they may be less accessible to immediate conscious disclosure by the patient. In such circumstances exposure to the feared situation in conjunction with therapist-directed questioning probing the use of such responses is recommended. Particular attention should be given to eliciting covert safety behaviours such as 'blanking out' or mental rehearsal of sentences before speaking as part of the assessment and conceptualisation process. The following questions should be used to determine safety behaviours:

- When you thought (feared event) was happening, did you do anything to prevent it? What did you do?
- If you hadn't done (safety behaviour), how much do you believe that (feared event) would have happened?
- Do you do anything else to control your symptoms/improve your performance/hide your problem?
- Do you do anything to avoid drawing attention to yourself?
- What is the effect of using your safety behaviour?
  - What effect does it have on your self-consciousness?
  - What effect does it have on your performance?
  - What effect does it have on how friendly/conspicuous you appear?
  - What effect does it have on your symptoms?

## Example of a behaviour test to elicit data

Exposure to analogue phobic situations offers a means of obtaining data for conceptualisation. The conceptualisation presented in Figure 7.2 was constructed from the following dialogue which was held after brief (5 minute) exposure to public speaking (to a group of four people) in the therapist's office. The dialogue illustrates the use of questions presented in the previous sections to determine automatic thoughts, symptoms, safety behaviours, and the nature of self-processing in the behaviour test.

T: What I'd like to do now is bring four people into the room and ask you to talk about yourself for 5 minutes to the group, to see what happens when you get anxious. How do you feel about that?

P: Oh no. I'm not sure I can do that.

T: Let's try it to see what happens.

P: What should I talk about?

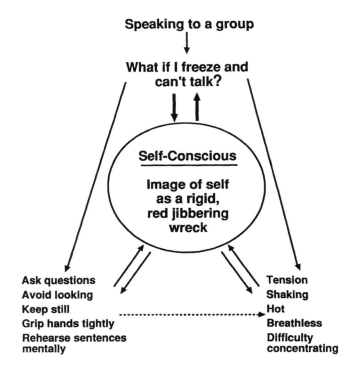

**Figure 7.2**   Individual case conceptualisation derived from a behaviour test

T: Anything at all. Tell us about your job or hobbies.

P: I feel nervous already.

T: (Brings four colleagues into room)
Okay. Can you stand up and talk to us for 5 minutes? It doesn't matter what you talk about. Off you go.

P: (Gives a brief talk)

T: Well done. I'll ask my colleagues to leave and then we'll discuss what happened. How did that feel?

P: Not too bad. I felt really anxious to start with.

T: What thoughts went through your mind to start with?

P: I thought I wasn't going to be able to do it.

T: What do you mean by that?

P: I thought I would freeze up and not be able to talk.

T: When you had that thought, what anxiety sensations did you notice?

P: I felt very tense, I was aware of feeling hot, and my legs felt shaky.

T: When you started talking what sensations did you notice?

P: My voice was a bit wobbly, I could feel my knees shaking and I felt hot and breathless, and had difficulty concentrating.

T: Did you do anything to control your anxiety or prevent yourself from freezing?

P: I asked questions, tried not to look at people, kept as still as I could, and tried to go over what I was going to say in my mind.

T: I noticed when you were talking that you were holding your hands tightly together. What was the reason for that?

P: I don't know what to do with my hands. I was trying to stop them shaking and stop my arms flying about all over the place.

T: When you were doing that, how self-conscious did you feel?

P: Very self-conscious.

T: What were you self-conscious of?

P: Trying to stay calm and look relaxed.

T: How do you think you looked during your speech?

P: Tense, probably.

T: What does that look like?

P: Well, you could probably see my knees trembling, see me shaking, and I looked flushed and rigid.

T: Do you have an image of that in your mind?

P: Yes, I can see it. But it wasn't as bad as it could be.

T: Do you ever get a worse image of yourself?

P: Sometimes, if I'm very anxious.

T: What does that look like?

P: I look like a red, jibbering wreck with my arms flying about all over the place.

In this example the initial perception of social danger is manifest as the negative automatic thought 'What if I freeze and can't talk'; this thought was associated with initial anxiety marked by the physical symptoms of tension, shaking, feeling hot, etc. The response to the thought was an attempt to reduce the chance of catastrophe by asking more questions, avoiding looking at people, keeping still, clasping hands tightly together, etc. Heightened self-consciousness consisted of a particular negative public self-image that did not resemble the patient's actual appearance.

### Fine grained analysis of the phobic situation

One of the difficulties in designing effective exposure experiments in social phobia is the wide inter-individual variability in the nature of situations that provoke anxiety. Subtle features of the situation determine whether or not anxiety is evoked. A fine-grained analysis of the situation is required in order to determine the modulating influences on fear, this is possible through use of questions like the following:

- When does anxiety occur?
- Are there similar situations when it doesn't occur?
- What marks out these situations as different?
- Are there times when a typical phobic situation is not a problem?

Only through detailed analysis is it possible to construct analogue situations or to specify real-life situations that evoke anxiety and provide a basis for constructing experiments that effectively challenge negative appraisals.

## SOCIALISATION

Conceptualisation and socialisation proceed by tracing recent episodes of social anxiety within the context of the model. Guided discovery is used to elucidate elements of the model and guide the patient to an understanding of the significance of these elements and in their interaction in maintaining the problem. The conceptualisation is shared with the patient and the role of *safety behaviours* and *self-focused attention* on symptoms and performance is discussed initially and illustrated by in-session experiments. Useful questions in socialisation explore where the patient's evidence for negative appraisals come from. The aim is to demonstrate that most of the evidence is generated from internal (interoceptive) information. Key socialisation questions are presented below:

- What is the evidence that (e.g. everyone is looking at you)?
  — How do you know people think that about you? Where does your evidence come from?
  — What thoughts went through your mind at the time?
- Did you do anything to change what happened (e.g. what people might be thinking about you)?
  — Did you do anything to control your anxiety/symptoms?
  — What would happen if you didn't do that—could anything bad happen? How do you know that will happen?
- What happens to your performance when you engage in safety behaviours?
  — What happens to your consciousness of yourself when you engage in these behaviours?
  — Do you think you are able to find out what really happens so long as you avoid situations or do things to save yourself?
- If you could be less self-conscious in social situations, do you think that would help? How would it help?

## Selling self-processing

Guided discovery is preferred over didactic presentation of the model since patients often believe they have good evidence to support their fear of negative evaluation and are initially reluctant to accept that the problem is primarily one of negative self-evaluation. The following extract of guided exploration illustrates the use of verbal techniques to sell the self-processing aspect of the model.

P: I feel uncomfortable in the situation. Like everyone is paying attention to me.

T: So your impression is that everyone is looking at you?

P: Yes, it's awful. I feel so self-conscious. I just don't want to be there when I feel like that.

T: What makes you think that everyone is looking?

P: Well I know they are. It's not normal to shake like this is it?

T: How do you know that they're looking at you. What's your evidence?

P: Well they must be looking, it must be obvious there's something wrong.

T: Have you ever looked around to see if people are looking at you?

P: No. I tend to avoid looking at them. If I saw someone looking that would make it worse.

T: So, if you're not looking at other people how do you know they're paying attention to you?

P: Well it just feels as if I am conspicuous, and people are looking.

T: Okay, that's an important discovery. What you're saying is that because you feel conspicuous and self-conscious you assume that other people are looking at you. It seems that you are assuming things based on your feelings rather than on facts.

This dialogue was followed by a discussion of the role of self-focused attention in increasing awareness of feelings and the mistaken attribution that such feelings must be attracting attention. It transpired that the patient had an image of herself 'shaking uncontrollably' which she mistakenly assumed reflected the way she must have looked to others. In subsequent objective tests of her appearance while actually shaking it transpired that the symptoms were not as apparent as she had imagined.

## Behavioural experiments in socialisation

Behavioural experiments should be used to illustrate components of the model. Experiments in social phobia should focus on demonstrating the effects of safety behaviours on physical symptoms, on social performance, and on self-consciousness. Typically, this involves social performance under two contrasting conditions. In the first condition patients are asked to practise all of their safety behaviours in an analogue or actual feared situation, and in the second condition they are instructed to enter the situation while dropping all safety behaviours. The effect of safety behaviours on the perception of symptoms and on performance fluency can then be reviewed by contrasting the two conditions. Patients should also be instructed to perform socially under conditions of increased self-focus, and under decreased self-focus in which they are instructed to process features of the environment or other people. The effects of attention on symptom intensity and on performance can thus be demonstrated. Three examples follow:

1. J presented with a six-year history of being unable to drink in public for fear of shaking and making a fool of himself. His main cognitions were that he would shake uncontrollably and would spill his drink or drop the cup. In the first therapy session he was asked to drink from a cup and saucer, first, while using all of his safety behaviours which were specified in detail, and then while abandoning all of his behaviours. When the two conditions were contrasted with appropriate questioning by the therapist, J realised that when using safety behaviours his behaviour was much less fluent, tremor was more noticeable, and self-consciousness was greater. The experiment was repeated a third time in which J was asked to walk around the therapist's office carrying a cup and saucer while observing and memorising the objects in the room. This procedure was intended to

reduce his self-consciousness. He discovered, contrary to his prediction, that he spilled very little of his drink and that the shaking was barely present. A discussion followed concerning the role of safety behaviours and the role of self-focused attention in maintaining his problem.

2.  P reported difficulty making conversation in a group. She feared her mind 'going blank' or getting her words wrong and people thinking she was stupid. Her safety behaviours included talking quickly, sitting on the edge of the chair, playing with her jewellery, rehearsing sentences in her mind, and avoiding eye contact. The therapist worked with a colleague to construct a small informal gathering of three people in which conversation was to be sustained for ten minutes. Under increased safety behaviour conditions the patient found conversation difficult, noting that it was difficult to keep track of people's comments and that it was difficult to think of things to say. The belief that she would be unable to talk fell little from 70 per cent to 60 per cent. In contrast the reversed safety behaviour condition consisting of sitting back in the chair, observing and listening closely to others comments, and making statements without mental rehearsal was much easier. The belief that she would be unable to speak fell to 10 per cent. However, she still believed that she had not presented herself in an interesting or coherent fashion. In subsequent sessions the therapist worked with video-tape feedback to correct this faulty self-appraisal.

3.  M's primary concern was sweating in group meetings. He feared that others would pay much attention to this and think he was 'odd'. His safety behaviours included sitting with his arms folded, keeping still, wearing a jacket, hiding his face with his hands, and gripping a handkerchief. A social interaction was planned under increased, and abandoned safety conditions. M was able to discover that his safety behaviour exacerbated his sweating and the behaviour was probably more noticeable and 'odd' than the sweating itself. The manipulation was followed by practising social interaction under no-safety and external attention instructions which seemed to moderate symptom intensity and provided a framework for subsequent disconfirmatory strategies in treatment.

## SEQUENCING OF TREATMENT INTERVENTIONS

We saw in the chapters on panic and hypochondriasis how treatment emerges as a sequence of procedures ranging from conceptualisation of cross-sectional details of the problem to modifying negative appraisals, and then assumptions and beliefs. Within this framework behavioural experiments are used as early as possible in treatment to facilitate assessment, socialisation and testing of predictions based on patients' negative thoughts. While this general sequence is preserved in the treatment of social phobia, there are several reasons to propose that a more specific sequence in treatment strategies may be of particular value. First, the overall model is rather complex and comprises elements which are novel to the patient. This necessitates presenting the model in stages and reframing patient experiences in terms of the model.

Second, effective disconfirmation of belief in negative appraisals is moderated by the patient's behavioural *and* attentional responses in situations (Wells & Matthews, 1994, 1997). Moreover, safety behaviours not only prevent disconfirmation but also provide confirmatory evidence. For example, some behaviours impair performance, make the person more conspicuous or exacerbate physical symptoms. Self-focus reduces the opportunities for observing the real rather than imagined aspects of the social situation, and thereby interferes with processing of disconfirmatory experiences. Thus social phobics should initially acquire skills of shifting attention to external processing, and dropping safety behaviours in order for exposure experiments to produce optimal belief change.

Third, patients are often only willing to engage in exposure experiments if they have some means of reducing the distress associated with their symptoms. (This should not, however, become another safety behaviour.) **External attentional strategies and decreased safety behaviours present a means of moderating symptoms** *while* **maximising disconfirmatory processing**.

Fourth, manipulations targeted at reducing negative anticipatory processing may be an important prerequisite for exposure tasks in order to prime disconfirmatory processing and maintain control over disconfirmatory strategies (e.g. focus of attention).

## MODIFYING SELF-PROCESSING

Following socialisation to the general model the next stage of treatment consists of modifying the content of self-processing. This is the next step because it is the main source of evidence used by the social phobic to make inferences about the content of other people's appraisals, and it maintains low self-confidence.

The principal strategy for modifying the content of self-processing is exposure to the true observable self. This is accomplished with audio and video-feedback. However, feedback should be managed in a particular way to maximise change in self-image. A problem is that observing the self on video is prone to activate self-consciousness and the processing of internal information which contaminates objective appraisal of the observability of symptoms. A further difficulty is that some social phobics discount the accuracy of feedback, claiming that recording devices are insensitive, or that their symptoms were 'not as bad as usual'.

To overcome these difficulties the therapist should ask the patient to run a 'mental' video first and operationalise the conspicuousness of symptoms and behaviours in observable terms. An example follows (the patient was video-taped while making conversation with the therapist's colleague):

T: I'd like you to think back to the image of yourself in the conversation that you have just had. Describe to me how you think you looked.
P: I was stumbling over my words, my hands were shaking, and I felt flushed.
T: How noticeable are these things in your image?
P: Very noticeable, my hands are shaking and I look very red.
T: Okay. Can you show me how visible the shaking was?
P: (Patient makes her hand tremble)
T: Okay. Let me catch that on the video as well. I have some pieces of red card here. Can you show me how red you think you looked?
P: As red as that (points to a card).
T: In your image is the redness all over your face?
P: Yes, I'm red from top to bottom.
T: Okay. I'd like us to review the video of your conversation now, so that you can see how observable your symptoms were.

In this case the video was reviewed and the patient discovered that, contrary to her self-generated image, her symptoms were largely inconspicuous. In view of this the therapist asked her to repeat a conversation with a colleague while deliberately trying to exaggerate her symptoms. Even when she attempted to make the symptoms worse than they would normally be they were less conspicuous than predicted by her self-generated image.

Several video-feedback demonstrations are typically required in which the patient is recorded in various anxiety-provoking situations in order to challenge the validity of negative self-processing. Once a more accurate impression of the self is established, the patient should be encouraged to use the more accurate replacement self-image whenever the negative distorted self-impression becomes activated. Patients can also use rational self-statements based on the corrective feedback to challenge the validity of negative appraisals and to maintain control over attention (i.e. reduce self-consciousness). Examples of self-statements include: 'My symptoms feel worse than they look'; 'Even though I feel a tremor its hardly noticeable to others'; 'I look calm even when I don't feel it'; 'I know I look okay no matter what they say'.

## VERBAL REATTRIBUTION

Negative self-appraisals, negative thoughts concerning the reaction and thoughts of others should be targeted for reattribution.

The primary strategy for challenging belief in negative automatic thoughts consists of a detailed review of the evidence that the social phobic has for negative automatic thoughts. The evidence typically stems from self-appraisal rather than from objective events, and this conclusion can be sought through guided discovery. However, in some cases tangible evidence does exist, and the 'goodness' of the evidence is then collaboratively reviewed with an aim of: (1) disputing its validity; (2) reframing it in more realistic terms (e.g. generating alternative explanations for evidence, and modifying any thinking errors in interpretation of it); (3) considering strategies for changing the situation if the evidence is considered to be entirely reasonable (e.g. if the social phobic does appear socially inappropriate in some way, strategies for overcoming this should be taught).

Examples of questions useful for challenging specific NATs in social phobia are as follows:

| | |
|---|---|
| *Negative thought:* | *'He/she doesn't like me.'* |
| *Questions:* | • What's the evidence? |
| | • What's so bad about that? |
| | • What's the counter-evidence? |
| | • Is it possible to be liked by everyone? (why not?) |
| | • What does it mean if someone doesn't like you? |
| | • If one person likes you and one doesn't, who's right? |
| | • Can you think of very special people who were disliked by some people? What about Jesus? |
| *Rational responses* | 'I don't have to be liked by everyone.' |
| | 'If someone doesn't like me it's not my fault.' |
| | 'I'm mind reading—I don't know what he/she thinks.' |
| | |
| *Negative thought:* | *'He/she thinks I'm boring.'* |
| *Questions:* | • What's the evidence? |
| | • What would that mean? |
| | • Is your thinking based on facts or are you mind reading? |
| | • If one person thinks you're boring and one doesn't who's right? |
| | • If a person thinks you're boring, does that mean you are boring? |
| | • What is it that makes someone boring—are you like that? |

| | |
|---|---|
| *Rational responses:* | 'It's okay to be boring some of the time.' |
| | 'If someone thinks I'm boring it doesn't mean I am boring.' |
| | 'If only you knew how interesting I really am.' |
| *Negative thought:* | *'I'm going to sound stupid.'* |
| *Questions:* | • What's the evidence? |
| | • What's the worst that could happen? |
| | • What's the best that could happen? |
| | • What's the most likely thing that could happen? |
| | • Are you taking events as they happen or trying to predict the future? |
| | • What's so bad about that? |
| | • Could you rescue the situation? |
| | • If a person does sound stupid does that write them off as a person? (Why not?) |
| | • How do you define 'sounding stupid'? |
| *Rational responses:* | 'Go with the flow—I sound okay.' |
| | 'What is stupid anyway?' |
| | 'I'm going to sound fine?' |

## The social balance sheet

To facilitate socialisation and processing of evidence capable of disconfirming belief in NATs a social balance sheet can be used. This consists of a three-column record of 'internal evidence', 'external evidence' and 'external counter-evidence' for negative thoughts. Initially in the early sessions of treatment this should be completed with the therapist. Typically there is internal evidence to support specific thoughts (e.g. feeling like the centre of attention), but little external evidence (e.g. several people staring at the patient). The social balance sheet can therefore be used to illustrate the role of self-processing in drawing inferences about the social situation. As treatment progresses and attention is shifted to processing the environment, external disconfirmatory evidence should be logged. A running log can be maintained throughout treatment and each time new evidence and counter-evidence becomes available this should be entered on the social balance sheet.

## Thinking errors

The predominant thinking errors in social phobia are *mind reading* (e.g. He/she thinks I'm boring); *fortune telling/catastrophising* (e.g. If I'm asked to sign my name I'll be unable to write); and *personalisation* (e.g. They're not talking to me, I must have said something wrong). Social phobics also engage in an error of *projected self appraisal* in which they assume that their own negative impression of themselves is also held by others (e.g. I sound really boring, they must think I'm boring). Educating patients to identify thinking errors is the strategy of choice in this context.

## Using rational self-statements

Once answers to negative thoughts have been generated and/or validated by behavioural and verbal strategies they can be used as self-statements in social phobic situations as a means of preventing full activation of self-focused processing and of maintaining stability of the self-concept. Inevitably self-statements may be used by the social phobic to control anxiety, which is acceptable to some extent since anxiety and self preoccupation can interfere with performance. However, if the self-statements are used to avoid feared catastrophes in situations, then they become additional safety behaviours that can block disconfirmation of negative beliefs. In addition, questioning thoughts in-situ and using positive self-statements in a repetitive manner can be cognitively demanding, can increase the likelihood of performance decrements, and can reduce attention to external disconfirmatory information. As a result it is recommended that discrete positive self-statements are used in situations rather than more elaborate self-questioning of thoughts. The therapist should determine that self-statements are being used to enhance self-confidence and facilitate implementation of experiments rather than being used to prevent feared catastrophes.

Positive self-statements are an effective means of interrupting pre-event anticipatory worry, thereby reducing the priming of self-focused anxious processing. Moreover, they may be used both within situation and after exposure to difficult situations to prevent full activation of the post-mortem.

## Defining fears

Many of the fears expressed by social phobic patients are vague and ill-defined. For example, fears of acting foolishly, being stupid, losing control, and being unable to speak, offer little data concerning the idiosyncratic nature of the threat. What does the patient mean by 'being unable to speak'? The meaning of this can range from experiencing subjective difficulty in finding words to fear of actually being paralysed by anxiety. Belief in appraisals of this type are most effectively challenged when reattribution is directed at the precise idiosyncratic meaning of the thought. In some instances the patient will not have processed a more elaborated meaning and the act of doing so is capable of challenging belief in the fear. Once the belief is defined specific verbal and behavioural reattributions should be used if necessary.

## Dealing with anticipatory processing and the post-mortem

Anticipatory processing normally consists of worry concerning potential negative consequences in social situations. It may also be a component of safety-behaviours in which the patient actively attempts to rehearse social coping strategies. The advantages and disadvantages of engaging in this type of processing should be collaboratively reviewed. One of the key problems with anticipatory processing is that it is most often inaccurate and fails to depict events as they actually turn out. The patient's attention should be drawn to this factor and anticipatory processing is then banned.

The post-mortem consists of reviewing social encounters, and because the patient's anxious feeling and negative self-perceptions figure prominently in these encounters the post-mortem provides further incorrect support for social failure. The advantages and disadvantages of the post-mortem should be reviewed, and the distorted nature of the post-mortem should be established with the patient. The post-mortem is then banned.

## BEHAVIOURAL EXPERIMENTS

Verbal reattribution procedures have limited effectiveness if used alone in social phobia because social situations offer little exposure to unambiguous information concerning people's reactions to the social phobic. Moreover, if the social phobic has been functioning in a limited or highly controlled way in social situations there will have been few tests of the consequences of 'failed' social performance or of the consequences of showing anxiety.

### Interrogating the environment

Behavioural experiments should provide a means of testing the reactions of others in social situations, and are broadly based on strategies for 'interrogating the environment'. To successfully modify fear concerning negative evaluation it is necessary to devise strategies for assessing other people's thoughts and reactions. Other people's thoughts can be assessed in two ways: (1) by making predictions about specific observable behaviours that would be logically derived from particular appraisals (e.g. If someone thinks you are boring how will that person behave towards you? What will you see?); (2) by using probe questions that seek to determine what people noticed and what they thought in a situation.

Following identification of a means of assessing the reactions and thoughts of others, experiments consist of showing signs of anxiety, producing 'failures' in performance, or behaving in an 'unacceptable' manner. Thus, a social phobic who fears shaking and spilling drinks is asked to shake and spill some of his/her drink deliberately in a social situation, while observing the reactions of others. Similarly, the social phobic who fears being unable to speak in situations is asked to produce a long pause in conversation or deliberately 'forget' what he/she had to say. The individual who fears sweating is asked to dampen the clothing around his/her armpits and enter a social situation to test out predicted reactions of other people. Some patients find this type of behavioural experiment initially too anxiety-provoking to implement. The therapist should then model the behaviour in the feared social situation while the patient observes the proceedings. When patients observe that feared events do not occur they should then attempt the experiment for themselves.

One of the difficulties in implementing behavioural experiments that involve behaving in an 'unacceptable' fashion can stem from the therapist's own reluctance to implement these procedures. The therapist may have to work on his/her own social concerns in implementing this treatment. Initially it is important that the therapist accompanies the patient to a social situation so that the experiment is performed collaboratively. As we have seen this may involve the therapist in modelling the behaviour first. Subsequently, patients are instructed to practise experiments of this type for homework. A hierarchical approach to performance of these experiments can be adopted to facilitate compliance. Ultimately these procedures should lead to 'shame attacking' or 'bandwidth' experiments (see later).

## Overcoming avoidance

Avoidance of particular social situations is an obstacle to reattribution at negative automatic thought, and schema levels. A central objective of treatment is reduction and ultimate elimination of patient avoidance. Exposure experiments consisting of exposure to situations with concurrent dropping of safety behaviours, and external processing of disconfirmatory information are *crucial components* of cognitive therapy of social phobia. The continuation of counter-productive safety behaviours and avoidance should be monitored throughout treatment with the Social Phobia Rating Scale and

Avoidance Questionnaire (see Chapter 2). Continuous attention should be devoted in treatment to implementation of exposure experiments.

The experiments discussed in this section are applicable to the modification of underlying assumptions. In particular, experiments involving deliberate 'failures' of performance offer a means of increasing patients' assumptions concerning the 'bandwidth' of acceptable behaviour. Bandwidth experiments are discussed later in the section on modifying assumptions.

## WORKING WITH CONDITIONAL ASSUMPTIONS AND BELIEFS

In the present model schema content is divided into core social self-beliefs, conditional assumptions and rigid rules linked to social phobia. These will be considered in turn.

### Conditional assumptions

The techniques outlined previously for modifying negative automatic thoughts should be used to modify conditional assumptions as well. The first step in modifying assumptions is the generation of a clear *definition* of concepts represented in the assumptions, and their *operationalisation* in a testable format. Once this is accomplished, evidence and counter-evidence should be reviewed and this should be followed by disconfirmatory behavioural experiments. An example follows:

*Example*

P was a 36-year-old male computer operator who presented with anxiety making conversation with work colleagues. He avoided social outings after work and avoided taking lunch with his colleagues. His central fear was that he would 'blank out' and be unable to speak. While this appraisal, and related situational negative appraisals were effectively dealt with in the first few sessions of treatment, it was clear that P had a number of unhelpful assumptions concerning effective and desirable standards of social performance. These assumptions were:

(a) 'I must always speak fluently or people won't take me seriously.'
(b) 'If they see I'm nervous they'll think I'm weird.'

The first step in challenging these assumptions was to define them precisely. (What does P mean by *fluency*? What is fluent and what is not? What is meant by being *taken seriously*?) It was necessary to define these concepts as clearly as possible, and once defined to generate concrete and observable examples of them. These steps allowed **operationalisation** of the assumptions in a manner that became testable. For example, the negative outcome of 'not being taken seriously' required translation into a form such that its presence or absence could be evaluated by the patient. In P's case it was agreed that a sign of not being taken seriously would be being ignored by his colleagues, or being laughed at when he had something important to say. Given this operational definition P was equipped to conduct a number of behavioural experiments in which he said more and made deliberate errors in speech while actively searching for the presence or absence of these reactions in his colleagues.

Social phobics' assumptions typically represent a combination of mind reading and fortune telling. When assumptions contain a mind-reading element—that is, they imply knowledge of another person's subjective—experience they are difficult to falsify. We saw in the previous case how operationalisation of other people's thoughts and feelings in concrete observable terms offers a means of overcoming this difficulty. Another method which is more direct, but can be more readily discounted by the patient, involves getting the patient to ask interaction partners to comment on the patient's behaviour in situations. In this instance the therapist and patient work together to determine specific probe questions that may be used, and to role-play using these probe questions. For example, patients may be encouraged to comment on their own performance/symptoms and ask a probe question about the significance to others: e.g. 'I noticed I didn't say very much during that conversation—how did that seem?'. 'I felt quieter than usual in today's meeting—did you notice anything different?'.

### Generating alternative evidence

Counter-evidence is not typically apparent to social phobics due to their failure to process disconfirmatory information in the environment and because of their concealment of problems. Nevertheless, counter-evidence can be reviewed with reference to hypothetical scenarios and to situations in which the patient has observed the behaviour of others. For example, a social phobic feared that showing anxiety would attract attention. The socratic dialogue was used to explore general reactions of individuals to nervous behaviour as follows:

T: So if you see that someone is nervous when talking to them, do you stare at them more?
P: No, if anything I would look at them less.
T: So you would pay less attention?

P: Yes, otherwise they may feel more uncomfortable

T: Let's assume someone is acting really oddly. Someone is walking along the street shouting strange things and making strange noises. Would people pay a lot of attention to them?

P: Well, they might do, in case the person was dangerous.

T: Even if they think the person is dangerous will they stare?

P: No, I don't suppose they will.

T: Why not?

P: Because they don't want to get involved with the person.

T: So even if someone does appear nervous, or is acting very oddly, are people likely to pay more or less attention?

P: When you look at it that way they're probably going to notice, but then they'll pay less attention.

T: So, in the long term, if you don't want to be noticed is it better to be anxious or confident?

Some suggested strategies to guide the search for counter-evidence in the context of particular negative assumptions are as follows:

*Assumption: If people see me shaking they'll think I'm stupid.*
*Strategy:* Look at alternative explanations for someone shaking (e.g. construct a pie chart, Figure 7.3). Conduct a mini-survey. Run an experiment.

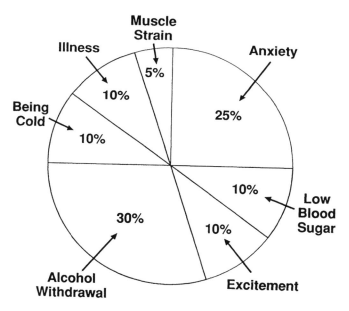

**Figure 7.3**   A pie chart of 'reasons for shaking'

*Assumption:If I get my words wrong people will think I'm inadequate.*
*Strategy*: List all the things that make someone inadequate: How many characteristics does the patient have? What is the relative importance of 'getting words wrong' among the other characteristics? Conduct a mini-survey. Run an experiment.

*Assumption: I'll vomit and everyone will reject me.*
*Strategy*: Examine a range of possible reactions of others to vomiting and reasons for the reactions. Explore how the patient would react if a friend vomited in public. Conduct a mini-survey to elicit people's reactions. Practise rushing out of the room in company to evaluate people's reactions.

*Assumption: I'll blush and everyone will laugh at me.*
*Strategy*: Examine the range of all reactions in the past when blushing occurred. Explore the meaning of the laughter: list all possible meanings. Conduct a mini-survey. Run a behavioural experiment to test it out.

## Rigid rules: increasing the 'bandwidth'

Social phobics often have rigid rules about the acceptable boundaries of behaviour in a social context. These rules operate in a wide range of social situations and are not specific to feared situations. Rigid rules are reflected in assumptions such as: 'I mustn't draw attention to myself'; 'I must always fit in'; 'I must not inconvenience anyone'; 'I should always behave properly'. A useful metaphor for conceptualising these assumptions, and the conservative behaviours that stem from them, is that of a *bandwidth*. The social phobic may be seen as operating socially within a highly restricted and narrow bandwidth of behaviour. Social phobics assume that if they remain within the bandwidth, which they may have succeeded in doing for a long time, situations will be 'safe'. The aim is to increase the bandwidth in which the social phobic operates, and this is accomplished by experimenting with the acceptable boundaries of 'risky behaviour'. Risky behaviour in this context means different things to different people. The methods here superficially overlap with the concepts of 'shame attacking' exercises. However, unlike shame attacking, 'bandwidth expansion' is geared to modifying long-standing restricted social patterns, and to providing evidence that a wide range of individual behaviours are acceptable, and unimportant to others, even if they break social convention. Examples of bandwidth expanding experiments include: making mistakes; disagreeing with people; making complaints; trying ten pairs of shoes and not buying any; 'accidentally' knocking some products off the supermarket shelves, etc.

## Unconditional negative self-beliefs

Unconditional negative self-beliefs of social phobics are similar to negative beliefs observed in other emotional disorders such as depression. Examples of social phobic beliefs are as follows: 'I'm different'; 'People are intolerant'; 'I'm boring'; 'Other people are better than me'; 'I'm weird'; 'People will ridicule me'; 'I'm stupid'; 'Everyone is more relaxed than me'; 'I'm unlikeable'; 'People always exploit your weaknesses'.

In addition to the strategies already reviewed in this chapter, other strategies used for challenging beliefs include: continua; positive data logs; flashcards; and interpersonal strategies. The use of continua and flashcards was outlined in Chapter 4 and the reader is referred to the relevant section there.

## The positive data log

Because dysfunctional beliefs distort processing and introduce biases in attention, the social phobic rarely processes information that is inconsistent with his/her dysfunctional belief system. The positive data log provides a means of accumulating evidence in support of replacement positive beliefs with the aim of strengthening them, and of counteracting negative cognitive bias. The technique requires that the patient compiles a daily log of events and experiences that contradict negative beliefs and support positive beliefs. For example, one patient believed that she was 'unlikeable' and this was supported by the fact that people seemed to ignore her. As a homework assignment she was asked to complete a daily log of different types of attention that she received from people including: eye contact, smiles and other non-verbal gestures, verbal greeting, compliments, invitations and so on. After four days of completing the positive data log she felt that she had no need to continue with it, as she realised that many people did not ignore her. She discovered that the converse was true; moreover the more she attended to others, the more attention she received in return. As a result, the belief that she was 'unlikeable' was severely eroded and a replacement belief, 'I am likeable', was introduced.

## Interpersonal strategies

In social phobia negative beliefs about the self or others influence interaction styles, and these styles may in turn perpetuate belief. A social phobic who believes that he/she is 'unintelligent' may try to appear more intelligent, and an individual who believes he/she is 'boring' may attempt to be 'interesting'. Such compensatory strategies can become over-compensations (cf. Young, 1990) that have a deleterious effect on social interactions. Compensatory strategies may be viewed as a form of safety behaviour, and the patient should be encouraged to abandon them. However, when overcompensatory behaviours or in-situation withdrawal behaviours have been long-standing strategies it is necessary to generate and practise new '*scripts*' for social interaction. This should be accomplished through education and role-play. Strategies that may be practised include: handling criticism, making complaints, dealing with arguments, initiating conversation, turning down requests, giving and receiving compliments, etc.

## CONCLUSIONS

The cognitive model of social phobia presented in this chapter asserts that an individual's self-appraisals, attentional strategies and safety behaviours maintain social phobia through a number of feedback loops. A central component of the model is the concept that social phobics use interoceptive information to construct a public impression of themselves, and use this to infer what other people see and think about them. In addition, safety behaviours contaminate the social situation and increase the likelihood of negative reactions from others. The social phobic is prone to ruminate about social situations before entering them and to dwell on negative aspects of situations afterwards (the post-mortem), factors that prime and maintain distorted negative appraisals.

We have seen how treatment based on this model is structured as a sequence in which conceptualisation and socialisation are followed by increased and decreased safety-behaviour manipulations plus shifting to external focused processing. Homework early in treatment consists of practise in dropping safety behaviours and shifting to external focus in problematic social situations. A primary aim of these strategies is to challenge belief in specific negative automatic thoughts. The next step in the sequence consists of modifying the content of self-processing via audio-visual feedback and standard reattribution techniques. Following this phase, or in conjunction, therapy focuses on operationalising and testing specific predictions (based on negative automatic thoughts and assumptions) through experiments in which the patient deliberately behaves in an 'unacceptable' fashion. Subsequent work focuses on underlying beliefs and assumptions that contribute to vulnerability to relapse.

The emphasis of intervention should be skewed in favour of behavioural experiments. Experiments should be introduced as early as possible in treatment so that the therapist may constructively use the social anxiety that exists in the therapy setting before familiarity sets in. Moreover, behaviour manipulations can offer a convincing display of factors maintaining social phobia, and provide a direct route to moderating symptom intensity in many cases.

# EXAMPLE TREATMENT OUTLINE

*Session 1*

1. Review recent social anxiety episodes and draw-out model.
2. Elicit model and illustrate components by creating analogue phobic situation.
3. Share model (begin socialisation).
4. Homework: complete the record of automatic thoughts

*Session 2*

1. Check homework : fit results to model.
2. Increased/decreased safety and external attention manipulation.
3. Begin testing specific negative automatic thoughts.
4. Homework: specific exposure plus dropping safety behaviours and shifting to external focus. Continue thoughts record.

*Session 3*

1. Check homework : fit results to model.
2. Conceptualise and introduce concept of self-processing.
3. Videotape performance in analogue feared situation (provide video-feedback).
4. Homework: exposure plus dropping safety and external focus.

*Sessions 4–9*

1. Check homework.
2. Testing specific negative thoughts (interrogating the environment).
3. Bandwidth experiments.
4. Ban anticipatory processing and post-mortem.
5. Homework: specific tests of predictions.

*Sessions 10–14*

1. Check homework.
2. Work on residual negative thought/self-appraisals.
3. Elicit and challenge assumptions and beliefs.
4. Overcome residual avoidance.
5. Develop therapy blueprint.

*Note.* Use sessional responses on the Social Phobia Rating Scale (SPRS) to guide the focus of treatment sessions.

Chapter 8

# GENERALISED ANXIETY DISORDER

Generalised anxiety disorder (GAD) is a common problem. The one-year prevalence rate in a community sample was approximately 3 per cent, and the lifetime prevalence was 5 per cent (DSM-IV; APA, 1994). The incidence among patients presenting at anxiety clinics is about 12 per cent. However, there have been few attempts to develop a specific cognitive model of GAD, possibly because the disorder only emerged from its status as a residual category in 1987 with the advent of DSM-III-R. Nevertheless, cognitive-behavioural interventions for GAD have been evaluated in a number of studies. These approaches have combined cognitive and behavioural methods without necessarily using a unifying-rationale or disorder-specific model. Even so, significant effects have been obtained (e.g. Butler, Cullingham, Hibbert, Klimes & Gelder, 1987) and studies show some superiority of cognitive methods over other forms of treatment (Durham & Turvey, 1987; Borkovec et al., 1987; Power, Jerrom, Simpson, Mitchell & Swanson, 1989; Butler, Fennell, Robson & Gelder, 1991). Borkovec and Costello (1993) compared applied relaxation with cognitive-behaviour therapy, and showed an advantage for the cognitive intervention. Durham et al. (1994) also report an advantage for cognitive therapy compared with analytic psychotherapy. In general, improved functioning is obtained in about half of the patients treated. There is clearly room for improvement in outcome. As specific cognitive models of GAD are advanced and drive treatment practises, treatment outcome should improve. This chapter outlines Wells's (1994a, 1995) model and the treatment derived from it.

Worrying is recognised as a predominant characteristic of GAD. According to DSM-IV (APA, 1994) GAD is defined as: Excessive anxiety and worry occurring more days than not for a minimum of six months about a number of events. The person should find the worry difficult to control, and should report at least three of the following symptoms: restlessness or feeling keyed up and on edge, easily fatigued, difficulty concentrating or mind going blank, irritability, muscle tension, and sleep disturbance (difficulty falling asleep, staying asleep, or restless unsatisfying sleep). The focus of anxiety and worry should not be confined to another Axis I disorder (e.g. worry is not about being embarrassed in public as in social phobia). The anxiety and worry should cause significant distress or impairment in functioning, and the disturbance should not be due to substance effects such as drug use or medical conditions such as hyperthyroidism, or occur only during a mood disorder or psychotic disorder.

Individuals with GAD report feeling anxious or apprehensive most of the time, this may be characterised by a general inability to relax or more specific symptoms such as muscle tiredness and feeling on edge. The worry component of the problem may be more or less marked at initial presentation. However, problematic worry is a key feature of the disorder. GAD should be conceptualised as essentially a disorder of worrying.

## THE NATURE OF WORRY

Worrying is both a normal phenomenon and an activity which occurs in association with a wide range of emotional disorders. The worries of GAD patients closely resemble in content the worries of non-patients. Craske, Rapee, Jackel and Barlow (1989) demonstrated that normal and GAD worries differed little in terms of their content, but GAD patients rated their worries as less controllable and less successfully reduced by corrective attempts compared with the worries of non-patients.

It may be useful to distinguish between different types of thought which may interact in significant ways in the development and maintenance of emotional dysfunction (Wells, 1994a, 1995). Worry appears to differ in form from negative automatic thoughts, and from obsessions (Wells, 1994a; Wells & Morrison, 1994). Borkovec, Robinson, Pruzinski and De Pree (1983a) define worry as a 'chain of thoughts and images, negatively affect-laden and relatively uncontrollable' (p. 10). Worry has been viewed as a problem-solving activity (e.g Borkovec et al., 1983a; Davey, 1994), and it is typically a more conceptual-verbal activity than an imaginal one (Borkovec & Inz, 1990; Wells & Morrison, 1994).

### The nature of worry in GAD

Patients with GAD report periods of chronic and repeated worrying on a variety of topics. The experience of worrying can range from a pervasive 'feeling' of being worried or, more typically in GAD, to discrete episodes of rumination lasting from minutes to hours. Worry is experienced as distressing and relatively uncontrollable, although people with GAD often report that the activity can be interrupted by distracting events. While worrying may be initiated by an involuntary intruding thought, it can also be initiated in a deliberate way. Wells (1994a) suggests that it is useful to distinguish the initiation of worry from its maintenance. While initiation may be relatively involuntary, continued worrying is amenable to conscious control. Wells (1994a) proposes that since GAD worries and normal worries differ little in content but differ more in their appraised uncontrollability, a model of abnormal worry in GAD should take account of patients' appraisal of the activity of worrying. This is a central feature of the cognitive model and treatment of GAD advanced by Wells (1994a, 1995) which is the focus of the remainder of this chapter.

## A COGNITIVE MODEL OF GAD

It follows that if the content of normal and GAD worries is similar, a main distinguishing feature of GAD is the form that worry takes and the subjects' appraisal of the significance of worrying. On the basis of this assertion, Wells (1994a, 1995) distinguishes between two types of worry termed Type 1 and Type 2 worries. Type 1 worries concern external daily events such as the welfare of a partner, and non-cognitive internal events such as concerns about bodily sensations. Type 2 worries in contrast are focused on the nature and occurrence of thoughts themselves—for example, worrying that worry will lead to insanity. Type 2 worry is basically worry about worry. The cognitive model of GAD asserts that abnormal varieties of worry such as that found in GAD are associated with a high incidence of Type 2 worries, in which GAD patients negatively appraise the activity of worrying. Negative appraisals or Type 2 worries reflect negative beliefs that patients hold about worrying: Examples are:

- My worries are uncontrollable.
- Worrying is harmful.
- I could go crazy with worrying.
- I could enter a state of worry and never get out.
- My worries will take over and control me.

Aside from negative beliefs the model asserts that GAD patients also have tacit positive beliefs about worrying, or the benefits of rumination as a coping strategy. Once worry has been triggered, for example, the person with GAD may feel compelled to reason-out the worry in order to find a solution or to prevent catastrophe. Similarly, there may be a specific belief that it is important to worry in order to maintain an acceptable degree of subjective safety. The use of worry as a safety strategy is illustrated by a patient who constantly worried about being mugged when walking alone in the street because he believed that worrying offered a means of *always being prepared* to deal with such a problem. Unfortunately his preoccupation with being mugged and how he could deal with it heightened his sense of vulnerability as he generated an increasing range of negative scenarios. It is unlikely that repeated worrying actually increases safety; a preoccupation with worrying thoughts in a situation may distract from actual vigilance for threat. Examples of positive worry beliefs are:

- Worrying helps me cope. ('If I worry about the worst and I can see myself coping then I probably will cope if it happens.')
- If I worry I can prevent bad things from happening.
- Worrying helps me solve problems.
- I wouldn't do anything if I didn't worry.
- If I worry I can always be prepared.

Unfortunately the use of worry as a coping or processing strategy generates its own problems. Worrying increases sensitivity to threat-related information, and generates an elaborated range of possible negative outcomes and scenarios each of which is capable of sustaining a worry in its own right. Thus, the magnitude and breadth of worrying is liable to increase. Furthermore, the initial belief that worry is intended to challenge (e.g. I can't cope) remains unchanged in the long term because new negative scenarios which could provide evidence of not coping are likely to be generated during the course of the worry episode.

According to this model the development of GAD can be seen over a time course. Many patients report that they have a long history of worrying. It appears that some people initially used worry in order to deal with real or imagined problems in life. This strategy may have evolved from the influence of a parent who modelled the use of worry as a means of dealing with problems, or from the reinforcement of the 'benefits' or worrying. At some point, however, worrying becomes the focus of negative appraisal. This may result from new information such as a parent experiencing mental health problems associated with worrying, or worry may be negatively appraised because practise of the activity has led to a degree of automatisation of worry triggers to the extent that it has become an increasingly disruptive influence in the person's life. Once worry about worry has been established a number of additional factors are involved in the escalation and maintenance of the problem: (1) behavioural responses; (2) thought control

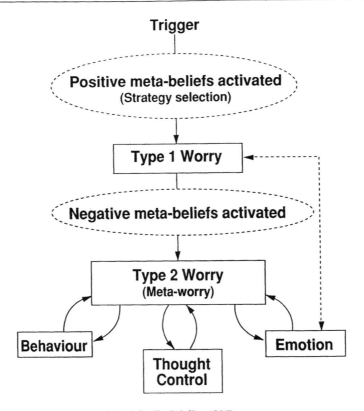

**Figure 8.0**   A cognitive model of GAD (Wells, 1995)

attempts; (3) emotional symptoms. This cognitive model of GAD is presented in Figure 8.0.

Figure 8.0 offers a schematic of the cognitive model that can be used for constructing idiosyncratic case formulations. In this model, the GAD patient uses worry as a processing strategy in response to a trigger. Triggers for Type 1 worrying vary, such as exposure to negative news material, an intruding thought such as an unpleasant image, exposure to a situation associated with a sense of subjective danger. The selection of worry (or rumination) as a coping strategy stems from the activation of tacit positive beliefs about the use of worry. Once the person with GAD is executing a worry routine, negative beliefs about worrying are activated. With repeated experience negative beliefs may be readily activated by the early signs of worrying, such as the initial intruding thought. Negative beliefs concern the uncontrollability, and dangers associated with worrying, and stimulate negative appraisal of worry (meta-worry). The negative appraisal of worry motivates the use of strategies intended to reduce the appraised danger. These strategies will now be considered in turn:

## Behavioural responses

Two types of behaviour are important: Avoidance, and reassurance seeking. The Type 1 and Type 2 worry distinction has implications for the way avoidance in GAD is conceptualised. What is it that GAD patients are avoiding? On one level GAD is associated with avoidance of a range of situations. There may be avoidance of social events, avoidance of unpleasant news items, or more pervasive avoidance resembling agoraphobia. Avoidance may be of external dangers (linked to Type 1 worry) believed to be inherent in a situation, such as the possibility of drawing attention to the self and humiliation. However, avoidance is also of the dangers of worrying itself (linked to Type 2 worry). The meta-cognitive model emphasises the importance of avoidance as a means of *preventing worry* and the dangers associated with it as well as a means of avoiding external threat. In summary, avoidance may therefore be linked to Type 1 and Type 2 worries and the beliefs from which they stem. Detailed analysis is required to determine the cognitions which motivate specific avoidance responses. Clearly, optimal cognitive modification procedures are those which manipulate key belief-linked behaviours. In the following example Type 1 and Type 2 worries and associated behaviours are evident:

*Example:* M was a 28-year-old engineer presenting with a four-year history of panic attacks and chronic worries. He met diagnostic criteria for panic disorder and GAD. His panic problem responded well to cognitive therapy and he became panic free following six sessions. The remaining five treatment sessions focused primarily on his remaining worry problem. He reported chronic worry about many life circumstances, such as failing to reach high standards of achievement at work, worries about contracting food-poisoning, and concerns that his partner could be involved in accidents. One of his central goals in treatment was to be able to worry less. He realised that his worries were unrealistic but believed that they were *uncontrollable*. As a result he attempted to avoid worrying by restricting his work, by carefully examining jars and tins of food in the supermarket to ensure that they were undamaged and sealed adequately, and by arriving home at the end of the day after his partner in case she may be late to return and this would lead to worrying.

In this example Type 1 worries are clearly evident and they concern:

(1) Failure.
(2) Contracting food-poisoning.
(3) His partner being involved in accidents.

Type 2 worries concern the uncontrollability of worry. It became clear during treatment that the patient reported arriving home after his partner in order to prevent worrying about her. This avoidance was clearly linked to Type 2 concerns since it was aimed at avoiding worry itself as opposed to some external danger. It also emerged that his avoidance of damaged food containers was primarily a means of preventing worry. When the patient was asked how likely it was that he thought he would contract food-poisoning from damaged containers he disclosed that he thought it was unlikely, but if he ate something from such a container he would not be able to stop worrying about it.

Other examples of overt avoidance serving to avoid the dangers of worry, rather than other danger, include avoidance of news items, television programmes, or uncertainty in order to avoid worrying.

Reassurance seeking is also evident in some cases of GAD. Reassurance seeking is aimed at interrupting worry cycles or preventing the onset of chronic worry. Unfortunately it can be a counter-productive strategy for worry control, since it may lead to increased ambiguity concerning Type 1 threat. For example, reassurance seeking can lead to conflicting responses across respondents which increases the range of stimuli that are worried about. In other situations, reassurance, such as having a partner telephone at regular intervals to say that he/she is safe, can temporarily prevent worry but this increases the propensity for worry if reassurance is not delivered on time. In other words, the search for reassurance can generate greater uncertainty, and a greater need to worry in order to plan coping options.


## Thought control

The use of thought control in GAD manifests in different ways. Since people with GAD have *positive* as well as *negative* beliefs about their worries, worry may be practised within strict limits or in special ways that are intended to exploit the benefits of worrying while, at the same time, avoiding the dangers. Thus worrying becomes a controlled rumination strategy used as a means of generating and rehearsing coping responses. In contrast, strategies may be used to suppress worries. Attempts not to worry are motivated by negative appraisal of the consequences of continued worrying. While the execution of Type 1 worry may be controlled in ways to meet personal goals, a disadvantage of suppression control attempts is that they may inadvertently increase the occurrence of unwanted thoughts, as demonstrated experimentally (e.g. Wegner, Schneider, Carter & White, 1987; Clark, Ball & Pape, 1991). The effect of thought control or suppression attempts may be to increase the frequency of worry triggers, an outcome likely to strengthen negative beliefs about thoughts such as beliefs about their uncontrollability.

A different perspective on thought control is presented by the concept that worry itself may serve a cognitive avoidance function. That is, some individuals may use worry or rumination to block-out other types of more distressing thought (e.g. Borkovec & Inz, 1990). According to this view, worry represents a form of cognitive-emotional avoidance. The use of worry to distract from more upsetting thoughts could lead to a failure to emotionally process and deal with more upsetting issues. Thoughts about such issues may continue to intrude as a sign of failure to emotionally process (Borkovec & Inz, 1990; Wells, 1995; Wells & Papageorgiou, 1995), and thereby strengthen meta-worries and negative beliefs.

Some patients report the use of distraction to avoid worries. This may take several forms such as absorption with work or hobbies. The distracting activity may then become a discriminative stimulus for worrying. The problem with attempts to suppress or distract from worry is that such attempts can prevent disconfirmation of negative beliefs about worry since it terminates exposure to the activity.

Thought control strategies in GAD are analogues to the concept of safety behaviours. Moreover, Type 1 worrying may itself be a safety behaviour to the extent that it is used to prevent appraised catastrophe. More specifically, it is a safety behaviour when it is used to generate and rehearse strategies for coping with future threats. Suppression strategies or attempts to control one's worries are safety behaviours intended to avert the appraised dangers of worrying, and are thus associated with Type 2 worries.

## Emotion

Type 1 and Type 2 worrying are associated with emotional responses. Type 1 worry can lead to initial increments in anxiety and tension, or decrements in anxiety if the goals of worrying are being met. However, with the activation of Type 2 worrying, anxiety escalates and emotional symptoms may be interpreted as evidence supporting Type 2 concerns. For example, symptoms of a racing mind, dissociation, and inability to relax may be viewed as evidence of loss of mental control. In some instances, where there are appraisals of immediate mental catastrophe, panic attacks may result. The model can account for the overlap between GAD and panic in this way.

## ELICITING INFORMATION FOR CONCEPTUALISATION

In some cases of GAD Type 2 worries (also termed meta-worries; Wells, 1994a) are highly apparent whilst in other cases they are less obvious. Since conceptualisation, socialisation, and treatment rely on the elicitation of Type 2 worry (meta-worry), the therapist should be skilled in the use of strategies for eliciting this material. Before considering in detail the process of building an idiosyncratic model, the next part of this chapter reviews verbal strategies for determining the nature and relevance of Type 2 worry (meta-worry).

## Verbal strategies for eliciting Type 2 worry

A range of strategies are available for eliciting Type 2 worry (meta-worry), these are: guided questioning; the advantages-disadvantages analysis; identifying control behaviours; experimental strategies; questionnaires.

### Guided questioning

One of the principal aims in the assessment and the socialisation process is the exploration of the role of appraisal of the worry process as a central determinant of problem level. Some examples of key questions for determining the content of meta-worry are as follows:

- What is it that bothers you most about worrying?
- As worrying is distressing for you, why don't you stop worrying?
- Could anything bad happen if you let yourself worry?
- How much control do you have over worry?
- What would it mean if you couldn't control worry?
- Could anything bad happen if you gave up worrying?
- Do you think it's normal to have worrying thoughts?
- What's the worst that could happen if you didn't try to control a bad worry episode?

In discussing the nature of the patient's problem the therapist should be sensitive to patient statements such as: 'The problem is I worry too much', 'I have periods when I worry about everything', 'I don't seem to be able to stop worrying', 'I worry all the time'.

These general statements about the *process* of worrying offer a pathway for accessing more specific Type 2 worries and concerns (note: these statements are manifestations of appraisal of worry itself, i.e. Type 2 worry). When these responses are encountered the therapist should determine the implications of worrying, determine the worst that can happen, and question why the patient doesn't stop worrying (this question can elicit appraisals of uncontrollability). Some examples follow.

*Example 1*
P: The problem is I worry too much.
T: Is it bad to worry so much?
P: Yes. I can't relax.
T: What's the worst that could happen if it carried on like this?
P: I'd be a wreck. I just couldn't function.
T: What do you mean by a wreck?
P: I'd go to pieces. Have a breakdown or something. (*A primary danger-related meta-worry.*)

*Example 2*
P: I can't stop worrying. (*A primary meta-worry concerning uncontrollability.*)
T: What will happen if you can't stop?
P: It's ruining my life. I'll feel bad all the time.
T: What do you mean by ruining your life?
P: I just want to be normal.
T: Do you think you're not normal?
P: It's not normal to worry like this.
T: So are you worried that you're abnormal in some way?
P: My aunt is schizophrenic and I sometimes think this could be the start of it for me. (*A primary danger-related meta-worry.*)

*Advantages–disadvantages analysis*

Use of the advantages–disadvantages strategy to elicit meta-worry consists of asking patients to consider, and list the advantages of worrying, and then list the disadvantages. The advantages given for worrying provide information relating to positive beliefs associated with sustained rumination/worrying. The disadvantages analysis provides a means of assessing the content of meta-worry and associated negative beliefs. In particular, the therapist looks for negative beliefs that relate to the *dangers* of worrying, and appraisals of *uncontrollability*. An advantages–disadvantages analysis of a 41-year-old male GAD patient who presented with a 12-year history of worry about illness/accidents, and social incompetence is presented in Table 8.0.

*Identifying control behaviours*

The existence of thought control behaviours is a marker for appraisals concerning the negative consequences of worrying. The function of control behaviours should be questioned to elicit meta-worry. The following dialogue illustrates the identification of control behaviours and elicitation of their idiosyncratic function:

**Table 8.0**   Results of an advantages–disadvantages worry analysis

| Advantages of worrying | Disadvantages of worrying |
| --- | --- |
| I won't become complacent | It makes me anxious |
| I'll be less likely to offend people | It stops me concentrating |
| I'll be prepared to deal with problems | I can't enjoy things |
| It helps me keep a check on my health | *It's harmful* |
| | It prevents me doing what I want to do |
| | *It's uncontrollable* |

T: When you had the distressing worry episode at the weekend, how did you deal with it?

P: I just spent hours worrying that my girlfriend could get attacked. There wasn't anything I could do about it.

T: It sounds as if you couldn't do much other than worry.

P: Well, I tried to do things, like tell myself there was nothing to worry about, but it didn't help.

T: Did you believe there was nothing to worry about?

P: I knew I was worrying unnecessarily. Other people don't get in a fix like this, I just couldn't help it.

T: When you say you couldn't help it, what do you mean?

P: Once I start worrying I can't stop, it's like I can't get it out of my head.

T: Did you do anything to try and get it out of your head?

P: Yes, I tried to work out how much risk there really was, I tried to reassure myself, but it seemed to make it worse.

T: It seems as if you tried not to worry some of the time and at other times you tried to reason with the worry. Why didn't you just let the worry happen without doing anything?

P: Then it would never go away, it would end up ruining the day and I'd be an emotional wreck.

T: What do you mean it would never go away?

P: I'd be out of my mind, I wouldn't be able to stop it.

T: So you tried to reason things out and tell yourself there was nothing to worry about in order to prevent that from happening. Is that right?

P: Yes, it's a terrible thing when it starts.

T: How much do you believe on a scale of zero to one hundred per cent that you could lose control of worry and be unable to stop it?

P: If I didn't do anything, I think it could happen 80 per cent.

T: How much do you believe that what you did at the weekend prevented loss of control or being out of your mind?

P: It would have been much worse if I'd not reassured myself, about 60 per cent.

In this example, detailed examination of the use of worry-control behaviours was used to prime information concerning the dangers of not using control. Here, control behaviours used by the patient consisted of telling himself not to worry, and self-reassurance by analysing the risks in the situation. Meta-worry focused on worry being uncontrollable, and worry leading to loss of mental functioning. The control behaviours were seen as preventing these negative events.

A similar analysis of avoidance and the aims of avoidance can be under-taken to determine meta-worry concerns. In this situation the consequences of not avoiding stimuli/situations should be questioned.

### Experimental strategies

When meta-worries and beliefs concern themes of loss of control, mental illness, and abnormality, individuals with GAD are often uncomfortable about disclosing this material. In some cases there is a fear that the therapist will confirm that particular presenting symptoms are a sign of mental illness or abnormality, and so these themes are avoided. In other cases these fears are readily accessible to the patient when in the worried/ruminatory mode, but are less apparent and tangible when not in this mode. During the course of treatment behavioural experiments in which the patient is encouraged to dwell on worry topics and engage in worry episodes can provide a means of determining meta-worries. However, worry induction tends to subjectively differ from 'naturally occurring' worry episodes. Nevertheless, discussion of the nature of this contrast can yield useful information.

## Questionnaire assessment

Self-report instruments for assessing dimensions of worry (including Type 2 worry) and beliefs about worry were reviewed in Chapter 2. The Anxious Thoughts Inventory (AnTI: Wells, 1994b) is particularly useful in the present context, since this measure of worry proneness has three subscales that assess Type 1 and Type 2 worry separately (see Chapter 2). The Meta-Cognitions Questionnaire (MCQ: Cartwright-Hatton & Wells, 1997) offers a measure of positive and negative beliefs about worry. Both measures are reproduced in the Appendix.

### Generalised anxiety disorder scale (GADS)

The GADS (reproduced at the back of this book) is a multi-component rating scale for measuring distress, positive and negative beliefs, behaviours, and control strategies considered important in the maintenance of GAD as predicted by Wells's (1995) cognitive model.

### Thought control questionnaire (TCQ)

The TCQ, developed by Wells and Davies (1994), is a 30-item instrument which assesses five empirically distinct types of strategies used to control unpleasant and/or unwanted thoughts: (1) distraction (e.g. 'I do something that I enjoy'); (2) social control (e.g. 'I ask my friends if they have similar thoughts'); (3) worry (e.g. 'I focus on different negative thoughts'); (4) punishment (e.g. 'I punish myself for thinking the thought'); and (5) reappraisal (e.g. 'I try to reinterpret the thought'). The questionnaire was initially devised as a research instrument but is useful for eliciting control behaviours and for measuring the extent of thought control attempts as a treatment outcome measure.

Two more general measures of worry that may be considered—although they do not provide separate information on meta-worry are the Penn-State Worry Questionnaire and the Worry Domains Questionnaire.

### Penn-State Worry Questionnaire (PSWQ)

The PSWQ is a 16-item questionnaire developed by Meyer, Miller, Metzger and Borkovec (1990) to evaluate an individual's tendency to worry in general, not related to specific worry topics. The items reflect a tendency to worry excessively and chronically. For example: 'I worry all the time'; 'Many situations make me worry'; 'Once I start worrying I cannot stop'. Responses are requested on a 5-point rating scale ranging from 'not at all typical' to 'very typical'. The scale shows good psychometric properties and initial data suggests that it is responsive to treatment effects (see review by Molina & Borkovec, 1994; Borkovec & Costello, 1993).

### Worry domains questionnaire (WDQ)

The WDQ was developed by Tallis, Eysenck and Mathews (1992), as a content measure of worry. Twenty-five items are used to tap five domains of worry: worry about relationships (e.g. 'that I will lose close friends'); lack of confidence (e.g. 'that I lack confidence'); aimless future (e.g. 'that I'll never achieve my ambitions'); work (e.g. 'that I don't work hard enough'); and financial (e.g. 'that I am not able to afford things'). Respondents are asked to indicate how much they worry about each of the items and make their responses on a scale of: 'not at all, a little, moderately, quite a bit, and extremely'. Total score provides a measure of frequency of worry, while individual items can be examined to determine the content of most salient concerns. For further information the reader should refer to Tallis, Davey and Bond (1994).

## FROM COGNITIVE MODEL TO CASE CONCEPTUALISATION

To construct a GAD conceptualisation a recent and specific problematic worry episode should be reviewed and the data needed to construct the model elicited. Several episodes may be sampled in a similar way to build-up the full range of data for an overall conceptualisation. The model is necessarily somewhat complex because it includes two types of worry and

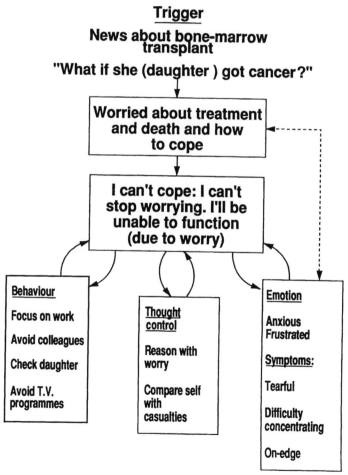

**Figure 8.1**  A cross-sectional idiosyncratic GAD case conceptualisation

belief, and feedback loops among them. However, it is simplified in practice by prioritising parts of the model. More specifically, the lower half of the model incorporating negative interpretation of worry (meta-worry) and resulting behaviours and affect should be formulated first. This serves in simplifying the model for socialisation. Later treatment sessions focus on eliciting the role of positive beliefs and the problems associated with the use of worry as a coping strategy.

An excerpt of the guided questioning used to construct the conceptualisation shown in Figure 8.1 is presented below:

P: I heard about that girl who is having the bone-marrow transplant, and I thought: That could happen to my daughter. What if she got cancer? I wouldn't be able to cope.

T: So your worry was triggered by having the thought that your daughter could get cancer. What happened next? Did you go on to think other things, or did you do anything about the worry?

P: I thought of all the bad things that could happen. All of the horrible treatment that she would have to go through, and what I would do if she died.

T: It sounds as if you rehearsed in your mind all the worst things that might happen. Is that right?

P: Yes, it's like I have to think of all the worst possibilities, and then somehow I'll be prepared if they do happen.

T: It's interesting that you've said that, and I'd like to come back to that idea later. For the moment though, can you tell me what you thought next?

P: I thought, Oh no, I'm worrying again, I must stop it.

T: Why must you stop it?

P: Because its making me feel bad, and it just makes me think that I can't cope.

T: What do you mean by can't cope?

P: Well, obviously I can't cope otherwise I wouldn't be worrying like this.

T: Maybe you think dwelling on these things is a way of coping?

P: Yes I suppose I do, but when I start worrying I can't stop.

T: How did you feel when you thought you couldn't cope or stop worrying?

P: I felt anxious and frustrated with myself.

T: So what did you do when you thought: Oh no, I'm worrying again? Did you do anything to try and stop it?

P: Yes, I tried to get on with my work and I avoided the people I work with in case I overheard them talking about it.

T: Did you avoid anything else?

P: No, I don't think so.

T: Did you do anything else to put your mind at rest?

P: I checked that my daughter was feeling well when I got home.

T: Did you try to control your thoughts?

P: I tried to talk myself out of it.

T: How did you do that?

P: I told myself it wouldn't happen.

T: If you had not tried to stop your worry could anything bad have happened?

P: Yes, I would have ended up embarrassing myself.

T: How would that have happened?

P: I would have started crying and been unable to function properly.

T: What do you mean by unable to function. What would have stopped you functioning?

P: I just wouldn't be able to concentrate on anything, and I wouldn't get my work done.

T: Do you get any other symptoms when you're worried?

P: Yes. I feel on-edge all the time, like I can't rest.

T: Because worrying is such a problem has it affected what you pay attention to? For example, are you more sensitive to certain types of information?

P: Yes. I'm sensitive to news about illness or accidents in the newspaper. And I avoid medical dramas on television. If I do see something I have to read it and work out if the people involved are like me. If they are, I worry more.

In this example the patient was worried that her daughter may become ill. There were some initial indications of worrying being used as a means of self-reassurance about coping. Type 1 worry consisted of worry about treatment and death. Guided questioning revealed specific meta-worries and associated behaviours, thought control strategies, cognitive biases, and emotional responses. Treatment initially focused on socialising the patient in this model and proceeded to challenge belief in negative meta-worries.

A complete idiosyncratic case formulation of a different GAD patient incorporating positive and negative meta-beliefs and maintenance cycles is presented in Figure 8.2 for guidance.

## SOCIALISATION

Dimensions of the formulation can be illustrated with in-session and homework experiments, and also with particular lines of questioning. Education in the role of worry about worry and counter-productive responses in maintaining GAD is a primary goal.

### Socialisation questions

The central component of the model, and that which it can be difficult for patients to grasp, is the concept that it is not only worry about external events or non-cognitive internal events that is the problem, but also worry

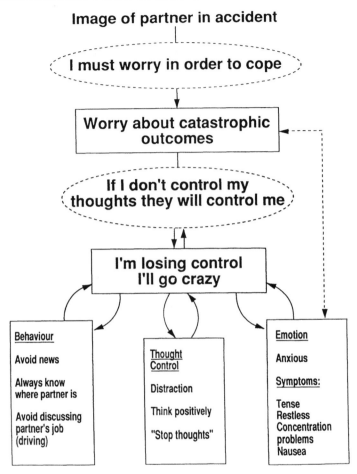

**Figure 8.2**  A full GAD case conceptualisation

about worrying. Later in treatment it is also necessary to convey that the problem is associated with the motivated use of worrying as a processing strategy, and this implies that some beliefs are held about the benefits of worrying.

## Selling meta-worry

To introduce the concept of meta-worry and provide a model for the patient to use in understanding the problem, the therapist should emphasise the shifting focus of worry content. In this strategy the therapist questions: 'If you were to stop worrying about X (a particular topic) would that solve your

problem?' The GAD patient usually concedes that he/she would find something else to worry about. This should be followed by the question: 'Is it
better therefore to try and deal with individual worry topics as they occur,
or to deal with factors that keep the tendency to worry going?' These questions help to establish that it is not the content of worry (Type 1 worry) that
is the problem, and the problem lies with factors that cause worry to be
repeatedly activated. Once this idea is in place the therapist should then
suggest that part of the problem may be what the patient thinks about
worrying. The role of negative beliefs (appraisals) and behaviour can be
illustrated with hypothetical scenarios. For example:

T: Most people worry. It's quite normal to do so. Some people worry a lot
and are not distressed by this while others are very distressed. Why do
you think some people who worry a lot are not bothered by it?
P: I don't know.
T: People who are not bothered do not worry about worry. Some of them
. think that worry is a good thing. Is your worry a good thing?
P: No. It's getting me down.
T: If you believed that your worry was a good thing—let's say you believed
that you had to worry in order to survive—would it get you down?
P: No. I'd be worried about not worrying.
T: So that suggests that worrying is a problem for you partly because you
worry about it.

As illustrated in this example, the fact that worry is a normal phenomenon can
be used to explore dimensions of worrying that are problematic for the individual. Here, the emphasis rests on questioning why it is that worry is a problem
for only some people when in fact almost everyone worries. The aim is the elicitation of negative appraisals of worry, and the problem should be framed in
terms of these negative appraisals (e.g. If you no longer believed that your worry
is uncontrollable, how much of a problem would be left? If you didn't believe that
your worries are harmful, how much would you be bothered by them?).

A different but related strategy consists of asking the patient to consider a
hypothetical situation in which they were able to think each time they worried: 'there's another worry, it doesn't really matter', and they believed this
thought. The therapist then questions how much of a problem worrying
would be in these circumstances.

## The worrying thoughts record (WTR)

The worrying thoughts record is a self-report protocol for recording a range
of data useful for increasing patients' awareness of meta-worries. It can be
used to facilitate socialisation in the model, and for structuring the use of

repeated reattributions. Eight response columns comprise the WTR, as illustrated in Table 8.1

In the first column day and date are recorded, and then a brief description of the situation in which worry occurred is given. The trigger for worry is the third entry in the WTR. The trigger may be internal, such as another intrusive thought (image) or external, such as hearing a particular news item. The content of the initial worry is then reported, and worry about worry, and emotional responses (including somatic state) are noted. The next column requires a response to worry about worry. The response is a rational response based on verbal reattributions made in therapy or it is an account of the conduct of, and results of, a behavioural experiment. The final column of the WTR can be used to record the outcome of answering worry about worry, re-rating emotion and making any other useful summary notes. Initially, some patients experience difficulty in identifying worry about worry and will record other responses to Type 1 worry. However, by examining these responses it is possible to determine the nature of worry about worry by questioning the need for responses or the consequences of not engaging in the responses noted.

## Socialising experiments

Having established the role of worry about worry, the therapist proceeds to examine—with the aid of discussion and experimental techniques—the role of counter-productive behaviours in worrying. This should proceed in accordance with the patient's idiosyncratic behavioural and thought control strategies. Two particular experiments are useful for demonstrating vicious cycle effects in the model: suppression experiments and 'what if' reasoning experiments.

### Suppression experiment

The literature on thought suppression shows how attempts 'not to think' certain thoughts can have a paradoxical effect of making the target thought more likely to intrude. This effect can be used to demonstrate the effect of trying 'not to think' or control unwanted thoughts in GAD. This should be presented as an open-ended experiment to determine what happens if the patient is asked 'not to think about' a thought (e.g. a white bear) for 'three minutes'. The procedure typically results in difficulty dismissing the thought completely or repeated intrusions of the thought. This effect is then discussed in terms of the patient's attempts not to think particular worries: 'If trying not to think a thought makes it occur more, what happens if you try not to think a worry, or try not to think about something that might trigger a worry?' Demonstration of the unhelpful effects of thought control is a prerequisite to banning control activities.

**Table 8.1**   The Worrying Thoughts Record (WTR)

| Date | Situation | Trigger | Description of worry | Worry about worry | Emotion (0–100) | Response to worry about worry | Outcome: Re-rate emotion |
|------|-----------|---------|----------------------|-------------------|-----------------|-------------------------------|--------------------------|
|      |           |         |                      |                   |                 |                               |                          |

*Instructions:* When you notice yourself worrying or feeling anxious, make a note of the situation in which it occurred. Write down the trigger for your worry (this may be another thought or image), and make a brief note of your worry. Try to be aware of negative thoughts you have about your worry and note these in the worry about worry column. Next write down your emotional reaction and rate its intensity (0–100). Make a note of your response to worry about worry (your therapist will explore new responses with you in treatment). Finally re-rate your emotion.

### 'What if' experiment

Some patients report extended worry in an attempt to solve problems and improve coping capacity. These strategies extend worry and increase the range of catastrophic possibilities that can be contemplated. The 'what if' experiment is intended to demonstrate how using a worrying style of thinking exaggerates problems. It can thus be used to socialise patients in the unhelpful effects of worry, and the counter-productive effects of trying to reason with worries as a control strategy. The therapist plays the role of the patient's 'What if . . . ' worrying style for a specified worry, and the patient is required to reason with and answer each 'what if' question. With each patient response the therapist presents a further negative 'what if' possibility representing the worst scenario. An example follows:

T: I'd like to try an experiment with you to see what happens when you try to reason-out all the possibilities in a worry. Let's start with your worry: 'What if my husband is involved in a road accident?' I'm going to be your worry and ask you a series of 'what if' questions and I'd like you to try and reason with them and give yourself a sense that you can cope. I'll start us off. What if my husband's involved in an accident?

P: It depends how serious it is.

T: What if it's serious?

P: He'll have to go to hospital.

T: What if he's seriously ill in hospital?

P: I don't know how I'd cope. I'd have to tell the children. I can see him lying in bed with tubes everywhere.

T: What if it were uncertain whether he'd live?

P: I'd be alone with the children and I'd miss him. I'd ask my parents to help.

T: What if he died and they become too old to help?

P: My life would be so depressing. I'd lose my nerves.

T: What if I lost my nerves?

P: I couldn't manage the children anymore.

T: What if I couldn't manage them?

P: They'd be taken away. They wouldn't have much life and there wouldn't be anything left for me. I'd probably end up in hospital.

T: OK. Let's stop at this point. What happened as we worried?

P: It just became more and more negative.

T: That's right, more and more negative possibilities were generated. How useful do you think that is in reducing stress and helping you cope.

P: Well, it's not useful at all. I can see how I'm just giving myself more to worry about.

In summary, this strategy can be used to demonstrate how the use of a 'what if . . . ' worrying style generates its own problems, and how trying to reason with worry prolongs rumination. It should be concluded that using worry to solve problems or cope, or trying to reason with worrying, can be counter-productive.

*Selling worry as a motivated strategy*

At a later stage in the treatment process, it is necessary to introduce patients to the concept that the use of worry to solve problems is supported by patients beliefs about worry. Typically, this stage follows modification of negative beliefs. However, some GAD patients ask why it is that they worry in the first place. At this juncture the role of positive beliefs should be discussed. Positive beliefs can be elicited with the advantages–disadvantages worry analysis as outlined earlier, and with reference to positive belief ratings on the Meta-Cognitions Questionnaire.

## MODIFYING META-WORRY AND NEGATIVE BELIEFS

We have seen how the overall formulation can be generated in stages. Treatment also proceeds in stages in which meta-worry and associated negative beliefs are the focus of the earlier sessions of treatment, and positive beliefs about worry become an increasing focus later on. In this section techniques for modifying belief in meta-worries and negative beliefs are presented. Treatment based on Wells's (1995) model shifts the emphasis of intervention away from teaching GAD patients ways of controlling worry characteristic of early anxiety management approaches, and it shifts away from purely challenging Type 1 worries. The primary aim is to challenge Type 2 worries, and negative and positive beliefs. A range of strategies for accomplishing this are reviewed here. The technique of controlled worry periods, originally developed by Borkovec, Wilkinson, Folensbee and Lerman (1983b) is discussed in the context of the present model. In this context it differs in subtle and important ways from its original implementation. The clinician should keep in mind that whichever procedures are used, they should be presented in a way that maximises disconfirmation of meta-worry and negative and positive worry-beliefs. Typically, treatment consists of challenging uncontrollability beliefs, challenging other meta-beliefs and meta-worries, challenging positive meta-beliefs, and practise in alternative processing strategies, in this sequence.

## VERBAL REATTRIBUTION

### Questioning the evidence

The evidence supporting meta-worry concepts can be questioned in several ways. Questioning typically opens with the standard line: 'What makes you think that (idiosyncratic catastrophe, e.g. worrying can make you crazy)?'. This is followed by probes for other sources of evidence. Responses to this line of questioning will reveal either no evidence, in which case elicitation of counter-evidence should follow, or the patient provides some evidence to support meta-worry. If evidence is presented, the quality of the evidence should be questioned and *alternative explanations for the evidence* elicited. The following extract illustrates this principle:

T: How much do you believe that worry can make you go crazy?
P: I'm sure it can. Eighty per cent.
T: What makes you think that worry can cause you to go crazy?
P: I don't know. It just feels so unpleasant.
T: It feels unpleasant when you worry. But is that evidence of going crazy?
P: It could be I suppose. I don't know. You tell me, what is it like to go crazy?
T: It depends what you mean by crazy. What do you mean?
P: Losing your mind, thinking all weird thoughts, like what happened to my mother.
T: What happened to your mother?
P: Well she gradually got worse, and finally she had a breakdown and was taken to hospital.
T: Do you think that will happen to you?
P: Well, she always worried a lot, and then it just took her over.
T: Is that what makes you think worry could make you crazy?
P: Yes it is. I think that could happen to me.
T: How do you know that it was worry that caused her problem?
P: I suppose I don't really.
T: Are there other reasons that she might have had a breakdown?
P: She was depressed a lot.
T: OK. So do you have good evidence that worry will make you go crazy?
P: No, I don't really have evidence it can make you crazy. But, surely it can't be very good for you.
T: Let us look at the evidence that suggests it's bad. What makes you say that?

This line of questioning was followed by a review of evidence supporting the idea that worry is harmless. It may have been equally effective if the therapist had followed up with a consideration of the mechanism by which worry may cause mental breakdown (see below). The line of questioning was followed by a behavioural experiment in which the patient tried to go crazy during a worry episode.

## Questioning the mechanism

Questions directed at the causal mechanism by which worry could lead to catastrophe offers a means of eroding the validity of belief in meta-worry.

Often, the person with GAD will not have thought through possible mechanisms, and difficulty specifying a causal pathway loosens belief. In some cases, when a mechanism is articulated, the evidence supporting the mechanism and the counter-evidence is reviewed. For example, if a hypothesised mechanism for worry causing 'mental breakdown' is stress, discussion may focus on evidence showing that stress does not cause *mental breakdown* (e.g. soldiers do not tend to experience mental breakdown even though they have intense stress and worry: individuals taking examinations suffer stress but not mental breakdown). The evolutionary perspective may also be evoked in this type of context: Humans evolved from highly stressful primitive conditions on earth. How could we have survived if stress caused mental breakdown?

## Challenging uncontrollability appraisals

Since worry is a complex attentionally demanding mental activity, it is generally displaceable by competing mental activities. Modulators of worry are those events or activities that naturally interrupt or stop the perseveration of worry. When identified, the presence of modulators in the patient's experience can be used to illustrate that worry is controllable, thus counteracting appraisals of uncontrollability. (Note, however, that it is important to look beyond appraisals of uncontrollability and at the consequences of non-control as well.)

In the following example discussion of modulators is used to challenge belief in uncontrollability:

T: On a scale of zero to one hundred per cent, how much do you believe that you have no control over your worrying?

P: I don't have much control. I believe 70 per cent I can't control it.

T: When was the last time you were seriously worried?

P: This morning I was worried, because I sent my son to school and I think he's catching a cold.

T: Was that worry controllable?

P: No, I couldn't stop thinking about it all morning.

T: Did you try to stop thinking about it?

P: Yes, I told myself he would be OK but it didn't help much.

T: What eventually stopped you worrying?

P: A neighbour called and I forgot about it for a while. It didn't seem so bad after that.

T: Something happened to take your mind off the worry. If it was uncontrollable would taking your mind off it make it go away?

P: No, it would be there all the time.

T: That's right. Can you think of other times when doing something, or when something happened it interrupted the worry?

P: Yes, sometimes if I read or do something interesting I stop worrying.

T: OK. So what do you make of that?

P: It means that I can learn to control it.

T: There are problems with trying to control worry. I would like to talk about that in a minute. I was thinking that perhaps its not out of control in the first place. What do you think?

P: Yes, I can see that it can be interrupted, so it must be controllable.

T: How much do you believe it's uncontrollable?

P: I believe it less, say, 20 per cent.

### Education (normalising worry)

Worry is a normal phenomenon. Most people worry on a weekly basis. For example, in a study by Wells and Morrison (1994), 38 individuals were given a diary in which to record their first two worries and first two intrusive thoughts over a two-week period. Thirty subjects returned their diaries. All of these subjects reported experiencing worries over the two-week period.

If we assume that the non-respondents did not worry and therefore did not think it worth while to return their diaries, then this conservative estimate suggests that at least 79 per cent of people report worrying over a fixed two-week period.

The type of data reviewed above is useful for normalising the occurrence of worrying. Individuals with generalised anxiety are prone to assume that worrying is abnormal, and if they disclose that they worry they will be negatively evaluated by others. Data on the natural occurrence of worrying can be used to correct such distortions. In a similar vein, worriers may assume that worry is damaging or indicative of mental illness. Data on the frequency of worry offers a potentially useful reference for challenging these appraisals and beliefs (e.g. if 79 per cent of people worry over a given two-week period, does that mean 79 per cent of people are mentally ill?). Therapists should present corrective data when this is necessary, and follow up with a behavioural experiment such as a mini-survey to reinforce new information.

### Dissonance techniques

The co-existence of positive and negative beliefs about worry provides an opportunity to induce cognitive dissonance with a view to loosening belief

systems and enhancing motivation for change. Heightened cognitive dissonance is achieved when two incompatible and contradictory beliefs or appraisals are activated and held to be true at the same time. In the present
model the dissonant state can be heightened by eliciting both positive and
negative beliefs and emphasising that they cannot co-exist. For example, the
belief that worry is harmful contradicts the belief that it is helpful, or the
belief that it can cause illness contradicts the belief that it keeps the individual safe.

An illustration of use of dissonance induction to challenge belief is presented below:

T: I'd like us to focus on your belief that worry is harmful. How much do
you believe that?

P: If I continued to worry I'm sure it would affect my mind and body. I'll
say 60 per cent.

T: If you believe it's harmful why continue to worry?

P: I can't help it. It's as if I've got to find something to worry about.

T: What do you mean by that?

P: Once I start worrying I've got to work it through in my mind until I feel
better, and then I think I'll be better able to cope in the future if anything
bad happens.

T: So you seem to be saying that prolonging worry helps you cope in the
future?

P: Yes. I suppose that's right, I do think that.

T: It sound as if you have conflicting beliefs about your worry. On the one
hand you think it helps you cope, on the other hand you think it's
harmful. I'm not sure both can be true; which one will you go for?

P: I see what you mean. Maybe worrying isn't that harmful then.

T: How much do you now believe it's harmful?

P: About 20 per cent.

T: What's keeping your 20 per cent belief going?

P: Although worrying might not be as harmful as I first thought, I suppose
it could be a problem if you do it too much.

T: But if you do it even more, won't that help you cope even better?

P: Even good things can be harmful if you do too much of them.

T: Maybe we should run an experiment to see if you can actually harm
yourself with worry.

In this example the elicitation of dissonance through guided questioning
weakened the negative belief. The result may have gone in the opposite
direction of weakening the positive belief while maintaining or
strengthening the negative belief. No matter in which direction the change

occurs the outcome is desirable since treatment aims to modify both types of belief. However, if the negative belief remains unchanged or strengthened the therapist should continue with verbal and behavioural reattributions directed at the negative belief.

## Imagery techniques

Although definitions of worry emphasise that it is a predominantly verbal-ruminative activity, it may partially consist of images during the course of the worry episode, or images may serve as a trigger for worry periods. The role of images in worrying should be explored. Often images represent frozen aspects in time in which negative and catastrophic events occur. Moving events on in time in which the patient images coping effectively with negative scenarios can be used as an alternative to verbal problem-solving (worry-based) strategies. However, imagery modification should not become a source of self-reassurance or safety that prevents the disconfirmation of dysfunctional beliefs. It should be used in a context that facilitates belief change. Thus, imagery modification should not become a means of preventing feared events associated with continued worrying. That is, imaging should not be used as a means of stopping worry when appraised dangers of worrying are still present. (Refer to 'Strategy shifts', p. 232, for further discussion.)

## BEHAVIOURAL EXPERIMENTS

In this section the use of behavioural strategies in cognitive therapy of GAD are considered. Some of these techniques may be familiar to therapists who have used behaviourally-based treatment approaches to worry. However, the cognitive model presented here leads to changes in the emphasis, aims and implementation of some procedures.

## Controlled worry periods

Stimulus control applications to the treatment of worry have been devised by Borkovec et al. (1983b). This technique is based on theorising that worry is learned as a coping response to an initial fear reaction, and it represents cognitive reactions whose aim is to avoid future trauma. Moreover, Borkovec et al. (1983b) assumed that worry is uncontrollable and therefore becomes associated with a wide range of environmental circumstances thereby leading to poor discriminative control of the activity. Stimulus control treatment is intended to restore discriminative control, and to make use of worry periods in which individuals engage in alternative strategies of problem solving in an attempt to eliminate their worries. The stimulus control procedure, as originally advocated (Borkovec et al. 1983b), involves the following elements:

1. Identifying worrisome thoughts.
2. Establishment of a 30-minute worry period to take place at the same location each day.
3. Catching oneself worrying, postponing the worry period and replacing it with attending to present-moment experiences.
4. Using the 30-minute worry period to worry about one's concerns and engage in problem solving to eliminate those concerns.

Worry control periods are highly effective strategies in the present treatment. However, the cognitive model of GAD outlined in this chapter modifies the aim and emphasis of worry control strategies in a number of important ways. First, the emphasis shifts away from concepts of diminished control over worrying and shifts towards distorted beliefs about uncontrollability and beliefs about the negative and positive consequences of worrying. Second, the present model implies that worry itself is used as a problem-solving strategy in some cases. Therefore, it may not be useful to encourage a worry period plus problem solving as a means of eliminating rumination. This encourages rumination about topics and reinforces beliefs about the need to ruminate on one's concerns. Third, the emphasis of the present model on meta-appraisal suggests that worry control strategies are prone to reinforce beliefs about the need for control by preventing exposure to situations that can disconfirm dysfunctional meta-worries and beliefs. For example, if GAD patients believe that if they fail to control worry this will lead to mental illness, the use of control within a stimulus control framework is likely to establish greater subjective control but is not likely to modify the meta-belief that worry causes mental illness.

In view of these considerations, worry control procedures based on the cognitive model should be designed to challenge belief in *idiosyncratic meta-worries* and *beliefs*. In this context control procedures can serve as powerful behavioural experiments, although their implementation differs from the stimulus control method. In the present treatment worry control is modified and used in a way to challenge beliefs about uncontrollability, and challenge beliefs about the dangers of worrying. The precise application in each of these contexts is outlined below.

## Challenging uncontrollability beliefs

Worry control experiments can be used to modify patients' belief in the uncontrollability of worrying. Here the rationale should be:

> Worrying is a demanding and complex thought process. Although it may seem uncontrollable this is not the case, as is evident from occasions when you have stopped yourself from worrying or when something has happened to take your mind away from worrying. In order for you to find out more about your worrying I would like you to try the following:
>
> 1. When you first notice that you are worrying, postpone your worry by telling yourself that you will give yourself time to think about your problem later in the day.
> 2. Think of a time in the day when you will allow yourself 15 minutes to worry.
> 3. When the time arrives, and only if you feel it is necessary to do so, allow yourself to worry for 15 minutes only. (Make a note of why you felt it was necessary to worry.)

When this procedure is practised patients typically report that they were successful in postponing their worries and often did not use the specified worry period. Belief in uncontrollability of worries should be rated before and after this procedure (note the differences between this procedure and the Borkovec et al. (1983b) stimulus control application).

## Loss of control experiments

Postponement strategies offer only one means of challenging uncontrollability cognitions. Specified worry periods can be used for attempting to 'lose control' over worrying thereby establishing that loss of control is not possible. Paradoxically, when the individual tries to lose control of worrying, loss of control seems less likely and worry appears better regulated than initial appraisals suggest. Variants of paradoxical experiments should be used to challenge related catastrophic beliefs concerning loss of behavioural control, mental illness, humiliation, performance failure, etc., resulting from failure to control worrying. Thus patients should be encouraged to 'push their worrying' to the limit and attempt to lose control of their mind or behaviour. It is often necessary to practise this several times and with each attempt the patient tries harder to cause the feared catastrophe.

## Pushing worry limits in-situ

In order to challenge meta-worries and beliefs concerning the consequences of worrying, experiments should culminate in individuals exaggerating their worries to test out feared consequences during problematic worry episodes rather than only in planned worry periods. The individual may be asked to engage in heightened catastrophising, to deliberately have crazy thoughts, or to try to lose mental control. By observing the impact of these strategies on the reaction of others, on the situation, or on oneself, specific dysfunctional beliefs can be disconfirmed.

### Abandoning thought control

We have seen how suppression strategies, distraction, and attempts to main-tain control, such as keeping control of one's mind, are among the be-haviours that the individual uses to avert feared consequences of worrying. Behavioural experiments in which the patient is encouraged to worry with-out using these safety behaviours should be used to promote full disconfir-mation of dysfunctional beliefs.

Once the problems inherent in using control have been established the use of control strategies should be banned.

### Surveys

Other negative meta-worries and beliefs, in particular those concerning the abnormality of worrying or potential negative responses of others towards worriers, can be challenged by survey techniques. Here the patient is asked to question friends and colleagues to determine if they worry and how they would react to someone who was worrying. Specific questions geared to-wards disconfirming the patient's fears can be generated and these should be added to the patient's survey schedule.

## MODIFYING POSITIVE BELIEFS ABOUT WORRY

Standard verbal reattribution techniques offer effective means of modifying positive beliefs about worrying. For example, the *evidence* supporting the value of worry as a strategy can be questioned, and any *supporting evidence reinterpreted. Counter-evidence*, suggesting that worry is *disadvantageous*, can also be reviewed. Typical counter-evidence includes: worry is a cause of distress; it is a waste of time; it interferes with concentration; it is unrealistic and so provides no advantage for coping in the real world, etc. A particularly effective technique consists of generating examples of situations when worry was not used, and events turned out positively. These occurrences can be used as evidence that it is not necessary for the individual to worry in order to be adequately prepared, or to deal with situations effectively.

## Mismatch strategies

Implicit in the use of worry as a means of anticipating future problems and rehearsing coping options, is the assumption that worries offer accurate depictions of the world and of future events. The ability to question the accuracy of one's worries and generate equally, if not more plausible, alternative mental scenarios is an important therapeutic goal. If worries can be shown to be inaccurate representations of situations, their credibility as a means of coping and positive beliefs about the value of worry are diminished. To achieve this goal the mismatch between the content of worries and the actual events of worried-about situations should be explored. This can be achieved both retrospectively and prospectively.

### Retrospective mismatch

In this procedure the patient is asked to think of a recent time when anticipatory worry occurred, such as before participating in an important social event, or entering an unfamiliar situation. Having identified a situation, the content of the worry is described in as much detail as possible which includes thoughts and images of negative outcomes. Once salient aspects of the worry scenario are noted the patient is then asked to recall the actual events observed in the situation. These are then compared with the events predicted in the worry scenario. The resulting mismatch is used to challenge the accuracy of worries and their usefulness as a coping strategy.

### Prospective mismatch

The mismatch strategy reviewed above relies on memory for events and is therefore somewhat restricted. A similar strategy, which can enhance motivation for reversing avoidance, requires entering worried-about situations and contrasting the content of anticipatory worry with the actual events encountered. In collaboration with the therapist the content of worry should be noted in detail *prior* to entering the situation. If naturally occurring worry cannot be identified, the patient can be instructed to deliberately engage worry about a situation, and the content is noted. For homework, the patient enters the worried-about situation and afterwards writes out a detailed description of the situation to compare against the description depicted in the worry scenario. Belief in the extent to which worries are accurate and useful should be tracked across these procedures.

## Worry abandonment experiments

Experiments in which the person with GAD is encouraged to give-up worrying to determine if negative events occur, provide a means of challenging particular positive beliefs. For example, beliefs that worry protects against the dangers of surprise, or worrying prevents the individual from being punished, can be challenged by banning worry for a fixed period of time in which it is thought that the feared event is likely to happen.

## Worry enhancement experiments

We saw earlier how paradoxical worry enhancement strategies were used to challenge negative beliefs. Experiments in which the individual is encouraged to increase worrying are also effective for challenging positive beliefs. For example, the belief that worry increases mental efficiency or performance can be challenged by increasing the amount of effort and time invested in worrying over a specified time period. The quality of performance for this period should then be compared with the performance for a normal period or non-worry period. No change in performance, or a decrement in performance when worry is intensified, goes against the prediction (based on the belief) that increased worry enhances performance.

## MODIFYING COGNITIVE BIAS

Individuals with GAD are hypervigilant for external threat which is consistent with their Type 1 worries, and are hypervigilant for internal sources of cognitive information which may be consistent with Type 2 meta-worries. Hypervigilance for external sources of threat includes searching for information that is consistent with worries. For example, a person with GAD who was fearful of being attacked scanned the local newspaper for evidence of attacks in his town, and then proceeded to worry at great length about how he could be assaulted, and how he could take precautions to prevent this. The patient reported a tendency to search for information consistent with his worries rather than considering inconsistent evidence. The value of the repetitive nature of this activity was questioned (why not assess risk and plan coping just once rather than repeatedly engage in this activity?) and the therapist introduced a new strategy of scanning the real environment for evidence of *reduced* risk.

The patient's threat-monitoring strategies should be modified in the course of treatment. More specifically, patients should be encouraged to process information that is inconsistent with Type 1 worries. However, this strategy should not become a means of averting feared events associated with worrying; in contrast it offers a means of challenging the validity of Type 1 concerns. Manipulation of the intensity of threat-monitoring strategies as a behavioural experiment also provides a pathway for demonstrating that changes in thinking style do not increase the probability of dangerous events. Hypervigilant threat-monitoring strategies may otherwise maintain a subjective sense of vulnerability.

## STRATEGY SHIFTS

### New endings for old worries

We have seen how worry is used as a coping strategy and it involves chains of negative thought in which worst possibilities are contemplated. In this sense it is a form of negative cognitive rehearsal. Owing to long-standing use of worry strategies some patients have limited experience of contemplating uncertain and mildly stressful events in a positive way. Strategy shifting requires individuals to examine more positive scenarios in association with initial worries and to give at least equal subjective probability to more positive outcomes as they would to catastrophic ones. The initial generation of less catastrophic and more 'positive' outcomes may be problematic at first, and this process should be therapist assisted. The aim of this procedure is to free-up entrenched negative thinking styles and facilitate more flexible thinking in worrying situations.

### Letting go of worries

The antithesis of controlling worries, or using hypervigilant threat monitoring, and trying to reason with worry, is passive 'letting go' of the activity. To some degree this is a requirement of worry control techniques such as the postponement strategies reviewed earlier. Letting worries go is a general strategy shift in which patients are encouraged to acknowledge the presence of a worry to themselves without doing anything with the worry. This may be facilitated by a simple self-statement such as 'Here's another worry—it doesn't mean anything—let it go'; or 'I'm worrying—it doesn't help me—let it go'. The essence of this procedure is the development by the patient of an increased awareness of worrying, and development of new strategies for dealing with worry that are less problematic. This type of procedure is better introduced later in therapy when it is not likely to be used as a control strategy that prevents modification of belief in meta-worries.

### Avoidance

Since avoidance in GAD may relate to Type 1 or Type 2 worries, analysis of the precise function of avoidance is necessary in the planning of effective counter-avoidance strategies. Exposure experiments should be targeted at testing predictions based on both types of worry.

## THE PROBLEM OF CO-MORBIDITY

Worry is a characteristic of most emotional disorders. For example, social phobics worry before entering social situations, health-anxious patients worry about the occurrence of bodily symptoms, obsessional patients worry that they have contaminated food or they may cause a catastrophe by failing to perform an action, and panic-disorder patients worry that the next panic attack could be catastrophic. The model of GAD presented in this chapter asserts that preoccupation and overconcern with worrying is a central feature of GAD. However, GAD patients, like many others, often present with multiple problems. In such cases treatment targets should be prioritised (see Chapter 2). In cases where demoralisation and depression have set in, initial interventions should be targeted at improving mood, counteracting depressive inertia, and restoring a sense of hope. For further information on treating depression see: Beck, Rush, Shaw and Emery (1979) and Burns (1980). In general, when GAD is the primary problem, Type 2 worries and beliefs should be challenged first. The therapist can then assess the contribution of other anxieties to the patient's remaining problem. For example, in some cases, when worry about worry subsides and GAD symptoms improve, there is 'residual' avoidance of situations. This type of avoidance may be a marker for other worries such as social-phobic concerns, or agoraphobic fears that should be conceptualised and treated.

## CONCLUSION

This chapter presents a cognitive model of GAD and the treatment derived from the model. In this framework GAD is conceptualised as a problem of perseverative worry maintained by positive and negative beliefs about the meaning and significance of worrying. Given the interaction of different types of belief and appraisal in the maintenance of the problem, and the primacy of negative beliefs and meta-worry in determining immediate distress, a treatment sequence is advocated. Meta-worry and negative beliefs are modified first in treatment, and then positive worry beliefs and residual Type 1 worries are treated. The habitual nature of worrying for some individuals requires training in strategy shifts in which alternative strategies for dealing with thoughts are practised. However, it is important that these strategies do not become behaviours that patients believe prevent feared catastrophes associated with continued worrying.

An initial target of meta-worry modification is the belief that worry is uncontrollable. This may be challenged by reviewing evidence for individual control, and worry postponement experiments should be used. Controlled worry periods offer a containment strategy when rumination is severe; however, it is crucial that control strategies do not prevent disconfirmation of fears concerning the consequences of worrying. The use of worry-postponement experiments may seem to conflict with the theme that thought-control strategies are counter-productive. However, postponement strategies do not represent attempts 'not to think about' a triggering thought, but are strategies of postponing the conceptual-ruminative process of worrying in response to initial intruding thought. Moreover, postponement experiments are specifically designed to challenge beliefs, whereas naturally occurring suppression strategies preserve dysfunctional beliefs.

Paradoxical experiments in which patients are encouraged to worry more in order to determine the true effects of worrying, and thus challenge negative and positive beliefs, are central techniques for belief change. Avoidance in GAD requires detailed analysis since it may be tied to Type 1 or Type 2 worries. Specific exposure exercises should be similarly linked to disconfirming belief in worries at the respective Type 1 or Type 2 level. Avoidance and other behaviours (e.g. reassurance, evidence seeking) may be subtle, but they should not be overlooked in treatment.

## EXAMPLE TREATMENT OUTLINE

*Session 1*

1. Review a couple of recent worry episodes, and construct a model.
2. Share model.
3. Socialise by questioning the effects of meta-worry, and use a suppression experiment.
4. Homework:
   (a) Complete Worry Thoughts Record (WTR).
   (b) Ban control attempts if appropriate.

*Session 2*

1. Check homework. Fit result to model.
2. Emphasise need to examine negative beliefs about worry and counter-productive control attempts.

3. Verbal and behavioural reattribution of specific negative beliefs (e.g. uncontrollability, danger).
4. Homework:
   (a) Continue WTR.
   (b) Postponed worry experiments.
   (c) Paradoxical experiments (e.g. try to lose control/go crazy).

*Session 3*

1. Check homework. Fit results to model.
2. Elicit negative beliefs and belief level, and challenge (continue paradoxical experiments).
3. Explore nature of avoidance.
4. Homework:
   (a) Behavioural experiments to test predictions (surveys, pushing worry limits, etc.).
   (b) Reverse worry avoidance behaviour.
   (c) Continue thought-control ban.
   (d) Postponed-worry experiment.

*Sessions 4–10*

1. Check homework.
2. Continue challenging specific negative beliefs.
3. Elicit and challenge positive beliefs.
4. Continue exposure experiments.
5. Homework:
   (a) Specific tests of predictions.
   (b) Introduce concept of 'letting go' of worry (ban use of worry as coping).
   (c) Reverse avoidance.

*Sessions 11–14*

1. Check homework.
2. Work on residual negative and positive beliefs.
3. Conceptualise and work on additional problems (e.g. social fears: cognitive therapy of Type 1 worries).
4. Check for residual avoidance and modify.
5. Training in alternative processing strategies.
6. Develop therapy blueprint.

*Note.* Use sessional responses on the Generalised Anxiety Disorder Scale (GADS) to guide the focus of treatment sessions.

Chapter 9

# OBSESSIVE-COMPULSIVE DISORDER

The primary feature of Obsessive-Compulsive Disorder (OCD) is the occurrence of recurrent obsessions or compulsions that are time consuming (take more than one hour a day) or cause marked distress or impairment (DSM-IV; APA, 1994). Obsessions are persistent thoughts, impulses, or images that are experienced as intrusive and inappropriate. For example, a religious person may have persistent blasphemous thoughts, or a mother may have thoughts of harming her new-born child. The most common obsessions concern thoughts about contamination (e.g. becoming contaminated by touching money), doubting (e.g. wondering whether one has locked a door or whether one has unknowingly collided with someone while driving the car), aggressive or horrific impulses (e.g. the urge to shout-out in church, or to hurt one's child), and sexual imagery (e.g. a recurrent pornographic image). Obsessions can be differentiated from other types of intrusive thoughts such as worry (Wells, 1994a; Wells & Morrison, 1994).

A compulsion is a repetitive behaviour that is overt or covert. Overt compulsions include hand washing, checking, ordering or alignment of objects. Covert compulsions are mental acts such as praying, counting, or repeating words. The goal of these acts is to prevent or reduce anxiety or distress. From a cognitive perspective they are intended to neutralise or prevent feared events. In some instances individuals perform stereotyped acts according to idiosyncratic rules, and are often unable to indicate why they are doing them.

In order to meet diagnostic criteria (DSM-IV) for OCD individuals must have recognised at some time during the disorder that the obsession or compulsion is excessive and unreasonable. 'The ability of individuals to recognise that obsessions or compulsions are excessive or unreasonable occurs on a continuum' (DSM-IV; APA, 1994, p. 421). In some cases the obsession may be of delusional magnitude, for example a person may believe that he/she has caused the death of someone by thinking negative thoughts about them. Delusions are beliefs that are held with complete conviction in the presence of contradictory evidence.

If another Axis I disorder is present the obsession or compulsion is not restricted to it. For example, in depression ruminating or brooding on being worthless is a mood-congruent aspect of depression and is not considered an obsession because it is not ego-dystonic. If recurrent distressing thoughts exclusively concern the fear of having, or the idea that one has, a serious illness as in hypochondriasis, then hypochondriasis should be diagnosed. However, if there are concurrent rituals or checking an additional diagnosis of OCD may be indicated.

## PREVALENCE OF OBSESSIONS AND COMPULSIONS

Obsessions and compulsions occur as normal phenomena, differentiated from their OCD counterparts by the distress or disruption they cause. Normal obsessions occur in 80–88 per cent of individuals, and the content of normal and abnormal obsessions are similar (Rachman & de Silva, 1978; Salkovskis & Harrison, 1984). Estimates of the prevalence rates of OCD vary. The Epidemiological Catchment Area survey indicated that the lifetime prevalence of OCD was 2.5 per cent, and the six-month prevalence rate was 1.6 per cent, making it the fourth most common psychiatric disorder in the USA (Karno, Golding, Sorenson & Burnam, 1988).

## COGNITIVE MODELS OF OCD

A wide range of concepts have been evoked in the development of cognitive theoretical models of OCD. Different perspectives have emphasised the role of perfectionistic beliefs (McFall & Wollersheim, 1979), inflated responsibility (Rachman, 1976; Salkovskis, 1985), cognitive deficits or abnormalities in decision making (Reed, 1985; Persons & Foa, 1984; Sher, Mann & Frost, 1984), thought action-fusion (Rachman, 1993) and meta-cognitive beliefs (Clark & Purdon, 1993; Wells & Matthews, 1994).

A diversity in theoretical concepts, lack of a generally agreed framework, and limited research on cognitive dimensions of obsessions contribute to the underdevelopment of cognitive models of obsessive-compulsive disorder. Patients presenting with OCD continue to present a considerable challenge to the therapist. Behavioural treatment consisting of exposure to obsessional stimuli and prevention of ritualistic behaviour (Meyer, 1966) shows consistent positive results (e.g. Foa, Kozak, Steketee & McCarthy, 1992; Marks, Hodgson & Rachman, 1975). The addition of cognitive therapy has yet to show that it consistently improves outcome over and above exposure and response prevention alone.

## The Salkovskis model

A comprehensive cognitive analysis of OCD, and one based within Beck's cognitive theory, has been presented by Salkovskis (1985). Salkovskis's original formulation integrated important cognitive and behavioural concepts in the cognitive formulation of obsessional problems. It combined features of earlier models such as the concept of inflated responsibility (e.g. Rachman, 1976), beliefs about thought and action (e.g. McFall & Wollersheim, 1979) with behavioural principles. One of its most influential contributions is the delineation of the importance of appraisal of intrusions as the major source of distress, rather than the content of the intrusion itself, and an emphasis on the concept of such appraisals relating to the concept of responsibility. More recently, Salkovskis (1989) has elaborated further the role of appraised responsibility in obsessional problems. According to his model, obsessional patients interpret the occurrence of intrusive cognitions as an indication that they may be responsible for harm unless they take action to prevent it. The appraisal of the significance of intrusions is determined by underlying beliefs such as: 'Having a thought about an action is like performing the action; not neutralising when an intrusion has occurred is similar or equivalent to seeking or wanting the harm involved in that intrusion to happen; one should (and can) exercise control over one's thoughts.' Negative appraisals of intrusions occur as negative automatic thoughts and are amplified by states of depressed mood because of the increased accessibility of negative schemata. Once negative appraisals of responsibility occur, the second process characteristic of obsessional problems is the initiation of neutralising responses, which may be internal (e.g. trying to think positive thoughts) or external (e.g. compulsive hand-washing in response to thoughts about contracting disease). Neutralising responses reduce responsibility and discomfort and are maintained by this association, and the recurrence of intrusions becomes more likely because responses to them result in such cognitions acquiring greater salience. The mechanism by which intrusions acquire 'greater salience' is not elaborated in detail. However, one possibility is that attempts to suppress unwanted thoughts leads to a rebound of unwanted thought (e.g. Wegner, Schneider, Carter & White, 1987).

In this model, overt or covert neutralising responses are motivated by beliefs concerning responsibility. Salkovskis, Richards and Forrester (1995) define neutralising as: 'voluntarily initiated and conducted activity which is intended to have the effect of reducing the perceived level of responsibility' (p. 285).

The Salkovskis (1985) model implies that cognitive therapy should concentrate on modifying automatic thoughts and beliefs concerning responsibility for harm. However, other theorists argue that this approach overemphasises the role of responsibility (Clark & Purdon, 1993), and meta-cognitive beliefs concerning the need to control thoughts should be given careful consideration in treatment. Wells & Matthews (1994, 1997) proposed that meta-cognitive beliefs concerning the danger and power of intrusive thoughts, and the attentional strategies used by obsessionals, are relevant in understanding the disorder. They view responsibility appraisals as emergent properties of meta-cognitive processing, and as markers for dysfunctional beliefs about the dangers and influence of thoughts which are more central to OCD.

## The Wells and Matthews meta-cognitive model

Wells and Matthews (1994) present a prototypical model of OCD mapped on a detailed cognitive processing framework of vulnerability to emotional disorder. They suggest that intrusions activate beliefs concerning the significance of the intrusion. These beliefs not only consist of information about intrusions but also consist of knowledge about behavioural responses. Beliefs about behaviour in OCD have received little attention in theoretical accounts. Greater consideration of such beliefs may facilitate conceptualisation of obsessive-compulsive problems.

In a meta-cognitive framework, beliefs about intrusions are relevant in understanding OCD. Rachman (1993) has introduced a useful new concept of 'thought–action fusion' (TAF) which represents meta-cognitive beliefs equating thoughts with actions (e.g. having a thought about harming my children means I am going to harm them). Meta-cognitive beliefs concern the consequences of thoughts (e.g. thoughts can cause actions/events) and the meaning of thoughts for past actions/events (e.g. if I think I have done something bad I probably have done it). Belief in TAF is likely to motivate particular behavioural responses such as trying to control actions or thinking. For example, if an individual believes that having a negative thought means that he/she has done something negative, the individual may engage mental or behavioural checking in an attempt to invalidate the intrusion. For instance a patient had the thought that she had stabbed her children and felt compelled to check her children's bedroom to reassure herself that she had not done so. Implicit in this response was the belief: 'Having this thought means I have probably carried out the action depicted in the thought.' In many cases the obsessional patient intellectually refutes such a belief. However, under triggering conditions, doubt concerning the invalidity of thoughts is likely to increase. At a superordinate meta-cognitive level one might suppose that these examples reflect the existence of a general-purpose belief that intrusive thoughts reflect reality. More specifically, some obsessional patients appear to be operating with a mental-model of experience that blurs important boundaries between internal (cognitive) and external events.

While some behavioural responses, such as covert neutralising or controlling one's mind, may be intended to prevent negative outcomes associated with intrusion, other behaviours are intended to relieve worry and discomfort. In the previous example the individual checked her children in order to terminate her rumination about having harmed them (not to prevent harm). The discomfort-reducing effects of such behaviours is likely to reinforce beliefs about neutralising/checking responses. The obsessional patient is prone to believe that neutralising is beneficial and not neutralising will have negative consequences of at least leading to perpetual worry and discomfort. However, neutralising behaviours and rituals themselves can become a source of distress as they become more time-consuming and are appraised as uncontrollable and dangerous. Two recent cases illustrates the use of checking behaviours to terminate worry–rumination cycles. In one case a 27-year-old sufferer of OCD reported recurrent thoughts that she had beaten up or mutilated her children or friends, and had dumped their bodies in the dustbin. These thoughts were followed by extended periods of rumination in which she attempted to reassure herself that this was not true; however, her doubts led her to check the dustbin in order to relieve her anxiety. In another case, a 36-year-old obsessional patient presented with problems of repeated checking during driving. He would drive his route home from work several times until he felt confident that he had not accidentally collided with someone. His checking was stimulated by intrusive images of having hit someone or by the thought 'What if I've knocked someone down?'. When asked what would happen if he did not check, he reported that he would not be able to 'get it off his mind'.

In summary, it is proposed that beliefs supporting the fusion of thought and action and positive and negative beliefs about rumination and neutralising strategies are relevant in conceptualising OCD. Once an intrusion has been appraised as dangerous, the individual is compelled to select a strategy for overcoming this danger. The strategy selected is determined by beliefs held concerning different strategies. In some instances, the individual will continue to ruminate and reprocess the intrusion, in order to challenge the intrusion's validity. This is likely to be associated with beliefs concerning the appropriateness of such a strategy. However, dwelling on the intrusion is prone to exaggerate rumination and worry, and can lead to secondary problems of fear of worry itself. Another possibility is to engage in neutralising or checking behaviours which can terminate the rumination cycle by mechanisms of distraction, activating 'superstitious' beliefs about safety, or by reality testing of intrusive thoughts. In this model, behavioural and cognitive neutralising and checking responses are aimed at reducing the *danger associated with the initial intrusion* or the *danger associated with sustained rumination* or worry about the intrusion. Overt neutralising can be seen as a behavioural form of rumination which itself can be subject to negative appraisal. In summary, a number of different feedback cycles may operate. With different combinations of cycles operating in different cases. The overall effect is an escalation of distress, and increasing amounts of effort and time required by combinations of negative appraisals and dysfunctional responses to them.

*Attentional strategies*

Apart from specification of meta-cognitive beliefs in OCD, Wells and Matthews (1994, 1997) suggest that the attentional strategies adopted by patients are likely to maintain OCD. More specifically, obsessionals are prone to focus on and monitor their thought processes, this heightened *cognitive self-consciousness* is likely to increase the detection of unwanted target thoughts, and it may even trigger intrusions. Wells and Mathews (1994) suggest that obsessionals have a tendency to assign priority to internally generated events rather than external events. Thus, even when sensory input confirms the execution of a behaviour, individuals focus excessive attention on fantasies concerning the consequences of not performing the action. This tendency to focus on doubts or internal fantasies reduces confidence in memory for actions/events and may contribute to checking behaviour. (Note, however, that checking is also likely to be stimulated by beliefs concerning the advantages of checking.)

# A GENERAL WORKING MODEL

An outline general working model of relationships between beliefs, behaviours and emotion in OCD is depicted in Figure 9.0. This model is intended to be a working template for clinically representing the relationships between key variables in the maintenance of obsessions with compulsions. It is presented as a model for developing individual case conceptualisations.

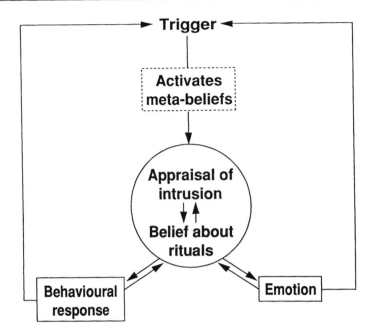

**Figure 9.0**   A cognitive model of OCD

In this model a trigger (most often an intrusive thought or doubt, although an intrusive feeling/emotion can also act as a trigger) activates beliefs concerning the meaning of the trigger. The beliefs relevant at this level include: beliefs about the dangers and meaning of thought encompassing themes of thought–action fusion and thought–event fusion; and beliefs about the consequences of emotion/discomfort. These beliefs influence the nature of appraisals of intrusions. A further influence on appraisals of intrusion results from beliefs that the individual holds concerning rituals and behavioural responses. Two types of belief are relevant here: positive beliefs (e.g. 'If I wash without thinking a bad thought, bad things won't happen'; 'If I don't perform my ritual the feeling will never end'), and negative beliefs (e.g. 'My rituals are out of control'; 'My mental rituals could damage my body'). Beliefs about the dangers and advantages of available responses influence the selection and implementation of behaviours, and influence the intensity of short-term emotional reactions. However, two feedback loops operate, as depicted in Figure 9.0. Anxiety and other negative emotional reactions resulting from the appraisal of intrusions may be subject to negative interpretation; for example, anxious symptoms may be misinterpreted as a sign of loss of control or a sign of other dangers associated with intrusions. Emotional responses increase the likelihood of further intrusions, as depicted by the feedback loop back to trigger. Emotional responses are likely to lower thresholds for the detection of obsessional stimuli. Moreover, the subjective emotional state may act as a trigger in its own right, such that some individuals believe that they will be overwhelmed with negative feelings or that feelings will be unremitting unless a ritual is performed.

The behavioural responses implemented by the OCD patient maintain the problem through two feedback cycles illustrated in Figure 9.0. Behavioural responses prevent disconfirmation of belief in dysfunctional appraisals of intrusions. The non-occurrence of catastrophic actions or events resulting from intrusions is attributed to the ritual and not to the fact that the appraisal of the intrusion is not valid. The feedback cycle back to triggers represents how behavioural responses exacerbate intrusions. Three main mechanisms are involved here: First, attempts to suppress thoughts can cause an enhancement of unwanted thoughts. Second, attempts to ruminate on intrusions or mentally neutralise them can maintain preoccupation with mental events, making intrusion more likely. Third, activities such as repeated checking or cleaning can set up associations between a range of stimuli and intrusions, such that a widening array of stimuli/actions can trigger intrusions. Different overt and covert behavioural responses can be identified, these include: overt checking, rituals, ordering, repeating, washing/cleaning, thought suppression, rumination, counting, focusing, controlling one's mind, distraction.

## DEVELOPING A CASE FORMULATION

In order to translate the preliminary model depicted in Figure 9.0 into an individual case formulation, it is necessary to elicit information concerning: (1) nature of the obsessional and compulsive symptoms; (2) triggering influences; (3) appraisals of the meaning and significance of obsessions *and* compulsions.

### Symptom profile and triggering influences

We saw in Chapter 2 that OCD symptoms can be assessed in terms of parameters such as frequency, duration and associated distress using subjective visual analogue ratings or diary measures. While these data provide information on base rates which is useful for monitoring treatment effectiveness, the data can be useful for discovering patterns in symptoms, and establishing triggers and relationships among affect, intrusive experiences and situational cues. Therapists should review with the patient a recent obsessive-compulsive episode and attempt to elicit triggers for overt and covert neutralising, checking behaviour, etc. Initially patient insight may be poor. An initial aim of treatment is to increase the patient's level of meta-cognitive awareness so that he/she is able to identify intrusive thoughts, doubts or feelings prior to the commission of behavioural responses. This task can be initiated through a detailed review of several recent episodes, through behaviour tests involving exposure to problematic situations, and through detailed self-monitoring.

## Eliciting dysfunctional appraisals

Therapists should aim to explore different categories of appraisals of intrusions, and of responses to intrusions. In assessing appraisals of intrusions, questions should be directed at eliciting dangers linked with intrusions, and the real-world validity of intrusions. The following questions and adaptations are suggested for this purpose:

### Appraisals of intrusions

- When you had (intrusion) how did you feel (e.g. anxious, afraid, guilty)?
- When you felt (e.g. anxious) what thoughts went through your mind?
- Did you have any negative thoughts about the intrusion?
- What did having the thought mean to you?
- What sense do you make out of having these intrusions? Do they tell you anything? What do they tell you about your actions or about events?
- Could anything bad happen as a result of having the intrusion? What could happen?
- Does the intrusion mean something bad has happened? What is that?
- Is it normal to have thoughts like this?
- What would happen if you couldn't get rid of these intrusions? What's the worst that could happen?

### Appraisals of behavioural responses

The present model presents a role for beliefs about behavioural responses in OCD. In developing cognitive conceptualisations of OCD it is useful to explore the appraisals and beliefs associated with the use of ritual behaviours. Some patients are fearful of giving up behaviours because of negative beliefs concerning the consequences of doing this. In other words they have positive beliefs about rituals. In some cases negative beliefs about rituals exist that contribute to distress. The occurrence of rituals in the absence of initial obsessions, suggests that the behaviour is not aimed at reducing a danger associated with a discrete intrusive thought. However, this does not necessarily mean that a danger-related appraisal is not present. In some instances of compulsive behaviour without obsessions, danger appraisals concern the *emotional consequences* of not engaging in the ritualised behaviour. For example, in a recent case of compulsive finger-nail cleaning, it was evident that the behaviour was triggered by subjective feelings of distress. The individual concerned believed that if she did not perform the behaviour her emotions would become 'overwhelming' and she would not be able to function. Furthermore, she believed that her negative feelings would become *permanent*. However, she also reported negative appraisals concerning *loss of control* of her ritual finger-nail cleaning. This negative appraisal contributed to her general level of distress, thus increasing the perceived need to engage in the ritual. Thus the patient was trapped in a vicious cycle of feeling compelled to perform the ritual to reduce distress but appraising the ritual in a way that contributed to distress. Use of the ritual behaviour to reduce the dangers associated with emotion prevented exposure to disconfirmatory experiences, such as the experience that emotion would naturally decay with time.

Examples follow of questions that are useful for eliciting appraisals associated with ritual behaviours. Note that for clinical purposes it is often necessary to elicit material by questioning the worst consequences of not engaging in a ritual behaviour, rather than only questioning about the benefits of engaging in behaviour.

- Do you do anything to prevent (catastrophe associated with intrusion) from happening? What do you do?
- Could anything bad occur if you continue to use the strategy? What is that?
- What's the worst that could happen if you didn't use the strategy?
- Are you bothered by (checking, neutralising, ruminating)? (If so) Why don't you just stop?
- How much control do you have over your (checking, neutralising, rumination)?
- What's the worst that could happen if you don't stop it?
- How does (checking, ruminating, neutralising) help?
- Does your (checking, ruminating, neutralising) keep you safe in some way? How does that work?
- Have you tried to stop?
- Is there a reason for not trying to stop?
- What happens to your feelings/thoughts when you are prevented from (neutralising, etc.)?

## CONCEPTUALISATION INTERVIEW: A CASE EXAMPLE

At this juncture it will be useful to illustrate how the basic questions presented previously are combined to elicit information for building an idiosyncratic case conceptualisation based on the model. An idiosyncratic conceptualisation is presented in Figure 9.1.

The person interviewed was a 24-year-old man with a seven-year history of OCD. His main presenting problem was the experience of repetitive

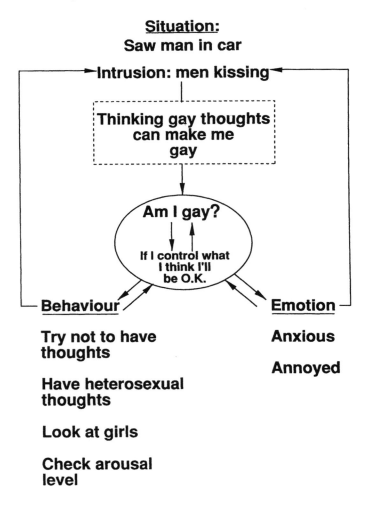

**Figure 9.1**   An idiosyncratic OCD case conceptualisation

intrusive thoughts and images of a homosexual nature. More specifically, he reported intrusive images of two men kissing, and whenever he noticed himself looking at a man in the street he had the intrusive doubt 'Do I find him attractive?'. These obsessions were accompanied by a range of self-reassurance strategies, neutralising strategies, and danger-limitation responses which became clear in the interview. The following abstract illustrates the elicitation of relevant material for constructing the conceptualisation presented in Figure 9.1.

P: The thoughts happen every day.

T: When was the last time you were bothered by these thoughts?

P: This morning I had the thought of men kissing. I was driving to work and I stopped at a junction. There was a young guy sitting in the car next to mine, I didn't want to look at him, but then I got the thought anyway.

T: How did you feel when you got the thought?

P: At first I felt annoyed at having it and I wanted to hit something, but then I felt scared.

T: What were you annoyed about?

P: I'm sick of having these thoughts, I know I'm not gay, so why do I keep having them?

T: If you were gay maybe it wouldn't be so bad to have the thoughts.

P: Yeah, maybe I'd want to have them. But that's not how it is.

T: You said you felt anxious about having the thought. What were you anxious about?

P: I don't know, I just don't want to think these things.

T: What would happen if you couldn't stop thinking them?

P: It scares me to think about that. It would be terrible.

T: What would be terrible about that?

P: Well it might mean that I am gay and I don't realise it.

T: Could it mean anything else bad?

P: Well to tell the truth, one thing that really bothers me is that maybe having these thoughts will make me gay.

T: So it sounds as if the thoughts are distressing because of what they signify, or what they might cause. You seem to be concerned that having the thought will make you gay, is that right?

P: Yes, I keep thinking 'Am I gay?' or something.

T: When you have that thought do you do anything to check that out or prevent it?

P: I don't know what you mean.

T: Do you do anything to prevent yourself from becoming gay?

P: I try not to have the thoughts. I tell myself I'm being stupid, and I think of my girlfriend instead.

T: Anything else?

P: I look at girls in the street to check that I still find them attractive. And I check that I still get turned-on when I'm with my girlfriend. But even that isn't as good lately.

T: What do you mean when you say it's not as good lately?

P: I seem to be getting less turned-on than before.

T: What do you make of that?

P: Well if I let it get to me I could worry about that in the same way.

T: So it sounds as if you try and control your thoughts, and try to stay heterosexually focused. Does that stop you becoming gay?

P: If I could control my thoughts then I'd be OK.

T: OK. Let's take stock of what we've covered so far. It sounds as if you keep getting gay thoughts, and these are bothering you because you interpret them as a sign that you are gay, or that they will cause you to become gay. That's something you don't want, and so you have been doing a number of things to reassure yourself that you're not gay, and some things to try and stop the thoughts from making you gay. Does that sound accurate?

P: Yes, that's exactly it.

T: I think it's very likely that some of the things you're doing right now are keeping your problem going. What do you think?

P: I think you're probably right. But what else should I do?

T: If you believed it was normal to have unwanted thoughts and you knew for sure they couldn't make you gay, do you think you would have a problem with them?

P: No, I wouldn't be too bothered by them.

T: So you see, the problem isn't just one of having gay thoughts, the problem is that you worry about having these thoughts. You have negative beliefs about them and you are using coping strategies that are making the thoughts more frequent, and are preventing you from overcoming your fear of them. How much do you believe that having gay thoughts will make you gay, on a scale of zero to one hundred per cent?

P: Eighty per cent.

T: What we need to do then, is change the way you're responding to gay thoughts and examine the accuracy of your beliefs about them. And that's what we'll be doing over the next few sessions.

This dialogue was followed by presenting the formulation in diagrammatic form (as in Figure 9.1). Socialisation in the model was continued by a behavioural experiment demonstrating the effect of behavioural strategies (thought suppression) on thought frequency and negative appraisals.

## SOCIALISATION

As usual, socialisation proceeds by sharing the conceptualisation with the patient. Socialisation begins in communicating the concept that negative beliefs about intrusions along with behavioural responses, and worry about intrusions are the main problem, rather than the occurrence of the intrusion alone.

Socialisation is facilitated with the use of questions like those in the therapy extract presented earlier. In particular, questions should be directed at determining the consequences in emotional terms of having intrusions if the individual no longer believed that they were harmful or were indicative of negative events.

Thought control experiments, like those discussed in Chapter 8, should be used to demonstrate how behavioural responses exacerbate intrusions and maintain the monitoring of thoughts. The impact of emotional reactions on intrusions (triggers) can be demonstrated by reviewing the effects of mood variation on the frequency of intrusions and doubts.

## GENERAL AIMS OF COGNITIVE THERAPY

The general aim of treatment based on the framework presented in this chapter is the modification of dysfunctional appraisals and beliefs concerning intrusive experience. While the concept of responsibility may be important in these appraisals, particular emphasis here has been directed at beliefs concerning the dangerous nature of intrusions, the fusion between thought and action, and beliefs about ritual/checking responses. In achieving these aims, it is necessary to manipulate the individual's behavioural and rumination strategies in a way that enhances the potential for belief change. A strategy that is effective early in treatment is the suspension of rumination or worry. (These techniques were discussed in Chapter 8 and the reader is referred back to them.) Behavioural experiments should be directed at challenging negative appraisals of intrusive experience, and beliefs about the consequences of not engaging in behavioural responses (rituals). The aim of treatment is the adoption by the patient of a *detached acceptance of intrusive thoughts as irrelevant for further action or processing*. In the remainder of this chapter some specific techniques for achieving these aims are reviewed. There is overlap in the treatment of GAD discussed earlier in this book and the treatment of OCD advocated in this chapter. While distinctions can be made in terms of the content of specific beliefs implicated in GAD and OCD, and in the behaviours employed by individuals, some of the treatment strategies for GAD may be used profitably in treating OCD.

## VERBAL REATTRIBUTION

### Defining the cognitive target and detached mindfulness

We have seen how models of OCD give special emphasis to the concept of appraisal of intrusions and behaviours in the maintenance of obsessional problems. These appraisals occur in the form of worry about intrusions and a differentiation between worry and obsessions is important since it is worry about intrusions that is the target for modification rather than the obsession itself. Initially the appraisal of intrusions in a worrying way can be managed by worry-postponement strategies. Here patients are encouraged to practise 'detached mindfulness' (Wells & Matthews, 1994, 1997) in which they do not engage with intrusions by ruminating on them or by using neutralising strategies. Instead they are encouraged to passively 'let-go' of intrusions—allowing them to occupy their own space without engaging with them. Reductions in distress accompanying this procedure can be used as evidence for the model that responses to intrusions rather than intrusions themselves are the problem.

Some patients are initially reluctant to disengage behaviourally or mentally from intrusions/feelings of discomfort. Failure to systematically implement disengagement strategies are linked to beliefs concerning the negative consequences of not responding to intrusions. These beliefs should be explored in detail, and verbal reattribution methods should be applied to weaken beliefs and enhance compliance with behavioural experiments. The presence of specific behavioural neutralising responses should be used to design behavioural experiments involving abandonment of these behaviours to test beliefs.

Once the role of negative appraisal (worry about intrusions) is established, the occurrence of obsessions should be normalised. That is, the obsessional individual should be educated about the occurrence of obsessions and informed that they are a normal event occurring in about 90 per cent of people. To substantiate these claims, patients may be shown research papers documenting the frequency of normal intrusions, and they may be encouraged to undertake a mini-survey for themselves consisting of asking ten people they know if they experience intrusive or worrying thoughts. These strategies should be followed by recording the content of worries about intrusions, and challenging them using a Dysfunctional Thoughts Record (DTR) specifically modified for obsessional problems. An example of a modified DTR is presented in Figure 9.2.

### The DTR in OCD

Separating intrusions from worries about intrusions on the DTR increases patient discrimination between types of thought and provides the focus for

| Date | Situation | Trigger | Intrusion: Thought/ Doubt/Feeling/ Behaviour Specify | Emotion (note intensity 0-100) | Worry about Intrusion | Answer to Worry | Outcome Emotion Intensity (0-100) |
|------|-----------|---------|--------------------------------------|----------------|-----------------------|-----------------|-----------------------------------|
|      |           |         |                                      |                |                       |                 |                                   |
|      |           |         |                                      |                |                       |                 |                                   |
|      |           |         |                                      |                |                       |                 |                                   |
|      |           |         |                                      |                |                       |                 |                                   |
|      |           |         |                                      |                |                       |                 |                                   |

*Instructions:*   *When you notice yourself having unwanted unpleasant thoughts or engaging in repetitive behaviours, make a note of the Situation where this occurred. In the Trigger column note the activity or event that triggered your unwanted thought or feeling (this may be another feeling or thought). In the Intrusion column describe your initial unwanted thought/image/doubt/discomfort/or behaviour. Specify and rate your emotional response under Emotion and then write in your main negative interpretation (Worry) about the intrusion. Make a note of how you responded to the intrusion in the Answer column, and finally re-rate your Emotion.*

**Figure 9.2**   A Dysfunctional Thoughts Record of OCD

treatment on worry about intrusions rather than on the intrusion itself. Standard verbal reattribution techniques can be applied to these worries, such as labelling the nature of cognitive distortions that they contain, questioning the evidence, and generating rational responses. The reattribution process should not become a rumination experience in its own right, and if there is a danger of this it is better to return to worry abandonment strategies, and challenge underlying beliefs and assumptions about intrusions through behavioural experiment. Repeated systematic use of DTRs is recommended to increase the patient's awareness of thoughts and the relationship between them in contributing to the problem. Specific in-session practise in completing the DTR may be necessary to overcome initial fear of self-monitoring, and for the patient to acquire sufficient discriminative insight and awareness.

## Thought–action defusion

While behavioural experiments provide one of the more powerful techniques for challenging beliefs of thought—action fusion (TAF), verbal methods should not be neglected. In this respect the therapist should aim to teach 'thought–action defusion'. Initially the concept of thought–action fusion is explained and the *mechanism* is questioned: '*How does thinking a thought cause an action . . .?* The *incongruence* of TAF beliefs should also be questioned: 'What sort of a person is likely to *worry* about thoughts of harming someone? Is it the sort who is likely to act on the thought? Are you the type of person who wants to act on the thought? Where's the evidence that you will?' A *historical review* of the occasions on which the patient has experienced an obsessional thought but was unable to neutralise it or otherwise prevent feared outcomes should be undertaken. The identification of these episodes can be used as evidence that thoughts do not lead to action.

The therapist should attempt to increase the patient's awareness of activation of TAF beliefs. This can be achieved by counting TAF appraisals or completing the DTR, and noting the content of recurrent TAF appraisals.

Behavioural experiments for challenging belief in TAF are reviewed in the behavioural reattribution section later in this chapter. In order to maximise the effectiveness of experiments detailed verbal pre-operationalisation of the effects that should be observable based on TAF beliefs, and following thought manipulation experiments should be undertaken.

In summary, verbal thought–action defusion is based on educating patients about the presence and effects of TAF beliefs. These beliefs can be challenged by questioning the *mechanism*, highlighting the *incongruence* of TAF effects, and by a *historical review* of disconfirmatory experiences. The modified DTR should be used for identifying and tracking the activation of TAF-related cognitions, and for monitoring verbal and behavioural challenges.

## Thought–event defusion

Beliefs concerning thought–action fusion (TAF) and thought–event fusion (TEF) are manifestations of an implicit belief in the validity of intrusive mental experience. Such beliefs are often tacit, and it is necessary for the therapist to increase patients' awareness of the influences of tacit knowledge. Patients typically *act as if* their intrusive thoughts are valid; for example, an individual driving his car has the thought: 'What if I knocked someone down, and I haven't realised?' The person who believes that such thoughts are valid will retrace his journey to check or is otherwise likely to be afflicted with prolonged worry, and preoccupation. Two aspects of this scenario are relevant to a conceptualisation of the problem. First, the individual is operating under the belief that intrusive thoughts reflect actual events and, second, the checking behaviour is intended to avoid protracted worry and distress. Clearly if the individual did not in the first instance believe that the thought was potentially valid no further action, and little distress, would result. For some individuals who realise that intrusive thoughts are unlikely to be true, it is less distressing to engage in a checking ritual than it is to run the risk of being unable to suspend worrying. Here the problem rests with negative appraisals of continued worry and distress.

An illustration of the influence of tacit beliefs concerning the validity of intrusive thoughts is evident in the case of a pregnant woman who had intrusive thoughts that the baby she was carrying was not her partner's, despite the fact that she had not had sexual relations with anyone else. The influence of tacit beliefs concerning the validity of the thought is apparent in her rituals which were attempts to invalidate the intrusion by reviewing her memories in detail for any evidence that she might have had extra-marital relations. Any absences in her memory of being with other men were interpreted as evidence that she may have had sex with one of them. If she did not have an accurate memory she would try to imagine having sex to determine if this 'felt real'. She also questioned details of the image, for example: 'What underwear was he wearing?' and if she could not 'remember' this was interpreted as evidence that the event did not happen. However, the fact that she was able to image sexual relations in the first instance was interpreted as evidence that something might have happened. In this case beliefs about the validity of the intrusive thought led to counter-productive attempts to disconfirm the thought through mental checking.

Thought–event defusion aims to challenge beliefs about the ecological validity of intrusions and teach patients alternative strategies for behaving in response to intrusions. The first step requires establishing the mental framework in which to build an alternative belief system. It is therefore necessary to socialise patients in the role of tacit beliefs. This is accomplished through guided discovery and the use of hypothetical examples. Many patients are operating at the level of how catastrophic it would be or how responsible they would feel if their intrusion were valid; however, this is operating at the Type 1 appraisal level not at the meta-cognitive level (Wells, 1995). The therapist should shift the patient to working at the meta-cognitive level; that is, focus on challenging the 'appraised' validity of the intrusion coupled with the abandonment of the patient's counter-productive invalidation strategies. Key questions for establishing the necessary framework are as follows:

- What prompts you to engage in your (overt/covert) checking behaviour?
- If you didn't believe your thought was realistic would you need to check?
- How responsible would you feel if you knew your thought was unrealistic? Is your problem one of responsibility or one of inflating the realism of your thoughts?
- Most people feel responsible for things but most people are not obsessional about those things—how can this be if the problem is one of responsibility?
- How does your checking behaviour/avoidance affect your confidence in your memory?
- How does your checking behaviour/avoidance affect your ability to discriminate between imagined and real events?

The last two questions should be modified to incorporate the patient's idiosyncratic behaviours (checking, ruminating, neutralising, rituals, avoidance, reassurance seeking, etc.). Through use of this form of questioning the therapist should help patients acquire a meta-cognitive model of their problem. The unhelpful nature of behavioural strategies for the long-term resolution of the obsessional problem should be highlighted. This can be achieved by asking patients why they continue to check/ritualise when past experience should tell them that their thoughts are not valid. An example follows:

T: How long have you been checking the power sockets at work?
P: About three years.
T: Have you ever discovered that you forgot to switch them off?
P: No. I go around systematically and switch them off. But that doesn't stop me driving back to work to check.
T: So even though you have many experiences telling you that your doubting thoughts are not true, you still believe that they are. What makes you believe that?
P: I don't know. Perhaps I haven't switched them off properly.
T: When you check is there any evidence of that?
P: No.
T: Yet you continue to check and you continue to have a problem. So how helpful is your checking in overcoming your problem?
P: Obviously it's not helping at all.
T: So why don't you stop checking?
P: I'd be too uncomfortable. It would ruin my weekend.

T: What do you mean by uncomfortable?

P: I'd be dwelling on the possibility that I'd not turned things off.

T: So you'd still be responding as if your thoughts were true. What if you responded to your thoughts differently, could that help?

P: Well, I already tell myself that it's stupid to think these things.

T: Does that stop you dwelling on the thought?

P: No. I go through my switching off routine in my head to see if I can remember all of it.

T: So you're still acting as if your thought is true. It sounds as if that might cause its own problems.

P: Sometimes it makes me feel better, but if I can't clearly remember switching off some of the appliances it means I'll feel worse and I'll end up checking.

T: So how useful is your behavioural or mental checking in the long run?

P: I can see it probably doesn't help. But I'd feel worse if I didn't check.

T: OK. We can explore that possibility in a minute, but I think we should do something about your strategies for dealing with your thoughts. It sounds as if your checking may be generating more doubts and keeping your problem going.

Once the basic framework and the role of counter-productive responses to intrusions is established the next step consists of developing an alternative set of responses to intrusions, and verbally challenging belief in thought–event fusion (TEF). This can be accomplished by questioning the *evidence* for TEF.

Rational responses that invalidate belief about intrusions should be formulated (e.g. 'This is just a thought not a reality; I don't need to reason with fantasy; let it go'), and detached mindfulness, in which patients are instructed not to engage with intrusions on a behavioural or mental level, should be practised. (Exposure and response prevention in which the patient deliberately holds the intrusion in awareness without engaging in rituals provides a means of practising detached mindfulness.)

Negative appraisals concerning the unremitting nature of discomfort or worry should rituals/checking be abandoned, should be challenged by questioning the evidence for this belief and by exposure and response prevention experiments to test this out. Detached mindfulness in combination with tracking of discomfort over time can also be used to disconfirm beliefs about perpetual discomfort.

## Identify images

Checking behaviour is often prompted by images such as an image of a door unlocking itself, or image of an electrical item not switched off properly. In these circumstances it can be helpful to question the evidence that supports the validity of the image. When 'feelings' predominate as evidence it can be useful to teach the concept of emotional reasoning, and have the patient label the feeling when it occurs as part of devaluing the validity of the intrusion. Imagery modification may also be practised in which the patient is encouraged to image having successfully completed an action after having completed it as a replacement for 'mentally undoing' the action in imagery or negative thought form. While this may serve as a temporary strategy for reducing the emotional salience of imagery and its effect on urges to check, this is not intended to become a covert ritual in its own right.

## BEHAVIOURAL REATTRIBUTION

In the following sections of this chapter behavioural techniques in the treatment of OCD are considered. The principles of exposure and response prevention are outlined first. While the learning theory, and cognitive theory applications of this technique appear superficially similar, a cognitive approach advocated here reconceptualises the aim of exposure and response prevention (ERP) as a behavioural experiment for challenging specific beliefs about intrusive thoughts and ritual behaviours. It also suggests a use for ERP in training in 'detached mindfulness', and for exposing to emotional discomfort in a way that challenges negative beliefs concerning the nature of discomfort. These new applications of ERP (exposure and response prevention experiments (ERP-E) are considered in subsequent sections.

### Exposure and response prevention: the behavioural perspective

Theoretical approaches to OCD have emphasised the role of the person's rituals and neutralising responses in the maintenance of the problem. The behavioural perspective is based on the principle that actions that relieve obsessive fear or discomfort are negatively reinforced, and thus become more widespread. Because they reduce distress they interfere with exposure to anxiety and with habituation of anxiety (e.g. Dollard & Miller, 1950; Mowrer, 1960). In order to overcome anxiety associated with obsessive stimuli it is necessary to expose the individual to the stimuli in the absence of rituals.

Exposure and response prevention procedures based on this principle offer the most successful procedures for reducing obsessions and compulsions. For example, an obsessional individual with contamination fears is exposed to a feared contaminant (e.g. urine) and prevented from washing for an extended time period so that anxiety habituates. The average improvement across studies varies but ranges from 40 to 75 per cent on target symptom measures (Steketee, 1993). The outcome of behavioural treatments for pure obsessions is less favourable than for obsessions with rituals, and obsessive compulsives that fail to make gains in exposure-based treatment may have higher depression levels, and show evidence of over-valued ideas (Foa, 1979); that is, they have greater belief that their thoughts are realistic. One possibility is that cognitive therapy may produce gains in these treatment failures. Salkovskis and Warwick (1985) treated a depressed over-evaluator who had intrusive thoughts about catching cancer. While the patient responded initially to behavioural treatment, she relapsed and was unresponsive to medication or behavioural treatment. The introduction of cognitive therapy resulted in a reduction of her belief from 98 to 40 per cent and an improvement in mood. Following this response the patient was engaged in behaviour therapy and the combined treatment resulted in almost complete recovery, which was maintained at six-month follow-up. The observation that pure obsessions respond less well to treatment than obsessions with overt compulsions has led some investigators to suggest that anxiety may be maintained in pure obsessions by covert or mental rituals. The interruption of an obsessional thought by mental rituals may interfere with exposure and habituation. This formulation suggests a treatment in which individuals should be exposed to anxiety-provoking thoughts while mental rituals are blocked. This technique, involving exposure to obsessions narrated on a *closed-loop audio tape*, has been demonstrated as effective across several studies (e.g. Headland & MacDonald, 1987; Salkovskis, 1983; Salkovskis & Westbrook, 1989).

## Exposure and response prevention: a cognitive reconceptualisation

The effects of rituals in problem maintenance have a different explanation in a cognitive model of OCD. In the present framework, overt and covert rituals act as behaviours that prevent exposure to information that can correct dysfunctional beliefs. Mental rituals in particular prolong rumination episodes and maintain preoccupation with thinking, thus extending the conscious accessibility of intrusions. Moreover, some mental rituals and mental control strategies may increase obsessions, as in examples of the paradoxical effects of attempts to suppress thoughts (e.g. Wegner et al., 1987). The overall effect is failure to revise, in a favourable way, dysfunctional beliefs about intrusive thoughts and rituals. Overt rituals are easier to identify and manage than mental rituals and thus the blocking of them is more readily accomplished—an effect possibly accounting for differences in treatment efficacy between cases of obsessions with, or cases without, overt rituals. In addition, mental rituals are likely to resemble rumination and this form of activity may deplete attention needed for executive meta-cognitive operations necessary for belief change—that is, individuals are unable to maintain a detached objective awareness of their intrusions and challenge their negative appraisals of them.

The cognitive perspective alters the rationale for exposure and response prevention. In a cognitive therapy framework, the rationale should emphasise exposure to thoughts, contaminants, or events as a means of *challenging beliefs* concerning the catastrophic nature of contact with such stimuli. Response prevention (or elimination of safety behaviours) then becomes a 'disconfirmatory manoeuvre' that facilitates attribution of the non-occurrence of catastrophe to the falseness of the original belief. As with preparing for exposure and response prevention used in a behavioural context, detailed examination of the full range of overt and covert strategies is required. The following gives an example of a rationale for introducing exposure and response prevention *experiments*.

> One problem is that you believe that having bad thoughts will lead to bad things happening. It is understandable that you should want to prevent these things, and so in order to do so you have developed a range of coping strategies or things that you do to keep the situation safe. It is important for you to understand that it is quite normal for people to have thoughts like yours. However, you are unable to discover that your thoughts are harmless and meaningless in the real world because you do things to prevent any harm. So long as you do these things your anxiety will remain. It is necessary for you to discover that your thoughts are harmless, and in order to do this you must not take safety precautions. By allowing yourself to have thoughts and by not taking safety precautions you will discover that your thoughts are harmless and do not mean anything.

Detailed analysis of covert and overt behaviours are required so that these may be abandoned during the exposure experiment. Such experiments should follow the PETS protocol presented in Chapter 2.

## Challenging specific beliefs

Different forms of exposure and response prevention experiment (ERP-E) can be used to challenge belief in negative appraisals and predictions arising from the patient's beliefs. These include, increasing the frequency or duration of unwanted thoughts in an attempt to cause a predicted catastrophe, or behaving in 'dangerous' ways (that actually have no danger in reality). For example, an obsessional patient had thoughts about harming herself in her sleep. In particular she believed that she might hang herself from the light cord while sleep walking. She also had obsessional thoughts about knives and would not allow them to be left on work surfaces in the kitchen. When people called at her home she had to check that all the knives were put away in the drawer and that the drawer was closed before answering the door. She feared that if this were not the case she might impulsively pick up a knife and attack a visitor. (*Note:* She had no desire to harm herself or others.) In order to challenge her belief in her thoughts about hanging herself during sleep, she was asked to sleep with a length of rope coiled on the floor at the foot of her bed. At first she was reluctant to engage in the experiment as she believed 100 per cent that she would harm herself. With careful explanation of the rationale for the experiment and with the use of a graded approach in which she practised sleeping with the rope in another room and then with it progressively closer to the bed, her belief declined to 20 per cent. Once her confidence had increased the next step involved sleeping with knives in the same room. Initially they were kept in a box, and then a knife was placed on the window-ledge in the bedroom. In this way the patient learned that her thoughts about harming herself or others were untrue.

This type of experiment can also provide a powerful means of demonstrating that unwanted negative thoughts of harming oneself or others in OCD do not lead to performance of these actions (thought–action defusion). In order to challenge beliefs concerning thought–action fusion (TAF), a modification of the procedure is required. Since TAF concerns the belief that one will act on one's thoughts, it is necessary to ask patients to deliberately increase the frequency of obsessional thoughts in 'risky' situations. For example, a patient is instructed to have thoughts of harming the therapist while holding a piece of rope or a knife.

Techniques of this kind can also be used to challenge beliefs about thought–event fusion (TEF), such as the belief that having intrusive thoughts can lead to bodily damage. In this scenario, the individual is asked to increase the frequency and intensity of intrusions in an attempt to 'damage' the body. In other cases, patients believe that having negative thoughts can lead to external events. One patient believed that thoughts about her husband being involved in a car crash would make the event happen. In order to challenge this belief she was initially asked to deliberately think about the therapist having a car accident. A week later she was asked to repeat the experiment with thoughts about her husband to determine if she could influence events in this way. This type of experiment is limited by time-course considerations. More specifically, some individuals believe that thinking 'bad' thoughts will only lead to negative events over a long time period. If these experiments are to be successful it is necessary to predetermine the time-course in influencing external events. Care should be taken to ensure that the person is not engaging in covert or overt rituals believed to avert negative events, during the experiment.

## Response prevention: contamination fears

In cases in which contamination fears are central, and individuals engage in excessive cleaning rituals, behavioural experiments consisting of exposure to contaminants are required. An innovative procedure used by Foa and colleagues consists of the manufacture of 'magical solutions' that can be used to contaminate objects and environments. The use of a contaminating spray has the advantage that the contaminant is widely dispersed and leaves no trace of its presence, thereby rendering neutralising by cleaning almost impossible. The 'magical' property of these solutions stems from the fact that when a single drop of contaminant (e.g. urine, saliva) is added to a volume of water (e.g. half litre) the water acquires contaminating qualities. Solutions can be produced for most contaminants such as soil or faeces, by adding a tiny grain of this material to water, or, in the latter case by using a drop of water from a toilet bowl. The solution is transferred to a hand-held spray and used to contaminate the home, and the self. In the home, furniture, carpets, curtains and the air may be contaminated. The individual can also be contaminated by spraying clothes, hair, skin and so on. As usual with behavioural experiments the therapist should ascertain specific predictions or beliefs that the procedure is intended to test. Following contamination the patient should not engage in overt or covert rituals that minimise appraised catastrophes associated with exposure to the contaminant.

## Absence of cognition

In some instances, cognitions associated with ritual behaviours are obscure and the patient reports a general feeling of distress associated with not performing the ritual, but no clear cognition seems available. The first step is to determine the nature of the distress reported, and the meaning and significance of the distress itself. There may be particular thoughts concerning an inability to 'cope' with the distress, in which case the concept of not coping requires definition. In other instances, there may be a fear that the emotional distress will not recede, or that it will lead to some other calamity. These concepts should be challenged with appropriate verbal and behavioural reattribution techniques.

Negative appraisals accompanying ritual behaviours may occur in the form of images or impulses, so it is important to check for the presence of these factors. The procedures outlined above can be adapted to challenge fears associated with images and impulses. For example, impulses can be intentionally intensified to demonstrate that strong feelings do not lead to loss of control. In a different context, ritual prevention can be used with the rationale of teaching greater tolerance and acceptance of emotional states.

In some instances mental preoccupations or rumination are the cause of distress, and the associated appraisals are 'I can't stand it' or similar. There may not be further appraisals concerning the consequences or meaning of not being able to 'stand it'. The preoccupation is experienced as aversive, and the strategy is to develop increased tolerance. One technique is to enhance the preoccupation rather than trying to eliminate it. In all likelihood the patient already attempts to eliminate the preoccupation without success. Moreover, attempts to control or eliminate a preoccupation can have the opposite effect of enhancing the preoccupation. This effect is similar to the paradoxical effects attributed to thought suppression. For example, a 24-year-old male patient with a five-year history of varying preoccupations (i.e. hyperalertness to background noise, various bodily sensations, intruding thoughts) tried to rid himself of these preoccupations. The harder he tried the more he felt overwhelmed and thought 'I can't stand it'. A treatment strategy consisted of focusing attention on the preoccupations, with the aim of developing acceptance of them. The therapist used a paradoxical instructional framework in which it was suggested: 'each episode of preoccupation is an opportunity to develop acceptance. It is essential that you continue to have preoccupations and practise accepting them in a relaxed way. Not having preoccupations would be most unhelpful at the moment.' Developing acceptance involved physical relaxation, not controlling the preoccupation, but maintaining attention on a preoccupying stimulus when it was triggered.

The closed loop tape offers another means of enhancing focus on preoccupying concepts. For example, the patient described above constructed a tape that repeated statements about his bodily sensations (e.g. My stomach is hurting, focus on the pain, it's uncomfortable, I can't stand it. My legs are weak, they're aching . . . ), and listened to the tape on a Walkman while physically exercising. In this way he developed an acceptance of his body-awareness and it became less aversive (this process may be likened to habituation training).

## ADDITIONAL CONSIDERATIONS

### Rituals and emotional avoidance

A subgroup of obsessive-compulsive individuals report overt or covert rituals in the absence of obsessions. They maintain that the rituals avert distressing or uncomfortable feelings, and they are unable to express negative thoughts that accompany such feelings. This variant of OCD is little understood; indeed, it is not clear if this should be conceptualised in the same way as other variants of OCD that involve clear obsessions. In some of these cases it seems that rituals are used to avoid unpleasant emotions, in a similar manner to which Borkovec and Inz (1990) suggest that GAD subjects use verbal rumination in the form of worry to avoid unpleasant affect. A potentially fruitful line of investigation in these cases involves exploration of the meaning and significance of not eliminating unwanted affect through the use of rituals. Individuals seem divided in response to this line of enquiry. Some claim that nothing bad would happen if they allowed the emotion to occur, but that it would feel unpleasant, while others express concepts of emotion running out of control or negative feelings becoming permanent. In these cases attempts should be made to decatastrophise the meaning of emotion, and exposure to feelings should be undertaken.

A further consideration when dealing with long-standing and pervasive behavioural rituals is their time-consuming nature. Some patients structure their daily experience around rituals; if asked to reduce the time spent in rituals, such individuals experience boredom, lack of structure or purpose in daily life. In such cases the therapist should work with the patient in establishing a new structure to daily living. Techniques such as activity scheduling, and encouraging patients to engage in new 'absorbing' activities such as hobby pursuits or exercise, can be helpful.

## Doubt reduction

The occurrence of compulsive checking has been linked to deficits in memory function in obsessive compulsives (e.g. Sher, et al., 1984, 1989). However, evidence of an actual memory deficit is inconclusive. It is more likely that checkers merely show reduced confidence in their memory. Techniques that make behaviour 'stand out' in memory should reduce the doubt that motivates checking. Tallis (1993) reports three cases of compulsive checking treated with a doubt reduction procedure that used distinctive stimuli. The procedure consisted of providing patients with a set of coloured cardboard shapes (star, square, triangle, circle, rectangle). Each particular shape was the same colour (e.g. all triangles were red, all squares were green, etc.) but each shape ranged in size forming a graded continuum of size. Patients were instructed to associate target behaviours (e.g. closing a door) with large figures first, and then to work through to the smallest figures. When subjects doubted an action, this was reduced by forming a mental image of the figure employed at the time. The use of graded reduction in stimulus size was intended as a 'fading' component to maintain treatment gains after the programme was completed. The procedure was effective in eliminating checking at twelve month follow-up. Tallis (1995) suggests also that psychometric tests may be used to show patients that their memory function falls within the normal range.

# CONCLUSION

Obsessive-compulsive disorder remains a complex disorder to model in a comprehensive cognitive framework, and a difficult disorder to treat. This chapter presents a new working model for representing relationships between cognitive, behavioural and mood variables, and the influences of meta-cognitive beliefs. The heterogeneous nature of obsessive-compulsive problems means that modification of the model will be necessary in representing the interactions between factors maintaining particular variants of OCD. In summary, the role of a range of beliefs concerning intrusive thoughts, ritual behaviours, and emotion in the maintenance of OCD have been delineated. The framework presented here emphasises working on meta-cognitive appraisals and beliefs, and introducing alternative strategies for dealing with intrusions that disconfirm beliefs in thought–action fusion, thought–event fusion, and positive and negative beliefs about rituals.

# EXAMPLE TREATMENT OUTLINE

*Session 1*

1. Develop idiosyncratic case formulation
2. Begin socialisation to model by:
   — thought suppression experiment
   — exploring historical effects of mood on intrusions
   — guided discovery: would there be a problem if believed thoughts invalid?
3. Introduce concept of worry about intrusions rather than intrusions as the problem.
4. Homework:
   (a) Modified DTR.
   (b) Ban suppression/rumination: controlled worry period.

*Session 2*

1. Review homework. Check DTR material fits model. If problems with DTR, go over in session.
2. Continue socialisation: reframe problem as one of reaction to thoughts, not a problem of thoughts themselves.
3. Verbal reattribution: challenge specific appraisals of intrusions.
4. Introduce 'detached mindfulness' and practise in-session.
5. Elicit and begin to modify beliefs about rituals. (Use these beliefs to suggest behavioural experiments.)
6. Homework:
   (a) Continue modified DTR.
   (b) Contain mental rituals/rumination: controlled worry periods.

    (c) Practise 'detached mindfulness'.
    (d) Mini-survey to 'normalise' intrusions.

*Sessions 3–6*

1. Fit results of homework to model.
2. In-session experiments to test *specific* beliefs about thought–action fusion, and thought–event fusion, e.g.
    — try to cause negative events by negative thoughts
    — increase intrusions and abandon rituals
    — exposure to contaminants plus ritual prevention
    — closed loop-tape experiment.
3. Develop answers to worry about intrusions (e.g. 'This is only a thought not a fact').
4. Homework:
    (a) Continue modified DTR.
    (b) Repeated behavioural experiments (as in 2 above).
    (c) Ban rituals/rumination: continue 'detached mindfulness'.

*Sessions 7–10*

1. Check on remaining use of overt/covert rituals. Use rituals/avoidance as a marker to explore beliefs about rituals.
2. Advantages–disadvantages analysis of remaining rituals/avoidance.
3. In-session experiments to challenge remaining beliefs.
4. Homework:
    (a) Further exposure and response prevention experiments.
    (b) If checking occurs reframe as an opportunity to invalidate intrusions (i.e. only one check required, focus attention on external data, further 'doubting' is disallowed).

*Sessions 10–14*

1. Work on remaining beliefs and behaviours.
2. Consolidate new strategies for dealing with intrusions:
    — act as if intrusions are invalid
    — detached mindfulness
    — ban rumination/doubting-questioning of actions
    — use urge to ritualise as cue to exaggerate intrusions and prevent rituals to test invalidity of intrusions
    — expose self to obsessional stimuli while abandoning rituals.
3. Develop therapy blueprint.
4. Homework:
    (a) Work on blueprint.
    (b) Continued experimentation.

Chapter 10

# FUTURE DEVELOPMENTS IN COGNITIVE THERAPY

The evolution of cognitive therapy in different anxiety disorders appears to follow a particular course. First, cognitive techniques are added to existing treatments such as exposure or relaxation therapies to determine if they improve outcome. The techniques selected are usually based on the general schema theory of emotional disorders, and thus techniques for challenging automatic thoughts and general beliefs are chosen. However, this may not be the best means of devising effective cognitive therapies for anxiety. Failure to find a superiority of treatments consisting of cognitive therapy components can be attributed to selection of suboptimal techniques, the use of some techniques that in combination could cause mutual interference in outcome, or the application of techniques to peripheral mechanisms that are not central to problem maintenance. The use of hybrid treatments combining unmodified cognitive and behavioural techniques are beset by problems of theoretical integrity, and in their extreme form offer little more than a 'shotgun' technique-based approach to treatment. Fortunately, cognitive models of particular anxiety disorders have evolved, and these models are capable of radically influencing the selection of treatment strategies, and influencing how strategies are revised for optimal effects within the context of an idiosyncratic case formulation. Outside of the research setting, new developments filter into clinical practice in a gradual way. However, in time, and as a result of demonstrable efficacy, old treatment strategies are abandoned or retuned. The result of this developmental sequence is that there is diversity among therapists in the practice of cognitive therapy within the schema tradition. A central argument in this book is that cognitive therapy should use specific treatments and techniques that are based on case conceptualisations, which in turn are based on specific models of anxiety. Cognitive therapists should be responsible for maintaining the theoretical integrity of treatment; that is, the techniques used should be logically derived from a model of the maintenance of a disorder. Cognitive therapy is *not* a technique-driven treatment, it should be driven by a clear case conceptualisation in which idiosyncratic data are entered into a basic model. While a wide range of techniques have been reviewed in this book, they are of limited use without an overall impression of problem maintenance and a structure to therapy capable of maximising necessary cognitive change.

This book presents specific cognitive models of anxiety disorder that offer direct implications for treatment. Particular models are more developed than others. Some models offer implications concerning the sequencing of cognitive modification, as in cases of social phobia and GAD. These models are based on a more detailed generic theory of emotional disorder that links schema theory with information processing (Wells & Matthews, 1994, 1997). Wells and Matthews (1994) have pointed out that schema theory considers only a narrow band of cognition and neglects broader aspects such as levels of control of cognition, attention, and meta-cognition. In the remainder of this chapter a model of emotional disorder integrating schema theory with information processing is reviewed, and the implications of such a model for the practice of cognitive therapy are discussed.

## THE SELF-REGULATORY EXECUTIVE FUNCTION MODEL

Wells and Matthews (1994) developed the self-regulatory executive function (S-REF) model to represent the interactions between appraisals, attentional control, and beliefs in the maintenance of emotional disorder. Figure 10.0 presents an outline of the model.

Three levels of processing are distinguished in the model: a level of automatic processing of external and internal stimuli, a level of controlled processing involved in the regulation of behaviour and thought, and a store of beliefs that guide the content and activities of the controlled processing system. Automatic processing is rapid and occurs outside of conscious awareness, although the output of automatic processing may intrude into consciousness. Highly practised activities acquire partial automaticity; for instance, the actions necessary for driving a car become more reflexive with practise, require less conscious involvement, and demand less attention. Fully automatised processing is not amenable to consciousness, and requires no attention, but it is unlikely that the processing that occurs in emotional disorder is ever fully automatised since it involves complex processing

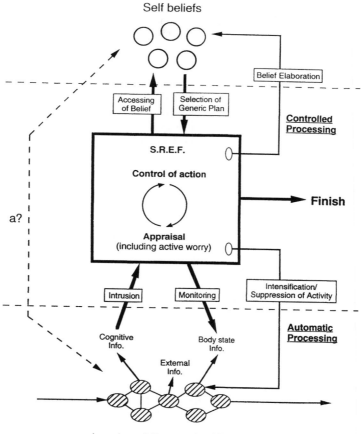

**Figure 10.0**  The S-REF model (Wells & Matthews, 1994)

operations that are influenced by changing patterns of internal and external information. Controlled processing is synonymous with attentionally demanding appraisals that are amenable to consciousness, although some patients report diminished awareness of such on-line appraisals initially. The execution of appraisals relies on the accessing of beliefs that shape the content and nature of appraisals and behavioural responses. For example, a social phobic may appraise the occurrence of sweating as an indication that he/she looks 'abnormal', while a non-phobic may appraise the same event as an indication that he/she looks hot. In each case the appraisals are based on beliefs concerning the meaning and significance of the bodily event. On the basis of these appraisals behavioural responses are tailored to deal with the situation, and are executed within the controlled processing system. Some of the behavioural and cognitive coping strategies executed are problematic because they prevent exposure to experiences that can disconfirm dysfunctional beliefs, or they affect the processing system in ways that maintain unhelpful modes of processing. For instance, the use of rumination or active worry as a coping strategy may drain the attention needed for processing disconfirmatory information, and can maintain preoccupation with, or increase attentional bias for threat. Verbal rumination may distract attention away from processing emotional information (intrusive images) such that emotional processing is retarded and symptoms of failed emotional processing, such as intrusive thoughts about stress, proliferate (e.g. Borkovec & Inz, 1990; Wells & Papageorgiou, 1995).

A benefit of articulating the dynamic interplay between levels of cognition in models like the S-REF is that it offers a preliminary working framework for understanding how cognitive processes and structures interact in the maintenance of disorder. Armed with this type of knowledge, predictions can be made concerning not only what should be done in cognitive therapy but also how cognitive change may be best achieved through manipulating interacting components of the system. In the S-REF model a particular mode of processing termed the S-REF is thought to be activated in emotional disorder. This mode consists of the activation of self-relevant beliefs, the appraisal of internal and external stimuli with respect to these beliefs, and the regulation of appraisal and behaviour intended to overcome any discrepancies between appraised actual and desired states of the self. Thus, S-REF processing serves a self-regulatory function. This function is partly metacognitive in its effect in that S-REF processing is capable of regulating and modifying aspects of the processing system, such as priming automatic processing, and the activation, deactivation, or assimilation of new information to existing beliefs. Some beliefs that are activated are primarily metacognitive in nature, such as beliefs that it is necessary to worry on an issue in order to cope, or the belief that having particular thoughts will lead to loss of control.

A particular mode of S-REF functioning is purported to underlie emotional disorder. A marker for this processing mode is chronic and intense self-focused attention. The mode comprises perseverative self-referent processing (worry or rumination), activation of dysfunctional self-beliefs and monitoring for threat. The exact content of active worry, beliefs, and the nature of intrusions from automatic processing varies across disorders. For example, threat monitoring in panic disorder includes selective attention to internal bodily events, in obsessional-disorder monitoring consists of selective attention for particular thoughts, while in social phobia there is self-monitoring of the publicly conspicuous aspects of self. Behavioural

responses exert an effect on the processing mode: perseverative S-REF processing is at least partially maintained by choice of coping strategy. We have
seen in previous chapters how safety behaviours may exacerbate symptoms,
block disconfirmation of belief, and generally maintain or increase discrepancies rather than decrease them over the long term. Some coping responses such as the use of worry or rumination to deal with imagined or
objective threat directly contribute to the dysfunctional mode of S-REF
activity.

Schema theory considers belief in the form of declarative knowledge such as
'I'm weak; I'm unattractive; I'm vulnerable; I'm a failure' stored at the
schema level. There is disagreement about how knowledge of this kind is
represented in the information-processing system, and some patients have
limited insight into the evidence that maintains negative appraisals. Thus,
Wells and Matthews (1994) propose that much of the self-belief system
exists in 'procedural' form, and declarative beliefs such as 'I'm a failure' are
the result of running particular processing routines. Hence, it is necessary in
cognitive therapy to modify the plan or blueprint for the processing routine
associated with emotional disorder. Modification of declarative beliefs alone
may only be partially effective if the individuals processing routine continues to generate patterns of attention and appraisal that generate dysfunctional knowledge. A panic disorder patient, for example, may be able to
concede that he/she rationally knows that he/she will not suffocate in a
panic attack, but selective attention, appraisal and safety behaviour responses may be activated during panic that override the reappraisal and
make danger tangible once again. The modification of declarative beliefs
may represent 'knowing with the head' while the introduction of new procedures will support 'knowing with the heart'. In order to generate and
effect changes in procedures it is necessary for the patient to acquire new
skills of processing. This will require repeated practise of new processing
routines so that new plans can be developed. The modification of attention
in treatment provides a central means of interrupting dysfunctional perseverative processing, increasing flexible control over processing, and facilitating the development of alternative processing routines.


## TREATMENT IMPLICATIONS OF THE S-REF MODEL

Models of social phobia and generalised anxiety disorder presented in this
book are based on concepts derived from the S-REF model. Moreover, treatment implications of managing the patient's processing configuration as a
prerequisite to disconfirmatory processing are clearly represented in the
sequential approach adopted in the cognitive therapy of social phobia

discussed in Chapter 7. The S-REF model offers a range of implications for cognitive therapy, which are briefly reviewed below.

## Managing on-line activity

In cognitive therapy, change in appraisals, belief, and lower level processing is achieved through the manipulation of conscious on-line appraisals and cognitive processes. The efficiency of cognitive change is influenced by the extent to which dysfunctional beliefs can be activated, alternative data processed, and the extent to which new data are used to revise beliefs. Perseverative self-focused processing reduces the attention available for processing new information that is incompatible with beliefs. Moreover, it leads to generating familiar patterns of information that maintain dysfunctional belief rather than modify belief. Early in treatment it is therefore necessary to interrupt perseverative self-focused processing cycles in order to configure the processing system to receive and assimilate new information. This can be achieved through abandoning rumination or worry, or use of worry-postponement strategies. Self-processing configurations can be interrupted with attentional training procedures that redirect the patient's attention away from the self. Attention training is not intended to be a distraction from affect, although it is likely to reduce the intensity of affect in some applications, but it is intended to redirect attention in a way that maximises belief change. On-line activity should be managed in a way that does not merely lead to the deactivation of belief but facilitates the modification of existing dysfunctional belief. In practical terms this means that the degree of affective arousal, rumination, and belief activation should be regulated. High levels of rumination may deplete attention for disconfirmatory processing, failure to activate arousal may lead to failure to prime dysfunctional processing routines, especially if arousal is a trigger stimulus for negative appraisal. Intense affect, on the other hand, may lead to severe attentional narrowing compromising cognitive change. A potential solution to the problem is to teach affect regulation strategies. However, these strategies have their own problems of contributing to safety behaviours, increasing self-focused processing, or draining attention needed for belief change. A recommended solution is to ban rumination early in treatment, and use attentional modification strategies in conjunction with exposure to feared situations. Feared situations are used to trigger dysfunctional beliefs and processing routines, and attentional modification is used to interrupt perseverative self-regulatory processing and guide attention towards processing threat-incongruent material. Patients should be encouraged to enter the most stressful situation they can manage in implementing this procedure. Thus level of affect can be regulated with a hierarchical exposure approach.

## Socratic dialogue

Verbal reattribution methods in existing cognitive therapy focus primarily on questioning the evidence for thoughts and beliefs, on identifying thinking errors, and reviewing counter-evidence. The S-REF model suggests that interrogating negative thoughts in the controlled processing system may not be the optimal way to modify belief in some circumstances. If patients are asked to interrogate their own thoughts in this way the process may contribute to active worry processes. Questioning of the evidence may be better employed as an initial belief-weakening manoeuvre conducted in therapy sessions, and as a means of setting up a cognitive set that augments belief change in conjunction with follow-up strategies. The procedure should be followed by exposure experiments involving behavioural and attentional manipulations that maximise belief change.

Further, the model assigns central significance to examining the individual's processing routine in problematic situations (i.e. when negative affect is activated). This goes beyond merely questioning the evidence for appraisals, and requires mapping of attentional, memory, and ideational processes in-situation. Wells and Matthews (1994, 1997) refer to this type of mapping as *meta-cognitive profiling* since it offers a means of objectifying the patient's procedural beliefs that guide activities of the processing system. Meta-cognitive profiling requires that the therapist asks a range of questions: Where does the patient's evidence for appraisals/beliefs come from? (e.g. self/external); What is the patient paying most attention to in-situation? Is appraisal predominantly verbal or imaginal? What beliefs about negative appraisals/intrusions (meta-cognitions) are activated on a conscious or implied level?; What memories are activated?; Is appraisal telegraphic or perseverative?; What are the key coping/safety behaviours?

## Developing new processing routines

Once dysfunctional routines are established, therapy should proceed to modify aspects of existing routines, such as the focus of attention in challenging negative appraisals and beliefs. A detailed analysis of the range of situations that trigger problems for the patient is required so that exposure to situations plus execution of modified routines can be executed in a way that challenges belief and leads to the formation of alternative plans for processing. Through repeated practise with new routines they may be triggered with reduced conscious intent by previously problematic stimuli. Some problems involve highly idiosyncratic combinations of internal and external stimuli to trigger problems such as anxiety. For instance, some social phobics are triggered by highly specific combinations of bodily sensations and external stimuli. It is necessary to understand the precise nature of triggering conditions so that exposure experiments that effectively activate dysfunctional processing routines are used in developing new strategies. New routines may exist of combinations of strategies such as: external attentional monitoring, selective attention to disconfirmatory evidence, abandonment of active worry, abandonment of safety behaviours, selectively recalling disconfirmatory experiences from memory, and perspective shifts in imagery.

A specific processing strategy suggested by Wells and Matthews (1994) is *detached mindfulness* in which patients are instructed to disengage ruminative appraisal or active worry from intrusive thoughts. This is a selective 'letting-go' of intrusions, in which awareness of the initial intrusion may remain but the patient is instructed not to engage with the intrusion on a mental or behavioural level. The process may be assisted through self-instruction such as: 'This is only a thought it isn't a reality; I don't need to give my time to this thought.' The intrusion should be allowed to decay in its own right. This technique is intended to offer patients new strategies for processing intrusive thoughts that overcome potential problems of blocked emotional processing and elaboration associated with active engagement with intrusions. In addition, detached mindfulness can be employed as a behavioural experiment to determine what happens to intrusions and the distress they cause if they are 'left to their own devices'. This is the antithesis of thought suppression attempts, and can be used to challenge beliefs about intrusions and the distress associated with them. On first impression, the practise of mental disengagement from thoughts may seem like sanctioning thought suppression, with all its inherent problems. However, detached mindfulness is not an attempt 'not to think' a thought; it is an attempt to disengage the elaborative ruminative or analytic processing from intruding thoughts.

A further aim of detached mindfulness is an increase in meta-cognitive awareness. More specifically, it is intended to prime meta-cognitive appraisals that allow subjects to objectively examine their ideational and attentional processes in response to stimuli in a detached intellectual way without activating the full S-REF dysfunctional-processing mode. The activity of the S-REF is time shared between dysfunctional processing and detached mindfulness. The latter augments the development of new meta-cognitive processing routines that can be used for self-appraisal and coping. For example, the health-anxious individual shifts from the processing mode 'I am seriously physically ill—I must examine my body' to the mode 'My problem is that I think I'm seriously ill—I must examine my thinking in a detached objective way'.

## Attention training

In view of the positive relationship between heightened self-attention and emotional disorder, and following a hypothesis that reduced self-focus may interfere with mechanisms maintaining anxiety disorder, Wells (1990) developed a procedure designed to reduce self-attention tendencies. Preliminary attempts to devise a procedure were based on visual attention exercises, however such exercises seemed to produce a limited overall effect on self-focus. The search for a useable strategy shifted to auditory attention manipulations, which appeared to produce more reliable effects. Attention training is designed to modify three conceptually distinct dimensions of attention, that could be relevant to problem maintenance: (1) intensity of self-focus; (2) attentional control; (3) breadth of attention. The procedure consists of auditory attentional monitoring that progressively increases in attentional demands as the procedure unfolds. Attention training is practised in treatment sessions and at least twice a day for homework. It is practised when the patient *is not* in a state of anxiety. It is not intended to be used as a distraction from anxiety responses. In an early single case study of a patient with panic disorder and relaxation-induced anxiety, the procedure was effective in eliminating panic and reducing subjective intensity of somatic responses (Wells, 1990). In a subsequent case series (Wells, White and Carter, in press) two panic disorder cases and a social phobic showed similar positive responses to the treatment. Moreover, the procedure reduced level of belief in key target negative appraisals in these cases. The effects of attention training appear to be stable with maintenance of treatment gains over twelve-month (Wells, 1990) and six-month periods (Wells et al., in press). It is premature to draw firm conclusions concerning the efficacy of attention training as a technique, and further evaluations are required. Nevertheless, preliminary results are promising and suggest that the periodic practise of attention control exercises that decrease self-focus has an effect on anxiety and belief levels in some cases. Attention training is not intended to be a treatment in its own right, but offers a strategy that may be used to partially modify affect and belief without directly challenging the content of cognition. The S-REF model predicts that heightened self-focus following treatment is a marker for continued vulnerability to emotional disorder. Attention training may offer a technique for reducing residual self-focusing tendencies and thus for reducing the likelihood of relapse following cognitive therapy. Future studies are needed to evaluate this possibility.

In the S-REF framework, attention training can be viewed as exerting an effect in at least two ways. First, it may decouple attention from negative beliefs, even though the beliefs remain latent in long-term memory. By attenuating self-focus the patient may subsequently be able to prevent full activation of the perseverative S-REF syndrome. Second, if we assume that negative beliefs are outputs of running particular self-focused processing routines, the amelioration of self-focused processing will lead to the production of modified outputs (beliefs). Thus, attention training increases the flexibility of attention such that new routines for processing can be developed.

Attention training represents one possibility for modification of cognitive processes in the treatment of anxiety disorders. Other possibilities for useful attention modification exist. We saw in the treatment of social phobia that instructions to shift to external-focused processing in conjunction with exposure experiments is a manipulation used early in the treatment devised by Wells and Clark (1995). In this context external attention helps to modulate aversive self-consciousness, and it is fundamental for configuring the social phobic's processing system to maximise disconfirmatory processing. The social phobic is unable to discover how other people are responding to them, and how much attention they actually attract if self-focus is maintained and there is resultant failure to interrogate the environment. External attention manipulations are therefore a means of facilitating the modification of appraisals. It is likely that specific attention modification strategies that direct processing towards information that modifies negative beliefs will be of benefit in other disorders as well.

## META-COGNITION AND ANXIETY DISORDER

Beliefs about cognition, and use of cognitive regulatory processes, are thought to play a role in vulnerability to emotional disorder (Wells & Matthews, 1994). We saw in Chapters 8 and 9 how meta-cognitive dimensions are specifically implicated in disorders of intrusive thoughts, namely generalised anxiety disorder (GAD) and obsessive-compulsive disorder (OCD). A meta-cognitive model of GAD (Wells, 1995) and treatment based on the model was outlined in Chapter 8. Treatment specifications based on this model differ in several respects from treatment of GAD based on the generic schema theory of anxiety. First, schema theory suggests that the content of Type 1 worries and the assumptions related to Type 1 concerns should be modified. However, the meta-cognitive model suggests that it is necessary to conceptualise and treat the mechanisms that contribute to distressing subjectively uncontrollable worry. In this respect Type 2 worries and meta-beliefs should be a focus of intervention based on the model. While dysfunctional meta-cognitive appraisals and processes are likely to play a role in the maintenance of other disorders characterised by unwanted intrusive thought, the S-REF model implies that particular meta-cognitive processing plans that are not directly amenable to consciousness are associated with general vulnerability to psychopathology.

Implications of the S-REF model and of meta-cognitive analysis in developing an understanding of obsessional problems are considered below.

## OBSESSIONAL PROBLEMS

Obsessive-compulsive disorder continues to present a challenge to cognitive theorists and therapists, perhaps more so than most of the other anxiety disorders reviewed in this book. James and Blackburn (1995) review fifteen studies of cognitive therapy of OCD and conclude that there is little evidence that the addition of cognitive therapy to existing treatments improves outcome. However, there is a high degree of variability in the nature of cognitive therapy across treatments. For example, some studies have used thought stopping as a treatment and have labelled the technique cognitive. Other studies have used rational emotive therapy techniques. In general, treatments have not been based on a specific cognitive model of the disorder. It is hoped that advances in theory will be used to develop more focused and effective interventions. In Chapter 9 Salkovskis's (1985, 1989) cognitive-behavioural model of OCD was presented. The model places appraised responsibility associated with intrusive thoughts in a pivotal role. Moreover, the obsessional patient's neutralising and thought control strategies are viewed as central in maintaining the problem, since they terminate exposure and exacerbate intrusions. Building on the concept of responsibility appraisals (Rachman, 1976), Salkovskis presents an influential model that emphasises the appraisal of the significance of intrusions, and provides specific implications for cognitive therapy. Salkovskis and colleagues continue to develop cognitive treatment based on this model. Meta-cognitive processing is clearly implicated in this approach to OCD. Other investigators have sought to elaborate on meta-cognitive content and processes in OCD. Clark and Purdon (1993) agree with Salkovskis that the appraisal of unwanted thoughts is a critical factor in the development of obsessions. However, they suggest that there is an overemphasis on appraisals of responsibility and blame, and they advocate that greater attention should be focused on dysfunctional beliefs about thought control. More specifically, it is suggested that schemas concerned with the need to control thoughts are a prerequisite for failure to control thoughts and the development of obsessions. Clark and Purdon (1993) also suggest that neutralising rituals may not play a definitive role in the development of obsessions. They assert that obsessions develop in response to a 'breakdown of mental control'. This breakdown results from obsessional individuals over-valuing the necessity for control, mood disturbance which makes suppression more difficult, and a concern to detect and prevent further occurrences of unwanted thought. What could motivate a need to control thoughts? In a cognitive analysis we should look at the beliefs held by the individual to answer this question. A promising and valuable concept concerning belief in OCD is advanced by Rachman (1993; Rachman, Thordarson, Shafran & Woody, 1995). He suggests that the belief that thoughts can influence events or are almost equivalent to actions—thought–action fusion (TAF)—is associated with the development of OCD. This is clearly a subtype of meta-cognitive belief and could provide a hitherto missing link between intrusions and appraisals of responsibility and need for control.

The meta-cognitive aspect of obsessional problems has been discussed by Wells and Matthews (1994) and was expanded in Chapter 9. They suggest that intrusive thoughts activate beliefs about the intrusion. The frequency of intrusions is increased by procedural beliefs such as monitoring for bad thoughts, and attempts to suppress or control thoughts or neutralise the dangers associated with them. The problem is that these strategies are counter-productive and maintain intrusions. Two feedback loops serve to maintain the problem. First, attempts to control thoughts lead to continued priming of automatic processing units for the detection of intrusions. Second, control and neutralising attempts affect beliefs by preventing disconfirmation of negative beliefs concerning the consequences of having an intrusion, and by leading to the encoding of an increasing range of stimuli and responses that may serve as future triggers for intrusion. It is suggested that negative appraisals of intrusions in the form of extended worry (rumination) episodes are problematic, since worry (as opposed to more fleeting negative automatic thoughts) about intrusions maintains activation of negative beliefs and continuously primes representations of the unwanted thought. The meta-cognitive beliefs thought to be important in OCD concern beliefs about the influence of thinking (e.g. 'My bad thoughts can make bad things happen'), beliefs concerning the uncontrollability of thought, and tacit meta-cognitive assumptions that lead to a blurring of boundaries between thought and the objective world. Wells and Matthews (1994) suggest that a particular meta-cognitive style could contribute to obsessional checking. Checkers are prone to question their memory for actions, and imagine negative consequences in situations. There is an attentional bias that favours the processing of internally generated negative scenarios as opposed to external aspects of a situation. In particular, obsessionals have a processing configuration characterised by heightened *cognitive self-consciousness* that contributes to increased doubting following the performance of actions, and leading to continued performance of neutralising and safety responses even in the absence of observable objective threat.

More specifically, the obsessional patient appears to assign attentional priority to an internal negative fantasy rather than the reality that is processed through objective senses. The process of acting as if the internal fantasy is valid strengthens this attentional configuration and maintains belief that the internal fantasy is valid. This strengthening process operates by preventing the encoding of disconfirmatory data. There are likely to be other biased processing operations which similarly distort information so that it is consistent with maintaining an unrealistic sense of validity associated with intruding thoughts. If this supposition is correct, treatment should focus on modifying the content of superimposed fantasies and shifting attention priorities to challenge the validity of negative ruminations. Strategies of detached mindfulness in which patients are encouraged to disengage from intrusions, and techniques for reducing heightened cognitive self-consciousness, should also prove helpful as additions to treatment.

## SUMMARY AND CONCLUSION

This book has presented a detailed review of cognitive therapy of anxiety disorders based on disorder-specific cognitive models of problem maintenance. Theoretical advances in the cognitive modelling of anxiety should stimulate further improvements in treatment effectiveness. The nature of cognitive therapy has evolved over time: from a general theory and the inclusion of cognitive techniques in behavioural treatment protocols, to the elaboration of more specific cognitive models embedded in a general theoretical framework. This has culminated in the generation of new, and fine-tuning of existing techniques based on new models. Attention is now returning to the basic generic model in an attempt to re-unite cognitive therapy with cognitive science.

Future developments of cognitive therapy should continue with improved models of anxiety disorder, and should increase the theoretical integrity of treatment, so that what therapists do in therapy is derived from an idiosyncratic cognitive case formulation that is based on a model of disorder. As theoretical and empirical advances occur, we can expect significant changes in the way cognitive therapy is practised. New models linking information processing with schema theory may offer new implications for the practise of cognitive therapy. The S-REF model represents one attempt to link schema theory principles to information processing, and suggests that it is important not only to modify cognitive content but cognitive processes in an endeavour to establish stable replacement beliefs in emotional disorder. An exciting possibility concerns the development of cognitive manipulations that do not directly target the content of appraisals but aim to manipulate the attentional and meta-cognitive dimensions that maintain dysfunctional processing operations and beliefs. Perhaps, armed with a more sophisticated model of cognition in emotional disorder, there will be a time when cognitive change can be efficiently accomplished through the manipulation of cognitive processes without the need to extensively verbally challenge the content of belief.

# RATING SCALES

## PANIC RATING SCALE (PRS)

1. How many panic attacks have you had in the last week? \_\_\_\_

2. How often in the past week have you avoided situations when you were afraid of having a panic attack?

| 0 | 1 | 2 | 3 | 4 | 5 | 6 | 7 | 8 |
|---|---|---|---|---|---|---|---|---|
| Not at all | | | | Half of the time | | | | All of the time |

3. People cope with anxiety in different ways. Place a number from the scale below next to each item to show how often you do the following when you are anxious.

| 0 | 1 | 2 | 3 | 4 | 5 | 6 | 7 | 8 |
|---|---|---|---|---|---|---|---|---|
| Not at all | | | | Half of the time | | | | All of the time |

Sit down \_\_\_\_          Use medication \_\_\_\_          Look for an exit \_\_\_\_

Control my breathing \_\_\_\_          Leave the situation \_\_\_\_          Move more slowly \_\_\_\_

Try to relax \_\_\_\_          Use distraction \_\_\_\_          Hold onto something/ \_\_\_\_

Control my mind \_\_\_\_          Check my pulse \_\_\_\_          someone

Try to be with someone \_\_\_\_

4. Below are a number of thoughts that people have when they feel anxious and nervous. Indicate how much you believe each one <u>when you are anxious</u> by placing a number next to each one from the scale below.

| 0 | 10 | 20 | 30 | 40 | 50 | 60 | 70 | 80 | 90 | 100 |
|---|---|---|---|---|---|---|---|---|---|---|
| Do not believe the thought | | | | | | | | | | Completely convinced the thought is true |

I'm having a heart attack \_\_\_\_          I'm going crazy \_\_\_\_

I'm dying \_\_\_\_          I'm having a stroke \_\_\_\_

I'm suffocating \_\_\_\_          I'm choking \_\_\_\_

I'm collapsing \_\_\_\_          I'm going blind \_\_\_\_

I'm fainting \_\_\_\_          I'm going to be paralysed \_\_\_\_

I'm losing control \_\_\_\_          I'm going to scream \_\_\_\_

I'm going to vomit \_\_\_\_          My panic attack will never end \_\_\_\_

Other thoughts not listed          Rating

1. _____          _____

2. _____          _____

3. _____          _____

## SOCIAL PHOBIA RATING SCALE (SPRS)

1. How distressing has your social anxiety been in the last week?

| 0 | 1 | 2 | 3 | 4 | 5 | 6 | 7 | 8 |
|---|---|---|---|---|---|---|---|---|
| Not at all | | | | Moder-ately | | | | Extremely—The worst I have ever been |

2. How much have you avoided social situations because of your anxiety in the past week?

| 0 | 1 | 2 | 3 | 4 | 5 | 6 | 7 | 8 |
|---|---|---|---|---|---|---|---|---|
| Not at all | | | | Half of the time | | | | All of the time |

3. How self-conscious have you felt in difficult social situations in the past week?

| 0 | 1 | 2 | 3 | 4 | 5 | 6 | 7 | 8 |
|---|---|---|---|---|---|---|---|---|
| Not at all | | | | Moder-ately | | | | Extremely self-conscious. The most I have ever felt |

4. People cope with their social anxiety in different ways. Place a number from the scale below next to each item listed to show how often you do the following when you are socially anxious.

| 0 | 1 | 2 | 3 | 4 | 5 | 6 | 7 | 8 |
|---|---|---|---|---|---|---|---|---|
| Not at all | | | | Half of the time | | | | All of the time |

| | | | | | |
|---|---|---|---|---|---|
| Say little | ____ | Control my thoughts | ____ | Hold my arms still | ____ |
| Take slow breaths | ____ | Try to relax | ____ | Focus on my voice | ____ |
| Grip objects tightly | ____ | Sit down | ____ | Avoid eye contact | ____ |
| Move slowly | ____ | Cover my face | ____ | Speak quickly | ____ |
| Use distraction | ____ | Wear certain clothes | ____ | Focus on my hands | ____ |

5. Below are a number of thoughts that people have when they are socially anxious. Indicate how much you believe each thought when you are socially anxious by placing a number next to each one from the scale below.

| 0 | 10 | 20 | 30 | 40 | 50 | 60 | 70 | 80 | 90 | 100 |
|---|---|---|---|---|---|---|---|---|---|---|
| Do not believe the thought | | | | | | | | | | Completely convinced the thought is true |

| | | | |
|---|---|---|---|
| I look bad | ____ | They'll notice I'm anxious | ____ |
| Everyone is looking at me | ____ | I'll drop and spill things | ____ |
| I'm losing control | ____ | I'm boring | ____ |
| I'll be unable to speak | ____ | I'm inadequate | ____ |
| I'll babble and talk funny | ____ | They think I'm stupid | ____ |
| I look abnormal | ____ | They don't like me | ____ |
| They won't respect me | ____ | I'll look foolish | ____ |
| Other thoughts not listed | | Rating | |
| 1. _____ | | _____ | |
| 2. _____ | | _____ | |
| 3. _____ | | _____ | |

## HEALTH-ANXIETY RATING SCALE (HRS)

1. How distressing/disabling have your health worries been in the last week?

| 0 | 1 | 2 | 3 | 4 | 5 | 6 | 7 | 8 |
|---|---|---|---|---|---|---|---|---|
| Not at all | | | | Moder-<br>ately | | | | Extremely—the<br>worst I have ever<br>been |

2. How often in the past week have you avoided activities because of worry about your health, place a number from the scale below next to each item.

| 0 | 1 | 2 | 3 | 4 | 5 | 6 | 7 | 8 |
|---|---|---|---|---|---|---|---|---|
| Not at all | | | | Half of<br>the time | | | | All of the<br>time |

(a) Physical exercise ____     (c) Thoughts about          (e) Magazine articles on
(b) Television                          illness        ____            illness            ____
    programmes    ____     (d) Strenuous                   (f) Other (specify):
                                              activity    ____          _____
                                                                         _____       ____

3. How many times in the past week have you checked your body?

| 0 | 1–5 | 6–10 | 11–15 | 16–20 | 21–25 | 26–30 | 30+ |
|---|-----|------|-------|-------|-------|-------|-----|
| Not at all | | | | | | | More than 30 times |

4. How often in the past week have you sought reassurance when you have been worried about your health?

| 0 | 1 | 2 | 3 | 4 | 5 | 6 | 7 | 8 |
|---|---|---|---|---|---|---|---|---|
| Not at all | | | | Half of<br>the time | | | | All of the<br>time |

5. Below are a number of thoughts people have about their health. Indicate how much you believe each thought by placing a number next to each one from the scale below.

| 0 | 10 | 20 | 30 | 40 | 50 | 60 | 70 | 80 | 90 | 100 |
|---|----|----|----|----|----|----|----|----|----|-----|
| Do not believe<br>the thought | | | | | | | | | | Completely<br>convinced the<br>thought is true |

I have a serious physical illness ____        I have AIDS                                    ____
I have a brain tumour              ____        I have cancer                                  ____
I have a serious heart problem     ____        I have a serious muscle disease ____

Other thoughts not listed                      Rating

1. _____                    _____
2. _____                    _____

## GENERALISED ANXIETY DISORDER SCALE (GADS)

1. How distressing/disabling have your worries been in the last week?

| 0 | 1 | 2 | 3 | 4 | 5 | 6 | 7 | 8 |

Not at all ... Moder-ately ... Extremely—The worst they have ever been

2. In the past week how much effort have you put into trying to control your worries?

| 0 | 1 | 2 | 3 | 4 | 5 | 6 | 7 | 8 |

None at all ... Moderate effort ... Full effort—I could not try more

3. Place a number from the scale below next to each item to show how often in the past week you have done the following in order to cope with your worry.

| 0 | 1 | 2 | 3 | 4 | 5 | 6 | 7 | 8 |

Not at all ... Half of the time ... All of the time

(a) Tried to distract myself _____
(b) Tried to control my thinking _____
(c) Tried to reason things out _____

(d) Asked for reassurance _____
(e) Talked to myself _____
(f) Tried not to think about things _____

(g) Looked for evidence _____
(h) Acted cautiously _____
(i) Planned how to cope if my worries were true _____

4. How often in the past week have you avoided the following in order to prevent worrying? Place a number from the scale below next to each item.

| 0 | 1 | 2 | 3 | 4 | 5 | 6 | 7 | 8 |

Not at all ... Half of the time ... All of the time

(a) News items _____
(b) Social situations _____

(c) Uncertainty _____
(d) Thoughts of illness _____

(e) Thoughts of accidents/ loss _____
(f) Other (specify):
_____
_____

5. Below are a number of thoughts that people have about their worries. Indicate how much you believe each one by placing a number from the scale below next to each one.

| 0 | 10 | 20 | 30 | 40 | 50 | 60 | 70 | 80 | 90 | 100 |

Do not believe the thought ... Completely convinced the thought is true

I could go crazy with worry _____
Worrying could harm me _____
Worrying puts my body under stress _____
If I don't control my worry it will control me _____
My worrying is uncontrollable _____
If I worry too much I could lose control _____

Worrying helps me cope _____
If I worry I'll be prepared _____
Worrying keeps me safe _____
Worrying helps me get things done _____
Something bad would happen if I didn't worry _____
Worrying helps me solve problems _____

# APPENDIX

## META-COGNITIONS QUESTIONNAIRE
*Developed by Sam Cartwright and Adrian Wells*

This questionnaire is concerned with beliefs people have about their thinking. Listed below are a number of beliefs that people have expressed. Please read each item and say how much you generally agree with it by circling the appropriate number. Please respond to all the items, there are no right or wrong answers.

Sex: _____  Age: _____

| | Do not agree | Agree slightly | Agree moderately | Agree very much |
|---|---|---|---|---|
| 1. Worrying helps me to avoid problems in the future. | 1 | 2 | 3 | 4 |
| 2. My worrying is dangerous for me. | 1 | 2 | 3 | 4 |
| 3. I have difficulty knowing if I have actually done something, or just imagined it. | 1 | 2 | 3 | 4 |
| 4. I think a lot about my thoughts. | 1 | 2 | 3 | 4 |
| 5. I could make myself sick with worrying. | 1 | 2 | 3 | 4 |
| 6. I am aware of the way my mind works when I am thinking through a problem. | 1 | 2 | 3 | 4 |
| 7. If if did not control a worrying thought, and then it happened, it would be my fault. | 1 | 2 | 3 | 4 |
| 8. If I let my worrying thoughts get out of control, they will end up controlling me. | 1 | 2 | 3 | 4 |
| 9. I need to worry in order to remain organised. | 1 | 2 | 3 | 4 |
| 10. I have little confidence in my memory for words and names. | 1 | 2 | 3 | 4 |
| 11. My worrying thoughts persist, no matter how I try to stop them. | 1 | 2 | 3 | 4 |
| 12. Worrying helps me to get things sorted out in my mind. | 1 | 2 | 3 | 4 |
| 13. I cannot ignore my worrying thoughts. | 1 | 2 | 3 | 4 |

| | Do not agree | Agree slightly | Agree moderately | Agree very much |
|---|---|---|---|---|
| 14. I monitor my thoughts. | 1 | 2 | 3 | 4 |
| 15. I should be in control of my thoughts all of the time. | 1 | 2 | 3 | 4 |
| 16 My memory can mislead me at times. | 1 | 2 | 3 | 4 |
| 17. I could be punished for not having certain thoughts. | 1 | 2 | 3 | 4 |
| 18. My worrying could make me go mad. | 1 | 2 | 3 | 4 |
| 19. If I do not stop my worrying thoughts, they could come true. | 1 | 2 | 3 | 4 |
| 20. I rarely question my thoughts. | 1 | 2 | 3 | 4 |
| 21. Worrying puts my body under a lot of stress. | 1 | 2 | 3 | 4 |
| 22. Worrying helps me to avoid disastrous situations. | 1 | 2 | 3 | 4 |
| 23. I am constantly aware of my thinking. | 1 | 2 | 3 | 4 |
| 24. I have a poor memory. | 1 | 2 | 3 | 4 |
| 25. I pay close attention to the way my mind works. | 1 | 2 | 3 | 4 |
| 26. People who do not worry, have no depth. | 1 | 2 | 3 | 4 |
| 27. Worrying helps me cope. | 1 | 2 | 3 | 4 |
| 28. I imagine having not done things and then doubt my memory for doing them. | 1 | 2 | 3 | 4 |
| 29. Not being able to control my thoughts is a sign of weakness. | 1 | 2 | 3 | 4 |
| 30. If I did not worry, I would make more mistakes. | 1 | 2 | 3 | 4 |

| | Do not agree | Agree slightly | Agree moderately | Agree very much |
|---|---|---|---|---|
| 31. I find it difficult to control my thoughts. | 1 | 2 | 3 | 4 |
| 32. Worrying is a sign of a good person. | 1 | 2 | 3 | 4 |
| 33. Worrying thoughts enter my head against my will. | 1 | 2 | 3 | 4 |
| 34. If I could not control my thoughts I would go crazy. | 1 | 2 | 3 | 4 |
| 35. I will lose out in life if I do not worry. | 1 | 2 | 3 | 4 |
| 36. When I start worrying, I cannot stop. | 1 | 2 | 3 | 4 |
| 37. Some thoughts will always need to be controlled. | 1 | 2 | 3 | 4 |
| 38. I need to worry, in order to get things done. | 1 | 2 | 3 | 4 |
| 39. I will be punished for not controlling certain thoughts. | 1 | 2 | 3 | 4 |
| 40. My thoughts interfere with my concentration. | 1 | 2 | 3 | 4 |
| 41. It is alright to let my thoughts roam free. | 1 | 2 | 3 | 4 |
| 42. I worry about my thoughts. | 1 | 2 | 3 | 4 |
| 43. I am easily distracted. | 1 | 2 | 3 | 4 |
| 44. My worrying thoughts are not productive. | 1 | 2 | 3 | 4 |
| 45. Worry can stop me from seeing a situation clearly. | 1 | 2 | 3 | 4 |
| 46. Worrying helps me to solve problems. | 1 | 2 | 3 | 4 |
| 47. I have little confidence in my memory for places. | 1 | 2 | 3 | 4 |

| | Do not agree | Agree slightly | Agree moderately | Agree very much |
|---|---|---|---|---|
| 48. My worrying thoughts are uncontrollable. | 1 | 2 | 3 | 4 |
| 49. It is bad to think certain thoughts. | 1 | 2 | 3 | 4 |
| 50. If I do not control my thoughts, I may end up embarrassing myself. | 1 | 2 | 3 | 4 |
| 51. I do not trust my memory. | 1 | 2 | 3 | 4 |
| 52. I do my clearest thinking when I am worrying. | 1 | 2 | 3 | 4 |
| 53. My worrying thoughts appear automatically. | 1 | 2 | 3 | 4 |
| 54. I would be selfish if I never worried. | 1 | 2 | 3 | 4 |
| 55. If I could not control my thoughts, I would not be able to function. | 1 | 2 | 3 | 4 |
| 56. I need to worry, in order to work well. | 1 | 2 | 3 | 4 |
| 57. I have little confidence in my memory for actions. | 1 | 2 | 3 | 4 |
| 58. I have difficulty keeping my mind focused on one thing for a long time. | 1 | 2 | 3 | 4 |
| 59. If a bad thing happens which I have not worried about, I feel responsible. | 1 | 2 | 3 | 4 |
| 60. It would not be normal, if I did not worry. | 1 | 2 | 3 | 4 |
| 61. I constantly examine my thoughts. | 1 | 2 | 3 | 4 |
| 62. If I stopped worrying, I would become glib, arrogant and offensive. | 1 | 2 | 3 | 4 |
| 63. Worrying helps me to plan the future more effectively. | 1 | 2 | 3 | 4 |

|  | Do not agree | Agree slightly | Agree moderately | Agree very much |
|---|---|---|---|---|
| 64. I would be a stronger person if I could worry less. | 1 | 2 | 3 | 4 |
| 65. I would be stupid and complacent not to worry. | 1 | 2 | 3 | 4 |

*Please ensure that you have responded to all items. Thank you.*

## Scoring key: Meta-Cognitions Questionnaire

| Factor: | 1 | 2 | 3 | 4 | 5 |
|---|---|---|---|---|---|
| Item number | 1 | 2 | 3 | 7 | 4 |
| | 9 | 5 | 10 | 15 | 6 |
| | 12 | 8 | 16 | 17 | 14 |
| | 22 | 11 | 24 | 19 | 20* |
| | 26 | 13 | 28 | 29 | 23 |
| | 27 | 18 | 43 | 34 | 25 |
| | 30 | 21 | 47 | 37 | 61 |
| | 32 | 31 | 51 | 39 | |
| | 35 | 33 | 57 | 41* | |
| | 38 | 36 | 58 | 49 | |
| | 44* | 40 | | 50 | |
| | 46 | 42 | | 55 | |
| | 52 | 45 | | 59 | |
| | 54 | 48 | | | |
| | 56 | 53 | | | |
| | 60 | 64 | | | |
| | 62 | | | | |
| | 63 | | | | |
| | 65 | | | | |

* Reverse scored items.

1 = Problem solving and positive worry beliefs.
2 = Beliefs about controllability.
3 = Meta-cognitive efficiency.
4 = General negative beliefs (including responsibility and superstition).
5 = Cognitive self-consciousness.

## ANXIOUS THOUGHTS INVENTORY (AnTI)
*Developed by Adrian Wells*

**Instructions:** A number of statements which people have used to describe their thoughts and worries are given below. Read each statement and put a circle around the most appropriate number to indicate how often you have these thoughts and worries.

Do not spend too much time on each statement. There are no right or wrong answers and the first response to each item is often the most accurate.

| | Almost never | Sometimes | Often | Almost always |
|---|---|---|---|---|
| 1. I worry about my appearance. | 1 | 2 | 3 | 4 |
| 2. I think I am a failure. | 1 | 2 | 3 | 4 |
| 3. When looking to my future I give more thought to the negative things than the positive things that might happen to me. | 1 | 2 | 3 | 4 |
| 4. If I experience unexpected physical symptoms I have a tendency to think the worst possible thing is wrong with me. | 1 | 2 | 3 | 4 |
| 5. I have thoughts about becoming seriously ill. | 1 | 2 | 3 | 4 |
| 6. I have difficulty clearing my mind of repetitive thoughts. | 1 | 2 | 3 | 4 |
| 7. I worry about having a heart attack or cancer. | 1 | 2 | 3 | 4 |
| 8. I worry about saying or doing the wrong things when among strangers. | 1 | 2 | 3 | 4 |
| 9. I worry about my abilities not living up to other people's expectations. | 1 | 2 | 3 | 4 |
| 10. I worry about my physical health. | 1 | 2 | 3 | 4 |
| 11. I worry that I cannot control my thoughts as well as I would like to. | 1 | 2 | 3 | 4 |

|  | Almost never | Sometimes | Often | Almost always |
|---|---|---|---|---|
| 12. I worry that people don't like me. | 1 | 2 | 3 | 4 |
| 13. I take disappointments so keenly that I can't put them out of my mind. | 1 | 2 | 3 | 4 |
| 14. I get embarrassed easily. | 1 | 2 | 3 | 4 |
| 15. When I suffer from minor illnesses such as a rash I think it is more serious than it really is. | 1 | 2 | 3 | 4 |
| 16. Unpleasant thoughts enter my head against my will. | 1 | 2 | 3 | 4 |
| 17. I worry about my failures and my weaknesses. | 1 | 2 | 3 | 4 |
| 18. I worry about not being able to cope in life as adequately as others seem to. | 1 | 2 | 3 | 4 |
| 19. I worry about death. | 1 | 2 | 3 | 4 |
| 20. I worry about making a fool of myself. | 1 | 2 | 3 | 4 |
| 21. I think I am missing out on things in life because I worry too much. | 1 | 2 | 3 | 4 |
| 22. I have repetitive thoughts such as counting or repeating phrases. | 1 | 2 | 3 | 4 |

*Please check that you have responded to all of the items. Thank you.*

Name: . . . . . . . . . . . . . . . . . . . . . . .      Date: . . . . . . . . . . . . . . . . . . . . . . . . . .

Scores:          S          H          M          Total

# Scoring key: Anxious Thoughts Inventory (AnTI)

| Subscale: | Social | Health | Meta |
|-----------|--------|--------|------|
| Item | 1 | 4 | 3 |
| | 2 | 5 | 6 |
| | 8 | 7 | 11 |
| | 9 | 10 | 13 |
| | 12 | 15 | 16 |
| | 14 | 19 | 21 |
| | 17 | | 22 |
| | 18 | | |
| | 20 | | |

# DIARY OF OBSESSIVE-COMPULSIVE RITUALS

Date:

Please record the daily occurrence of rituals, make a note of the time when the ritual occurred, the situation in which it occurred, and describe the type of ritual (e.g. washing, checking oven). Rate your discomfort on a scale of 0 (no discomfort/anxiety) to 100 (extreme/discomfort anxiety - the worst I have had) and put the number in the discomfort column.Record the length of time taken in your ritual. Finally, at the end of each day record the total number of rituals.

| Time | Situation | Description of ritual | Discomfort (0-100) | Duration of ritual |
|------|-----------|----------------------|--------------------|--------------------|
| A.M. | | | | |
| P.M. | | | | |

Total number of rituals today:

# DYSFUNCTIONAL THOUGHTS RECORD

DYSFUNCTIONAL THOUGHTS RECORD (DTR)

| DATE | SITUATION | EMOTION | AUTOMATIC THOUGHT | ALTERNATIVE THOUGHT | OUTCOME |
|------|-----------|---------|-------------------|---------------------|---------|
| | Note situation or thought/recollection leading to unpleasant emotion | 1. Note type of emotion (sad, anxious, angry etc) <br><br> 2. Rate intensity of emotion (0-100) | 1. Write automatic thought <br><br> 2. Rate belief in automatic thought (0-100) | 1. What's another way of viewing the situation <br><br> 2. Re-rate belief in automatic thought (0-100) | 1. Note type of emotion <br><br> 2. Re-rate intensity of emotion (0-100) <br><br> 3. What further action can I take |
| | | | | | |

# PANIC DIARY

| Date | Situation | Main bodily/mental sensations (e.g. dizziness, mind-racing, breathless, palpitations) | Negative thought (misinterpretation) | Answer to negative thought | Total number of panic attacks |
|------|-----------|------|------|------|------|
| MON | | | | | |
| TUES | | | | | |
| WED | | | | | |
| THURS | | | | | |
| FRI | | | | | |
| SAT | | | | | |
| SUN | | | | | |

*Instructions:*   *When you feel panicky make a note of the situation in which panic occurred (e.g. driving in a car) in the Situation column. Write down your main bodily sensation in the Main bodily sensation column. Write down the frightening negative thoughts that you had during your attack in the Negative thought column. Under the Answer to negative thought heading, write in your answer or rational response to your negative thought, this may be a verbal answer or a particular behaviour. Make a note of the total number of panic attacks you have each day in the Number of panic attacks column.*

## HEALTH ANXIETY THOUGHTS RECORD

| Date | Situation | Trigger for Health Anxiety | Emotion | Negative Thought (rate belief 0-100) | Response to Thought (include rational response rate belief 0-100) | Outcome (re-rate belief in negative thought) |
|------|-----------|----------------------------|---------|--------------------------------------|------------------------------------------------------------------|----------------------------------------------|
|      |           |                            |         |                                      |                                                                  |                                              |

**Note:** When you become concerned about your health, make a note of the situation where this occurred. Make a note of the "trigger" for your concern, this may be noticing a symptom, have a thought, or hearing about illness. Note your emotional response. Write down your main negative thought. In the "Response" column make a note of what you did in response to the thought and write a rational response (your therapist will guide you in responding differently in treatment). In the "Outcome" column, re-rate your belief in the negative thought, and make a note of anything that you found helpful.

# WORRYING THOUGHTS RECORD—GAD

| Date | Situation | Trigger | Description of worry | Worry about worry | Emotion (0–100) | Response to worry about worry | Outcome: Re-rate emotion |
|------|-----------|---------|----------------------|-------------------|-----------------|-------------------------------|--------------------------|
|      |           |         |                      |                   |                 |                               |                          |

*Instructions:* When you notice yourself worrying or feeling anxious, make a note of the situation in which it occurred. Write down the trigger for your worry (this may be another thought or image), and make a brief note of your worry. Try to be aware of negative thoughts you have about your worry and note these in the worry about worry column. Next write down your emotional reaction and rate its intensity (0–100). Make a note of your response to worry about worry (your therapist will explore new responses with you in treatment). Finally re-rate your emotion.

# DYSFUNCTIONAL THOUGHTS RECORD—OCD

| Date | Situation | Trigger | Intrusion:Thought/ Doubt/Feeling/ Behaviour Specify | Emotion (note intensity 0-100) | Worry about Intrusion | Answer to Worry | Outcome Emotion Intensity (0-100) |
|------|-----------|---------|------|------|------|------|------|
|      |           |         |      |      |      |      |      |
|      |           |         |      |      |      |      |      |
|      |           |         |      |      |      |      |      |
|      |           |         |      |      |      |      |      |
|      |           |         |      |      |      |      |      |

_Instructions:_    *When you notice yourself having unwanted unpleasant thoughts or engaging in repetitive behaviours, make a note of the <u>Situation</u> where this occurred. In the <u>Trigger</u> column note the activity or event that triggered your unwanted thought or feeling (this may be another feeling or thought). In the <u>Intrusion</u> column describe your initial unwanted thought/image/doubt/discomfort/or behaviour. Specify and rate your emotional response under <u>Emotion</u> and then write in your main negative interpretation (<u>Worry</u>) about the intrusion. Make a note of how you responded to the intrusion in the <u>Answer</u> column, and finally re-rate your <u>Emotion</u>.*

# REFERENCES

APA (1994). *Diagnostic and Statistical Manual of Mental Disorders*, Revised, 4th edn. Washington, DC: American Psychiatric Association.

Barlow, D.H., Craske, M.G., Cerny, J.A. & Klosko, J.S. (1989). Behavioural treatment of panic disorder. *Behaviour Therapy*, **20**, 261–282.

Bartlett, F.C. (1932). *Remembering: A Study in Experimental and Social Psychology.* Cambridge: Cambridge University Press.

Beck, A.T. (1967). *Depression: Causes and Treatment.* Philadelphia, PA: University of Pennsylvania Press.

Beck, A.T. (1976). *Cognitive Therapy and the Emotional Disorders.* New York: International Universities Press.

Beck, A.T. (1987). Cognitive models of depression. *Journal of Cognitive Psychotherapy*, **1**, 5–37.

Beck, A.T. & Freeman, A. (1990). *Cognitive Therapy of Personality Disorders.* New York: Guilford Press.

Beck, A.T., Brown, G., Steer, R.A., Eidelson, J.I. & Riskind, J.H. (1987). Differentiating anxiety and depression: A test of the cognitive content specificity hypothesis. *Journal of Abnormal Psychology*, **96**, 179.

Beck, A.T., Emery, G. & Greenberg, R.L. (1985). *Anxiety Disorders and Phobias: A cognitive perspective.* New York: Basic Books.

Beck, A.T., Epstein, N., Brown, G. & Steer, R.A. (1988). An inventory for measuring clinical anxiety: psychometric properties. *Journal of Consulting and Clinical Psychology*, **56**, 893–897.

Beck, A.T., Laude, R. & Bohnert, M. (1974a). Ideational components of anxiety neurosis. *Archives of General Psychiatry*, **31**, 319–325.

Beck, A.T., Rush, A.J., Shaw, B.F. & Emery, G. (1979). *Cognitive Therapy of Depression.* New York: Guilford Press.

Beck, A.T., Ward, C.H., Mendelson, M., Mock, J. & Erbaugh, J. (1961). An inventory for measuring depression. *Archives of General Psychiatry*, **4**, 561–571.

Beck, A.T., Weissman, A., Lester, D. & Trexler, L. (1974b). The measurement of pessimism: the Hopelessness Scale. *Journal of Consulting and Clinical Psychology*, **42**, 861–865.

Borkovec, T.D. & Costello, E. (1993). Efficacy of applied relaxation and cognitive—behavioural therapy in the treatment of Generalised Anxiety Disorder. *Journal of Consulting and Clinical Psychology*, **51**, 611–619.

Borkovec, T.D. & Inz, J. (1990). The nature of worry in Generalised Anxiety Disorder: A predominance of thought activity. *Behaviour Research and Therapy*, **28**, 153–158.

Borkovec, T.D., Mathews, A.M., Chambers, A., Ebrahimi, S., Lytle, R. & Nelson, R. (1987). The effects of relaxation training with cognitive therapy or nondirective therapy and the role of relaxation-induced anxiety in the treatment of generalised anxiety. *Journal of Consulting and Clinical Psychology*, **55**, 883–888.

Borkovec, T.D., Robinson, E., Puzinsky, T. & DePree, J.A. (1983a). Preliminary exploration of worry: some characteristics and processes. *Behaviour Research and Therapy*, **21**, 9–16.

Borkovec, T.D., Shadick, R.N. & Hopkins, M. (1991). The nature of normal and pathological worry. In: R.M. Rapee & D.H. Barlow (Eds.), *Chronic Anxiety: Generalised Anxiety Disorder and Mixed Anxiety Depression* (pp. 29–51). New York: Guilford Press.

Borkovec, T.D., Wilkinson, L., Folensbee, R. & Lerman, C. (1983b). Stimulus control applications to the treatment of worry. *Behaviour Research and Therapy*, **21**, 247–251.

Broadbent, D.E. & Broadbent, M.H.P. (1988). Anxiety and attentional bias: State and trait. *Cognition and Emotion*, **2**, 165–183.

Burns, D. (1980). *Feeling Good*. New York: New American Library.

Burns, D.D. (1989). *The Feel Good Handbook. Using the new mood therapy in everyday life*. New York: Morrow.

Butler, G. & Mathews, A. (1983). Cognitive processes in anxiety. *Advances in Behaviour Therapy*, **5**, 51–62.

Butler, G. & Mathews, A. (1987). Anticipatory anxiety and risk perception. *Cognitive Therapy and Research*, **91**, 551–565.

Butler, G., Cullingham, A., Hibbert, G., Klimes, I. & Gelder, M. (1987). Anxiety management for persistent generalised anxiety. *British Journal of Psychiatry*, **151**, 535–542.

Butler, G., Fennell, M., Robson, P. & Gelder, M. (1991). Comparison of behaviour therapy and cognitive behaviour therapy in the treatment of generalised anxiety disorder. *Journal of Consulting and Clinical Psychology*, **59**, 167–172.

Cartwright-Hatton, S. (1996). Uncontrollable thought: an experimental study of worry. Unpublished D.Phil. thesis, Oxford University.

Cartwright-Hatton, S. & Wells, A. (1997). Beliefs about worry and intrusions: the Meta-Cognitions Questionnaire and its correlates. *Journal of Anxiety Disorders* (in press).

Chambless, D.L. & Gracely, E.J. (1989). Fear of fear in the anxiety disorders. *Cognitive Therapy and Research*, **13**, 9–20.

Chambless, D.L., Caputo, G.S., Bright, P. & Gallagher, R. (1984). Assessment of fear of fear on agoraphobics. The Bodily Sensation Questionnaire and the Agoraphobic Cognitions Questionnaire. *Journal of Consulting and Clinical Psychology*, **52**, 1090–1097.

Clark, D.M. (1986). A cognitive model of panic. *Behaviour Research and Therapy*, **24**, 461–470.

Clark, D.M. (1988). A cognitive model of panic attacks. In: S. Rachman & J.D. Maser (Eds.), *Panic: Psychological Perspectives* (pp. 71–89). Hillsdale, NJ: Erlbaum.

Clark, D.M. (1989). Anxiety states: panic and generalise anxiety. In: K. Hawton, P.M. Salkovskis, J. Kirk & D.M. Clark (Eds.), *Cognitive Behaviour Therapy for Psychiatric Problems. A Practical Guide*. Oxford: Oxford University Press.

Clark, D.M. (1993). Cognitive mediation of panic attacks induced by biological challenge tests. *Behaviour Research and Therapy*, **15**, 75–84.

Clark, D.M. & Ehlers, A. (1993). An overview of the cognitive theory and treatment of panic. *Applied and Preventive Psychology*, **2**, 131–139.

Clark, D.A. & Purdon, C. (1993). New perspectives of a cognitive theory of obsessions. *Australian Psychologist*, **28**, 161–167.

Clark, D.M. & Wells, A. (1995). A cognitive model of social phobia. In: R. Heimberg, M. Liebowitz, D.A. Hope & F.R. Schneier (Eds.), *Social Phobia: Diagnosis, Assessment and Treatment*. New York: Guilford Press.

Clark, D.M., Ball, S. & Pape, D. (1991). An experimental investigation of thought suppression. *Behaviour Research and Therapy*, **29**, 253–257.

Clark, D.M., Salkovskis, P.M., Hackmann, A., Middleton, H., Anastasiades, P. & Gelder, M.G. (1994). A comparison of cognitive therapy, applied relaxation and Imipramine in the treatment of panic disorder. *British Journal of Psychiatry*, **164**, 759–769.

Clark, D.M., Salkovskis, P.M., Gelder, M., Koehler, C., Martin, M., Anastasiades, P., Hackmann, A., Middleton, H. & Jeavons, A. (1988). Tests of a cognitive theory of panic. In: I. Hand & H.V. Wittchen (Eds.), *Panic and Phobias* (vol. 2). Berlin: Springer.

Craske, M.G., Rapee, R.M., Jackel, L. & Barlow, D.H. (1989). Qualitative dimensions of worry in DSM-III-R. Generalised Anxiety Disorder subjects and non-anxious control. *Behaviour Research and Therapy*, **27**, 397–402.

Davey, G.C.L. (1994). Pathological worry as exacerbated problem solving. In: G.C.L. Davey & F. Tallis (Eds.), *Worrying: Perspectives on Theory, Assessment and Treatment* (pp. 35–60). Chichester: Wiley.

Dollard, J. & Miller, N.E. (1950). *Personality and Psychotherapy: An Analysis in Terms of Learning, Thinking and Culture*. New York: McGraw-Hill.

Durham, R.C. & Turvey, A.A. (1987). Cognitive therapy vs behaviour therapy in the treatment of chronic general anxiety. *Behaviour Research and Therapy*, **25**, 229.

Durham, R.C., Murphy, T., Allan, T., Richard, K., Treliving, L.R. & Genton, G. (1994). Cognitive therapy, analytic psychotherapy and anxiety management training for Generalised Anxiety Disorder. *British Journal of Psychiatry*, **165**, 315–323.

Ellis, A. (1962). *Reason and Emotion in Psychotherapy*. New York: Lyle Stuart.

Eysenck, H.J. & Eysenck, S.B.G. (1976). *Manual for the Eysenck Personality Inventory*. London: University of London Press.

Foa, E.B. (1979). Failure in treating obsessive-compulsives. *Behaviour Research and Therapy*, **17**, 169–176.

Foa, E.B. & Kozak, M.J. (1986). Emotional processing and fear: exposure to corrective information. *Psychological Bulletin*, **99**, 20–35.

Foa, E.B., Kozak, M.J., Steketee, G.S. & McCarthy, P.R. (1992). Imipramine and behaviour therapy in the treatment of depressive and obsessive-compulsive symptoms: immediate and long-term effects. *British Journal of Clinical Psychology*, **31**, 279–292.

Foa, E.B., Rothbaum, B.O., Riggs, D.S. & Murdock, T.B. (1991). Treatment of post-traumatic stress disorder in rape victims: a comparison between cognitive-behavioural procedures and counselling. *Journal of Consulting and Clinical Psychology*, **59**, 715–723.

Goldstein, A.J. & Chambless, D.L. (1978). A re-analysis of agoraphobia. *Behaviour Therapy*, **9**, 47–59.

Griez, E. & van den Hout, M.A. (1986). $CO_2$ inhalation in the treatment of panic attacks. *Behaviour Research and Therapy*, **24**, 145–150.

Hartman, L.M. (1983). A meta-cognitive model of social anxiety: implications for treatment. *Clinical Psychology Review*, **3**, 435–456.

Hartman, L.M. (1986). Social anxiety, problem drinking and self-awareness. In: L.M. Hartman & K.R. Blankstein (Eds.), *Perceptions of Self in Emotional Disorder and Psychotherapy* (pp. 265–282). New York: Plenum Press.

Headland, K. & MacDonald, R. (1987). Rapid audio-tape treatment of obsessional ruminations: a case report. *Behavioural Psychotherapy*, **15**, 188–192.

Heimberg, R.G., Mueller, G.P., Holt, C.S., Hope, D.A. & Liebowitz, M.R. (1992). Assessment of anxiety in social interaction and being observed by others: the Social Interaction Anxiety Scale and the Social Phobia Scale. *Behaviour Therapy*, **23**, 53–73.

Hibbert, G.A. (1984). Ideational components of anxiety: their origin and content. *British Journal of Psychiatry*, **144**, 618–624.

Hodgson, R.J. & Rachman, S. (1977). Obsessional compulsive complaints. *Behaviour Research and Therapy*, **10**, 181–189.

Hope, D.A., Gasler, D.A. & Heimberg, R.G. (1989). Attentional focus and causal attributions in social phobia: Implications from social psychology. *Clinical Psychology Review*, **9**, 49–60.

James, I.A. & Blackburn, I.M. (1995). Cognitive therapy with Obsessive-Compulsive Disorder. *British Journal of Psychiatry*, **166**, 444–450.

Karno, M., Golding, J.M., Sorenson, S.B. & Burnam, M.A. (1988). The epidemiology of obsessive-compulsive disorder in five U.S. communities. *Archives of General Psychiatry*, **45**, 1094–1099.

Kellner, R. (1986). *Somatization and Hypochondriasis*. New York: Praeger.

Layden, M.A., Newman, C.F., Freemen, A. & Morse, S.B. (1993). *Cognitive Therapy of Borderline Personality Disorder*. Massachusetts: Allyne & Bacon.

Lucock, M.P. & Morley, S. (1996). The Health Anxiety Questionnaire. *British Journal of Health Psychology*, **1**, 137–150.

MacLeod, C. & Mathews, A. (1988). Anxiety and the allocation of attention to threat. *Quarterly Journal of Experimental Psychology*, **38A**, 659–670.

MacLeod, C., Mathews, A. & Tata, P. (1986). Attentional bias in emotional disorders. *Journal of Abnormal Psychology*, **95**, 15–20.

MacLeod, A.K., Williams, J.M.G. & Bekerian, D.A. (1991). Worry is reasonable: the role of explorations in pessimism about future personal events. *Journal of Abnormal Psychology*, **100**, 478–486.

Marks, I.M. & Mathews, A.M. (1979). Brief standard self-rating for phobic patients. *Behaviour Research and Therapy*, **17**, 263–267.

Marks, I.M., Hodgson, P. & Rachman, S. (1975). Treatment of obsessive compulsive neurosis by in-vivo exposure. A two-year follow-up and issues in treatment. *British Journal of Psychiatry*, **127**, 349–364.

Mathews, A. (1988). Anxiety and the selective processing of threatening information. In: V. Hamilton, G.H. Bower & N.H. Frijda (Eds.), *Cognitive Perspectives on Emotion and Motivation*. Dordrecht: Kluwer Academic.

Mathews, A. & MacLeod, C. (1985). Selective processing of threat cues in anxiety states. *Behavioural Research and Therapy*, **23**, 563–569.

Mathews, A. & MacLeod, C. (1986). Discrimination of threat cues without awareness in anxiety states. *Journal of Abnormal Psychology*, **95**, 131–138.

Mathews, A., Richards, A. & Eysenck, M.W. (1989). The interpretation of homophones related to threat in anxiety states. *Journal of Abnormal Psychology*, **98**, 31–34.

Mattick, R.P. & Clark, J.C. (1989). Development and validation of measures of social phobia, scrutiny, fear and social interaction anxiety. Unpublished manuscript.

McFall, M.E. & Wollersheim, J.P. (1979). Obsessive-compulsive neurosis: a cognitive-behavioural formulation and approach to treatment. *Cognitive Therapy and Research*, **3**, 333–348.

Meichenbaum, D. (1977). *Cognitive-Behaviour Modification: An Integrative Approach*. New York: Plenum Press.

Meyer, V. (1966). Modification of expectations in cases with obsessional rituals. *Behaviour Research and Therapy*, **4**, 273–280.

Meyer, T.J., Miller, M.L., Metzger, R.L. & Borkovec, T.D. (1990). Development and validation of the Penn State Worry Questionnaire. *Behaviour Research and Therapy*, **28**, 487–495.

Miller, L.C., Murphy, R. & Buss, A.H. (1981). Consciousness of body: private and public. *Journal of Personality and Social Psychology*, **41**, 397–406.

Mogg, K., Mathews, A., Bird, C. & MacGregor-Morris, R. (1990). Effects of stress and anxiety on the processing of threat stimuli. *Journal of Personality and Social Psychology*, **59**, 1230–1237.

Mogg, K., Mathews, A. & Eysenck, M.W. (1992). Attentional bias to threat in clinical anxiety states. *Cognition and Emotion*, **6**, 149–159.

Mogg, K., Mathews, A. & Weinman, J. (1989). Selective processing of threat cues in anxiety states: a replication. *Behaviour Research and Therapy*, **27**, 317–323.

Molina, S. & Borkovec, T.D. (1994). The Penn State Worry Questionnaire: psychometric properties and associated characteristics. In: G.C.L. Davey & F. Tallis (Eds.), *Worrying: Perspectives on Theory, Assessment and Treatment*. Chichester: Wiley.

Mowrer, O.H. (1960). *Learning Theory and Behaviour*. New York: Wiley.

Ost, L.G. & Sterner, V. (1987). Applied tension: a specific behavioural method for treatment of blood phobia. *Behaviour Research and Therapy*, **25**, 25–30.

Ottaviani, R. & Beck, A.T. (1987). Cognitive aspects of panic disorder. *Journal of Anxiety Disorders*, **1**, 15–28.

Padesky, C. (1993). Title unknown. Paper presented at the EABCT London Conference.

Parkinson, L. & Rachman, S. (1981). The nature of intrusive thoughts. *Advances in Behaviour Research and Therapy*, **3**, 101–110.

Persons, J.B. & Foa, E.B. (1984). Processing of fearful and neutral information by obsessive-compulsives. *Behaviour Research and Therapy*, **22**, 259–265.

Power, K.G., Jerrom, D.W.A., Simpson, R.J., Mitchell, M.J. & Swanson, V. (1989). A controlled comparison of cognitive behavior therapy, diazepam, and placebo in the management of generalised anxiety. *Behavioural Psychotherapy*, **17**, 1–14.

Rachman, S.J. (1976). Obsessional-compulsive checking. *Behaviour Research and Therapy*, **14**, 269–277.

Rachman, S.J. (1993). Obsessions, responsibility and guilt. *Behaviour Research and Therapy*, **31**, 149–154.

Rachman, S.J. & de Silva, P. (1978). Abnormal and normal obsessions. *Behaviour Research and Therapy*, **16**, 233–238.

Rachman, S., Lopatka, K. & Levitt, L. (1988). Experimental analysis of panic 2: Panic patients. *Behaviour Research and Therapy*, **26**, 33–40.

Rachman, S., Thordarson, D.S., Shafran, R. & Woody, S.R. (1995). Perceived responsibility: structure and significance. *Behaviour Research and Therapy*, **33**, 779–784.

Razran, G. (1961). The observable unconscious and the inferable conscious in current Soviet psychophysiology: interoceptive conditioning, semantic conditioning, and the orienting reflex. *Psychological Review*, **68**, 81–147.

Reed, G.F. (1985). *Obsessional Experience and Compulsive Behaviour: A Cognitive Structural Approach*. London: Academic Press.

Robbins, J.M. & Kirmayer, L.J. (1991). Attributions of common somatic symptoms. *Psychological Medicine*, **21**, 1029–1045.

Salkovis, P.M. (1983). Treatment of an obsessional patient using habituation to audiotaped rumination. *British Journal of Clinical Psychology*, **22**, 311–313.

Salkovskis, P.M. (1985). Obsessional-compulsive problems: a cognitive-behavioural analysis. *Behaviour Research and Therapy*, **23**, 571–583.

Salkovskis, P.M. (1989). Cognitive-behavioural factors and the persistence of intrusive thoughts in obsessional problems. *Behaviour Research and Therapy*, **27**, 677–682.

Salkovskis, P.M. (1991). the importance of behaviour in the maintenance of anxiety and panic: a cognitive account. *Behavioural Psychotherapy*, **19**, 6–19.

Salkovskis, P.M. & Harrison, J. (1984). Abnormal and normal obsessions: a replication. *Behaviour Research and Therapy*, **27**, 549–552.

Salkovis, P.M. & Warwick, H.M.C. (1985). Cognitive therapy of obsessive-compulsive disorder – treating treatment failures. *Behavioural Psychotherapy*, **13**, 243–245.

Salkovskis, P.M. & Westbrook, D. (1989). Behaviour therapy and obsessional ruminations: can failure be turned into success? *Behaviour Research and Therapy*, **27**, 149–160.

Salkovskis, P.M., Clark, D.M. & Hackmann, A. (1991). Treatment of panic attacks using cognitive therapy without exposure or breathing retraining. *Behaviour Research and Therapy*, **29**, 161–166.

Salkovskis, P.M., Richards, H.C. & Forrester, E. (1995). The relationship between obsessional problems and intrusive thoughts. *Behavioural and Cognitive Psychotherapy*, **23**, 281–301.

Sanavio, E. (1988). Obsessional and compulsions: the Padua Inventory. *Behaviour Research and Therapy*, **26**, 169–177.

Sher, K.J., Frost, R.O., Kushner, M., Crews, T.M. & Alexander, J.E. (1989). Memory deficits in compulsive checkers: replication and extension in a clinical sample. *Behaviour Research and Therapy*, **27**, 65–69.

Sher, K.J., Mann, B. & Frost, R.O. (1984). Cognitive dysfunction in compulsive checkers: further explorations. *Behaviour Research and Therapy*, **22**, 493–502.

Spielberger, C.D., Gorsuch, R.L., Lushene, R., Vagg, P.R. & Jacobs, G.A. (1983). *Manual for the Stait-Trait Anxiety Inventory*. Palo Alto, CA: Consulting Psychology Press.

Steketee, G. (1993). *Treatment of Obsessive Compulsive Disorder*. New York: Guilford Press.

Sternberger, L.G. & Burns, L.G. (1990). Obsessions and compulsions: psychometric properties of the Padua Inventory with an American college population. *Behaviour Research and Therapy*, **28**, 334–345.

Stopa, L. (1995). Cognitive processes in social anxiety. Unpublished D.Phil. thesis, Oxford University.

Stroop, J.R. (1935). Studies of interference in serial verbal reactions. *Journal of Experimental Psychology*, **18**, 643–662.

Tallis, F. (1993). Doubt reduction using distinctive stimuli as a treatment for compulsive checking: an exploratory investigation. *Clinical Psychology and Psychotherapy*, **1**, 45–52.

Tallis, F. (1995). *Obsessive Compulsive Disorder. A Cognitive and Neuropsychological Perspective*. Chichester: Wiley.

Tallis, F., Davey, G.C.L. & Bond, A. (1994). The Worry Domains Questionnaire. In: G.C.L. Davey & F. Tallis (Eds.), *Worrying: Perspectives on Theory, Assessment and Treatment*. Chichester: Wiley.

Tallis, F., Eysenck, M.W. & Mathews, A. (1992). A questionnaire measure for the measurement of nonpathological worry. *Personality and Individual Differences*, **13**, 161–168.

Trandell, D.V. & McNally, R.J. (1987). Perception of threat cues in post-traumatic stress disorder: semantic processing without awareness? *Behaviour Research and Therapy*, **25**, 469–476.

van den Hout, M.A., de Jong, P., Zanderberger, J. & Merckelbach, H. (1990). Waning of panic sensations during prolonged hyperventilation. *Behaviour Research and Therapy*, **28**, 445–448.

Warwick, H.M.C. & Salkovskis, P.M. (1989). Hypochondriasis. In: J. Scott, J.M.G. Williams & A.T. Beck (Eds.), *Cognitive Therapy in Clinical Practice*. London: Gower.

Warwick, H.M.C. & Salkovskis, P.M. (1990). Hypochondriasis. *Behaviour Research and Therapy*, **28**, 105–117.

Warwick, H.M.C., Clark, D.M., Cobb, A.M. & Salkovskis, P.M. (1996). A controlled trial of cognitive-behavioural treatment of hypochondriasis. *British Journal of Psychiatry*, **169**, 189–195.

Watson, D. & Clark, L.A. (1984). Negative affectivity: The disposition to experience aversive emotional states. *Psychological Bulletin*, **96**, 465–490.

Watson, D. & Friend, R. (1969). Measurement of social-evaluative anxiety. *Journal of Consulting and Clinical Psychology*, **33**, 448–457.

Watts, F.N., McKenna, F.P., Sharrock, R. & Tresize, L. (1986). Colour naming of phobia-related words. *British Journal of Psychology*, **77**, 97–108.

Wegner, D.M. & Schneider, D.J., Carter, S.R. III. & White, T.L. (1987). Paradoxical effects of thought suppression. *Journal of Personality and Social Psychology*, **53**, 5–13.

Weissman, A.N. & Beck, A.T. (1978). Development and validation of the Dysfunctional Attitude Scale. Paper presented at the Annual Meeting of the Association for the Advancement of Behaviour Therapy, Chicago, Illinois.

Wells, A. (1990). Panic disorder in association with relaxation-induced anxiety: An attentional training approach to treatment. *Behaviour Therapy*, **21**, 273–280.

Wells, A. (1992). Cognitive therapy for anxiety and cognitive theories of causation. In: G.D. Burrows, Sir M. Roth. & R. Noyes (Eds.), *Handbook of Anxiety* (vol. 5). Amsterdam: Elsevier.

Wells, A. (1994a). Attention and the control of worry. In: G.C.L. Davey & F. Tallis (Eds.), *Worrying: Perspectives on Theory, Assessment and Treatment*. Chichester: Wiley.

Wells, A. (1994b). A multidimensional measure of worry: development and preliminary validation of the Anxious Thoughts Inventory. *Anxiety Stress and Coping*, **6**, 289–299.

Wells, A. (1995). Meta-cognition and worry: a cognitive model of Generalised Anxiety Disorder. *Behavioural and Cognitive Psychotherapy*, **23**, 301–320.

Wells, A. & Carter, K.E.P. (submitted). Tests of a meta-cognitive model of GAD.

Wells, A. & Clark, D.M. (1995). Cognitive therapy of social phobia: a treatment manual. Unpublished manuscript.

Wells, A. & Clark, D.M. (1997). Social phobia: a cognitive approach. In: D.C.L. Davey (Ed.), *Phobias: A Handbook of Description, Treatment and Theory*. Chichester: Wiley.

Wells, A. & Davies, M. (1994). The Thought Control Questionnaire: a measure of individual differences in the control of unwanted thoughts. *Behaviour Research and Therapy*, **32**, 871–878.

Wells, A. & Hackmann, A. (1993). Imagery and core beliefs in health anxiety: content and origins. *Behavioural and Cognitive Psychotherapy*, **21**, 265–273.

Wells, A. & Hackmann, A. (unpublished). Death Beliefs Questionnaire.

Wells, A. & Matthews, G. (1994). *Attention and Emotion. A Clinical Perspective*. Hove, UK: Erlbaum.

Wells, A. & Matthews, G. (1997). Modelling cognition in emotional disorder: The S-REF model. *Behaviour Research and Therapy* (in Press).

Wells, A. & Morrison, T. (1994). Qualitative dimensions of normal worry and normal intrusive thoughts: A comparative study. *Behaviour Research and Therapy*, **32**, 867–870.

Wells, A. & Papageorgiou, C. (1995). Worry and the incubation of intrusive images following stress. *Behaviour Research and Therapy*, **33**, 579–583.

Wells, A., Clark, D.M. & Ahmad, S. (1995a). How do I look with my mind's eye? Perspective taking in social phobic imagery. Paper presented at Annual Conference of the BABCP, Southampton University.

Wells, A., Clark, D.M. Salkovskis, P., Ludgate, J., Hackmann, A. & Gelder, M.G. (1995b). Social phobia: The role of in-situation safety behaviours in maintaining anxiety and negative beliefs. *Behaviour Therapy*, **26**, 163–161.

Wells, A., Stopa, L. & Clark, D.M. (unpublished). The Social Cognitions Questionnaire.

Wells, A., White, J. & Carter, K. (in press). Attention training: effects on anxiety and beliefs in panic and social phobia (submitted for publication).

Young, J.E. (1990). *Cognitive Therapy for Personality Disorders: A Schema Focused Approach*. Sarasota, FL: Professional Resources Exchange, Inc.

# INDEX